D0934426

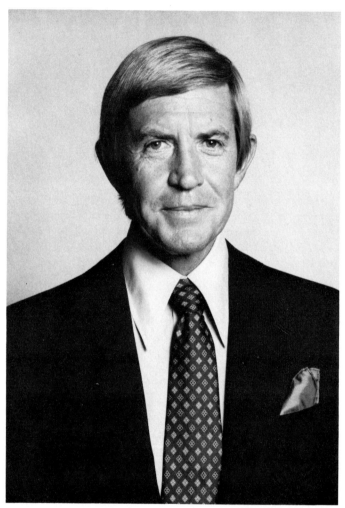

THOMAS D. REES, M.D., F.A.C.S.

VOLUME I

AESTHETIC PLASTIC SURGERY

THOMAS D. REES, M.D., F.A.C.S.

Clinical Professor of Surgery (Plastic Surgery),
  New York University School of Medicine;
Chairman, Department of Plastic Surgery,
  Manhattan Eye, Ear and Throat Hospital;
Attending Surgeon,
  New York University—Bellevue Medical Center

Illustrations by Daisy Stilwell

W. B. SAUNDERS COMPANY
Philadelphia   London   Toronto

W. B. Saunders Company: West Washington Square
Philadelphia, PA   19105

1 St. Anne's Road
Eastbourne, East Sussex BN21 3UN, England

1 Goldthorne Avenue
Toronto, Ontario M8Z 5T9, Canada

Aesthetic Plastic Surgery

ISBN   Volume I   0-7216-7519-0
ISBN   Volume II   0-7216-7521-2
ISBN   Set   0-7216-7522-0

Last digit is the print number: 9   8   7   6   5   4   3   2

This book is dedicated to my wife, Nan, and to Tom, David, and Liz, who have with equanimity borne my detachment on weekends and holidays and plane trips for too many years while preparing this book. I hope I can make it up to them.

CONTRIBUTORS

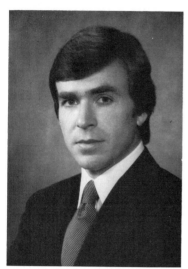

SHERRELL J. ASTON, M.D., F.A.C.S.

Assistant Professor of Surgery (Plastic Surgery), New York University School of Medicine; Attending Surgeon, Manhattan Eye, Ear and Throat Hospital; Associate Attending Surgeon, Institute of Reconstructive Plastic Surgery, New York University Medical Center, and Bellevue Hospital; Staff Member, Doctors' Hospital, New York

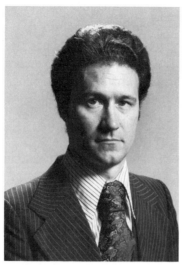

DANIEL C. BAKER, M.D.

Assistant Professor of Surgery (Plastic Surgery), New York University School of Medicine; Assistant Attending Surgeon, Institute of Reconstructive Plastic Surgery, New York University Medical Center; Associate Attending Surgeon, Manhattan Eye, Ear and Throat Hospital, New York

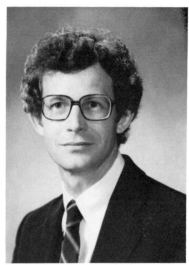

JOHN BOSTWICK, III, M.D., F.A.C.S.

Associate Professor of Surgery (Plastic and Reconstructive Surgery), Emory University School of Medicine; Attending Surgeon, Emory University Hospital, Crawford W. Long Hospital, and Grady Memorial Hospital, Atlanta, Georgia

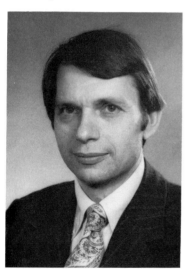

RICHARD J. COBURN, D.M.D., M.D.

Clinical Associate in Surgery, Mount Sinai School of Medicine; Attending Plastic Surgeon, Doctors' Hospital and St. Luke's Hospital, New York

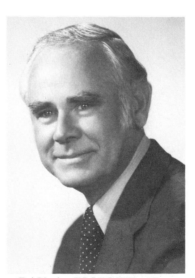

RAY A. ELLIOTT, JR., M.D., F.A.C.S.

Clinical Associate Professor of Plastic Surgery and Clinical Associate Professor of Orthopedics (Hand), Albany Medical College; Attending Plastic Surgeon, Albany Medical Center Hospital, Albany V.A. Hospital, Albany Memorial Hospital, and Child's Hospital, Albany, New York

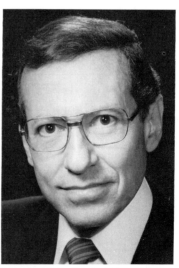

BERNARD L. KAYE, M.D., F.A.C.S.

Clinical Professor of Surgery (Plastic Surgery), University of Florida School of Medicine; Chief, Section of Plastic Surgery, Baptist Medical Center, Jacksonville, Florida

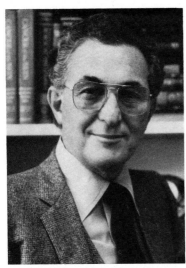

NORMAN ORENTREICH, M.D.

Clinical Associate Professor of Dermatology, New York University School of Medicine; Attending in Department of Dermatology, University Hospital, New York University Medical Center, New York

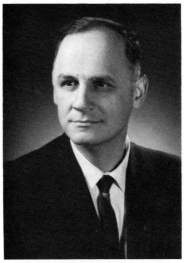

CHARLES P. VALLIS, M.D., F.A.C.S.

Instructor in Plastic Surgery, Tufts Medical School, Boston, Massachusetts; Senior Attending Surgeon, Lynn Union Hospital, Lynn, Massachusetts

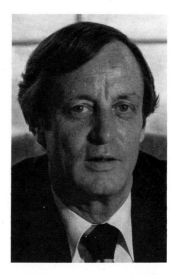

DONALD WOOD-SMITH, M.D.

Associate Professor of Surgery (Plastic Surgery), New York University School of Medicine; Attending Surgeon, University Hospital, New York University Medical Center, Bellevue Hospital, Manhattan Veterans Administration Hospital, New York Eye and Ear Infirmary, and Doctors' Hospital; Attending Surgeon and Surgeon Director, Manhattan Eye, Ear and Throat Hospital, New York

SIDNEY HOROWITZ, D.D.S.

Professor of Dentistry and Director of the Division of Orofacial Development, School of Dental and Oral Surgery, Columbia University, New York

SEAMUS LYNCH, M.D.

Chief of Anesthesiology, Central Suffolk Hospital, Riverhead, New York; Attending Anesthesiologist, Eastern L.I. Hospital, Greenport, New York; Consulting Anesthesiologist, Manhattan Eye, Ear and Throat Hospital, New York

FRANCES C. MACGREGOR, M.A.

Clinical Associate Professor of Surgery (Sociology), Institute of Reconstructive Plastic Surgery, New York University Medical Center; Consultant in Social Psychology, Plastic Surgery Department, Manhattan Eye, Ear and Throat Hospital, New York

FOREWORD

As the author and I have shared a close friendship for years, it is with both pride and pleasure that I write a few preliminary words about one of the leaders in the field of aesthetic surgery and the most recent record of his handicraft.

Aesthetic surgery is a highly sophisticated specialty that is dedicated not only to the return of the face and body to normal but to improvements that actually surpass the normal. Many of those who seek cosmetic surgery have exalted standards or illusionary expectations. Thus, the stakes are high, the margin of error is thin, and complications can be catastrophic. The cosmetic surgeon must be an aesthetic perfectionist with a sculptor's sense and a subtle ability to harness tension to his advantage while placing scars to the patient's advantage.

Thomas D. Rees, Clinical Professor of Surgery at the New York University Medical Center, is a talented plastic surgeon who has a special interest in aesthetic surgery. He is a second-generation Utahn of Welsh and Danish descent whose pioneer grandparents crossed America as children in wagon trains and pushcarts to settle in central Utah at the bidding of Brigham Young. His father was chairman of the Department of Life Sciences at the University of Utah for 35 years. Having inherited the drive and working ambition of his pioneer stock, he served as a hospital corpsman in the Navy, after which he graduated from the University of Utah Medical School in 1948, went East to train in general surgery in New York, graduated to a plastic surgery residency under Herbert Conway at Cornell University, and finally became a trainee with Sir Archibald McIndoe in England. A careful and conservative surgeon possessing both charm and style, Rees is portrayed in the words of Alfred Lord Tennyson, "A princelier-looking man never stemp thro' a prince's hall."

Always drawn to the West and to open spaces, Rees developed an interest in the possibilities of surgery in Africa. In 1955, Archibald McIndoe, Michael Wood, and Thomas Rees established the Flying Doctors Service of East Africa. They began with one small plane flying one surgical team, with Wood the surgeon and McIndoe and Rees joining him whenever they could. This organization has grown to ten airplanes, four surgeons, anesthesiologists, nurses, and pilots. The Flying Doctors have flown 1.5 million miles in the past twenty years and have treated many thousands of patients. Their emphasis now is on health education and preventive medicine, with a training center in Nairobi and satellite centers in the rural areas of Kenya, Tanzania, and the Sudan. During his travels, Rees has seen examples for the exotic color photographs portraying concepts of beauty from Africa, New Guinea, Mali, and Bali.

Aesthetic Plastic Surgery encompasses the *entire* field of aesthetic surgery and is a rewritten, improved, and expanded sequel to *Cosmetic Facial Surgery* by Rees and Donald Wood-Smith, which is now unavailable after several printings. It presents both standard and new procedures, primarily those that the author has found reliable over the past twenty years. The preoperative and postoperative photographs, being remarkably uniform, present an honest record, and the drawings of Daisy Stilwell are clear and classic, making this volume an excellent practical text for the younger surgeon.

Books often take years of thought even before the actual writing begins. Then there are the arduous years devoted to snatching spare hours for the writing, until the value of the work is inestimable. After four years of work, this book was almost totally completed, and it was carefully stored in the basement of the Rees' New York brownstone on 72nd Street. During street construction, Con Edison was ablating 72nd Street and in the process ruptured the water main, resulting in a four-foot water level in the surrounding area, including the Rees basement. For Tom there was the agonizing realization that four years of work was down the drain, and panic preceded the dash downstairs to the flooded basement. To his relief (and our joy), he found that his attractive wife, Nan, had stacked his manuscript high and dry on shelves well above the flood disaster. Although almost lost, this book is now a most vibrant, aesthetic, and educational work.

D. RALPH MILLARD, JR., M.D.

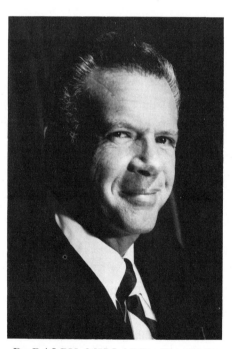

D. RALPH MILLARD, JR., M.D.

PREFACE

Historically, surgery has been performed for the treatment of organic disease. It was considered to be the ultimate tool for relieving human suffering when all other forms of therapy were exhausted. The concept that surgery can also be performed on an elective basis to improve the quality of life is a relatively modern idea that has grown at an accelerated rate throughout the world during the past decade. This extraordinary increase in public demand for a medical service was not predicted by anyone — certainly not by surgeons already practicing the profession.

Several factors converging at the same time in history are responsible for this boom in aesthetic surgery. The public has been continuously bombarded by the communications media. The general medical profession has become better educated about aesthetic surgery and has accepted the fact that it is safe. There is a growing awareness that the role of modern therapy should not be limited only to the treatment of organic disease but that it should alleviate human suffering in all its forms. Survival is no longer the only principal effort; improvement of the quality of life is also important.

It is impossible to measure human suffering. A minor physical irregularity can be of no consequence to one individual and yet can be of major significance to another. Vanity is a natural phenomenon not limited to Homo sapiens. Undergoing surgery to improve one's self-image can be the ultimate form of catering to vanity, but it is only one more modality in a long list since the beginnings of man that includes the constant changing of styles of clothes, hair, self-adornment, and even self-mutilation.

A bump on the nose may be unimportant to one individual; however, in another it can produce a range of problems from emotional discomfort to mental decompensation. The latter extreme is, of course, pathologic and bears little relationship to the physical problem. No one denies the tragic consequences of major facial disfigurement. Operations devised to improve such deformities are justified without question by all. Major surgery to correct significant craniofacial deformity is commonplace today. In the final analysis, these procedures are performed for aesthetic reasons.

Demand stimulates supply; however, there has been a woefully inadequate number of surgeons trained in these techniques to meet the need. It is hoped that this deficiency will be rectified in the near future as more and more residents graduate from programs well versed in the necessary skills.

This book was written expressly for the younger surgeon with a solid background in plastic surgery, in order to serve as a reference while he accumulates the experience required to season his judgment and surgical skill. Experience is still the best teacher in aesthetic surgery. If the older and more experienced surgeon finds some pearls herein, I will be pleased.

It was not intended that this book represent an encyclopedia of technique in aesthetic surgery. The literature is suffused with myriad solutions to every surgical problem. Many are useful and valid, but unfortunately, others provide many pitfalls for the inexperienced surgeon. As in the book that served as a precursor for this one (*Cosmetic Facial Surgery*), it is my intention to provide basic, practical, and tested surgical maneuvers that have withstood the tests of time. A few techniques of significant historical impact are also included. My contribution to this book is the result of personal experience gained in over 20 years in the practice of plastic surgery in New York City. It is a personal statement of an experience earned by observation, trial and error, and building upon the knowledge of those who taught me.

As each year passes, new techniques that promise to have an ultimate bearing on aesthetic surgery are introduced into the specialty of plastic surgery. The role of microvascular surgery with all the potential of free flaps has yet to be assimilated into aesthetic surgery. The implications of these techniques are not yet understood, except in breast reconstruction. Research in wound healing will eventually have direct application in aesthetic techniques and will eliminate some of the anxiety now associated with these procedures. The aging process is under intense investigation. It is doubtful that aging will be controlled; yet there is little doubt that human life will continue to be extended. The demand on aesthetic surgery will certainly increase—not to maintain eternal youth but to stave off the ravages of advanced years. Older people desire to look good in the same way that adolescents with physical defects do.

An effort has been made throughout this book to identify problems and pitfalls at the precise point in the procedure at which they can occur, and to indicate both the prevention and the treatment thereof. This dispenses with secondary problems throughout the text, but it seems to be a more practical approach than devoting an isolated section to secondary problems.

Our job as surgeons is to meet the needs of our patients with safety and perfection. It is the aim of this book to help provide the technical knowledge to meet this goal.

THOMAS D. REES, M.D., F.A.C.S.

ACKNOWLEDGMENTS

Cosmetic Facial Surgery (1973), co-authored with Donald Wood-Smith, can be considered the forerunner of this book. *Cosmetic Facial Surgery* was written because it was apparent that no work dealing specifically with cosmetic surgery had been produced for some years. In 1973, it seemed reasonable to assume that there would not be sufficient growth in the field of aesthetic surgery to warrant another edition for many years to come, to say nothing of a total rewrite. That assumption was wrong. *Cosmetic Facial Surgery* went into three printings and was well received. Its popularity can only be attributed to intense interest in the subject by surgeons throughout the world. The field of aesthetic surgery has grown at a surprising pace. A sufficient number of technical advances have occurred to justify this new book, which has been expanded to include the body as well as the face.

Much of the material was published previously in *Cosmetic Facial Surgery*. For the sake of completeness and to avoid repetitive references, this fact is hereby acknowledged.

Many of the illustrations and case studies are new or thoroughly revised to accommodate current changes and new developments. The authors make specific contributions based on their personal experience. Dr. Norman Orentreich, for example, invented the punch graft technique of hair transplantation and is an acknowledged expert on the subject of baldness.

I was particularly delighted that Dr. John Bostwick agreed to write the chapter on breast reconstruction. Postmastectomy patients present the most trying emotional handicaps imposed by a physical (aesthetic) deformity. Recent advances in techniques for reconstructing the female breast have improved the results dramatically. Thousands of women annually are seeking breast reconstruction. The contributions to improving the results in breast reconstruction utilizing myocutaneous flaps—pioneered by Dr. Bostwick and his associates, Dr. Louis Vasquonez and their mentor Dr. Josh Jurkiewicz—have revolutionized the technique. Breast reconstruction is clearly an "aesthetic" operation and as such deserves a prominent place in the repertoire of the plastic surgeon.

I am also very grateful for the contributions made by Drs. Richard Coburn, Sidney Horowitz, Bernard Kaye, Sherrell Aston, Richard Vallis, Seamus Lynch, and Ray Elliot. I realize very well the effort and the time put into preparing their chapters. I hope they will feel personally rewarded by the book, since I cannot adequately compensate their splendid effort in any other way.

The superb artwork is again the product of the mastery of Daisy Stilwell. Probably no other artist has her experience and knowledge of plastic surgery. Miss Stilwell translates the surgeon's thoughts and plans to paper with clarity and precision. Without her ability to interpret my scribblings and instructions, this book would probably never have been completed.

The photography is mostly the work of Don Allen in New York City, one of the best medical photographers in the world. His detail is brutal; this is the best way for a surgeon to evaluate his work.

I would also like to acknowledge Dr. Frances Macgregor, who contributed a chapter reflecting her deep commitment to the special psychosocial problems of those with physical irregularities. Dr. Macgregor has committed most of her professional life to working with patients undergoing plastic surgery. She has a profound knowledge and understanding of their problems. I recommend her chapter for intense study and reflection by the young surgeon, for it is this area of aesthetic surgery that is the least understood.

I would also like to thank Dr. Ralph Millard of Miami, Florida, and Dr. Ivo Pitanguy of Brazil, two surgeons of world renown, for their forewords. These two surgeons, legends in their own lifetimes, have been close friends and colleagues of mine throughout my training and experience in plastic surgery. We have often traded ideas, dreams, and experiences, as well as shared disappointments. I am envious of both Ralph and Ivo, as they both have extraordinary energy, multifaceted personalities, incredible skill, great charm, and considerable athletic prowess.

I owe much to my teachers, colleagues, and pupils over the years, who have prodded me, guided me, and stimulated me to search constantly for better answers and ways of doing things.

I offer sincere thanks for the endless help and encouragement from my staff and associates, who helped with secretarial work, gathering the case materials, and the manuscript. Special thanks to Miss Karola Noetel, Mrs. Charles (Sharee) Sorenson, Sandi Sledz (no task could be done soon enough), Mary Dean, Carole Cannataro, and Pauline Porowski.

I am also grateful to Mr. Al Meier, Ms. Jill Goldman, and Ms. Karen McFadden of W. B. Saunders Company, who guided this book through to the end, making the whole experience not only bearable but even fun.

THOMAS D. REES, M.D., F.A.C.S.

CONTENTS

VOLUME I

Introduction
CONCEPTS OF BEAUTY 1
Thomas D. Rees, M.D.

PART 1 GENERAL CONSIDERATIONS

Chapter 1
SELECTION OF PATIENTS 19
Thomas D. Rees, M.D.

Chapter 2
SOCIAL AND PSYCHOLOGIC CON-
SIDERATIONS IN AESTHETIC
PLASTIC SURGERY: OLD AND NEW
TRENDS 29
Frances C. MacGregor, M.A.

Chapter 3
ANESTHESIA 40
Seamus Lynch, M.D.

PART 2 RHINOPLASTY

Chapter 4
HISTORY 51
Thomas D. Rees, M.D.

Chapter 5
ANATOMY 53
Thomas D. Rees, M.D.

Chapter 6
PHYSIOLOGY 66
Daniel C. Baker, M.D.

Chapter 7
PREOPERATIVE CONSIDERATIONS..... 99
Thomas D. Rees, M.D.

Chapter 8
THE OSTEOCARTILAGINOUS VAULT. 114
Thomas D. Rees, M.D.

Chapter 9
SURGICAL APPROACHES TO THE
TIP... 177
Thomas D. Rees, M.D.

Chapter 10
THE LIP-TIP-COLUMELLA COM-
PLEX AND THE ALAR BASE.............. 243
Thomas D. Rees, M.D.

Chapter 11
CORRECTION OF THE DEVIATED
NOSE.. 284
Thomas D. Rees, M.D.

Chapter 12
POSTOPERATIVE CONSIDERATIONS
AND COMPLICATIONS 320
Thomas D. Rees, M.D.

Chapter 13
PROBLEMS IN RHINOPLASTY............. 387
Thomas D. Rees, M.D.

Chapter 14
THE NON-CAUCASIAN NOSE.............. 440
Thomas D. Rees, M.D.

INDEX... i

VOLUME II

PART 3 BLEPHAROPLASTY

Chapter 15
HISTORY 459
Thomas D. Rees, M.D.

Chapter 16
BAGGY EYELIDS.................................. 463
Thomas D. Rees, M.D.

Chapter 17
SURGICAL PROCEDURES..................... 470
Thomas D. Rees, M.D.

Chapter 18
POSTOPERATIVE CONSIDERATIONS
AND COMPLICATIONS.......................... 525
Thomas D. Rees, M.D.

PART 4 AESTHETIC SURGERY OF
THE NECK AND FACE

Chapter 19
HISTORY 583
Thomas D. Rees, M.D.

Chapter 20
PHYSICAL CONSIDERATIONS 587
Thomas D. Rees, M.D.

Chapter 21
PREOPERATIVE PREPARATION.......... 596
Thomas D. Rees, M.D.

Chapter 22
THE CLASSICAL OPERATION 600
Thomas D. Rees, M.D.

Chapter 23
THE SMAS AND THE PLATYSMA 634
Thomas D. Rees, M.D.

Chapter 24
ANCILLARY TECHNIQUES 684
Thomas D. Rees, M.D.

Chapter 25
POSTOPERATIVE CONSIDERATIONS
AND COMPLICATIONS 708
Thomas D. Rees, M.D.

PART 5   ASSOCIATED PROCEDURES

Chapter 26
FOREHEAD AND BROW 731
Bernard L. Kaye, M.D.

Chapter 27
CHEMABRASION AND
DERMABRASION 749
Thomas D. Rees, M.D.

Chapter 28
MENTOPLASTY 770
Richard J. Coburn, D.M.D., M.D.;
Thomas D. Rees, M.D.; and
Sidney Horowitz, D.D.S.

Chapter 29
OTOPLASTY 833
Donald Wood-Smith, M.D.

PART 6   TREATMENT OF BALDNESS

Chapter 30
PUNCH GRAFTS 865
Norman Orentreich, M.D.

Chapter 31
LATERAL SCALP FLAPS 875
Ray A. Elliott, Jr., M.D.

Chapter 32
STRIP GRAFTS 885
C. P. Vallis, M.D.

PART 7   BODY CONTOURING

Chapter 33
BREAST REDUCTION AND
MASTOPEXY 903
Sherrell J. Aston, M.D.; and
Thomas D. Rees, M.D.

Chapter 34
MAMMARY AUGMENTATION, COR-
RECTION OF ASYMMETRY, AND
GYNECOMASTIA 954
Sherrell J. Aston, M.D.; and
Thomas D. Rees, M.D.

Chapter 35
BREAST RECONSTRUCTION
AFTER MASTECTOMY 996
John Bostwick, III, M.D.

Chapter 36
ABDOMINOPLASTY 1007
Sherrell J. Aston, M.D.

Chapter 37
BUTTOCKS AND THIGHS 1039
Sherrell J. Aston, M.D.

INDEX i

Introduction

Concepts of Beauty

THOMAS D. REES, M.D., F.A.C.S.

An old adage says that "beauty is in the eye of the beholder." The evidence is clear that man's concept of beauty has changed through the ages, and it is likely to continue to do so for the rest of man's tenure on earth. The art of body adornment with paints or scarification dates from ancient times, probably from when primitive man first discovered the unusual effects that result from smearing his body with mud or painting it with pigments. He may have discovered this by looking at his image in the original looking glass — a pond of water.

Adornment of the self through the use of cosmetics, clothes, hairstyles, or jewelry is widely accepted today, but the ancient tribal customs of scarification and tattooing are generally unacceptable in modern culture. Scarification in our society is generally considered to be a form of self-mutilation, usually indicating psychopathology. Tattooing is still a widespread form of decoration, but it is considered to be in social bad taste in most so-called civilized countries. Just where the boundaries lie between self-mutilation and self-decoration is unclear. It is not difficult, therefore, to understand why self-mutilation is a common symptom of the neurotic or confused mind, for this type of activity may be nothing more than an attempt by the individual to call attention to himself.

Thus, primitive man incises, paints, and decorates himself as an acceptable social form of ego manifestation, whereas modern "civilized" man is permitted only lesser degrees of self-adornment, and he resorts to more severe forms of self-beautification (or self-mutilation) when he becomes frustrated, hostile, or aggressive and can perceive no other way of expressing inner feelings (Rees and Daniller, 1969).

Behavior similar to self-mutilation has been noted in other primates, such as the chimpanzee, following the production of a stressful or frustrating situation (Phillips and Muzaffer, 1961). Children and babies not uncommonly manifest frustration brought on by a delay in feeding or a reprimand by severely scratching or even mutilating their faces.

Phillips and Muzaffer define self-mutilation as a socially unacceptable alteration of physical form, but the term "socially unacceptable" clearly can mean different things in different cultures and to different people. Schedter (1962) reminded us that Greek mythology refers to a band of fierce women, the Amazones, who amputated their right breasts lest they interfere with drawing the bow. Atresia of the breast brought on by compression from tight chest binding was in vogue in ancient Hellenistic circles to improve élan and poise. It came into vogue again in Chaucer's day and again in the 1920's. The small firm breast as opposed to the voluptuous breast popularized by certain movie stars became fashionable again in the early 1970's, and it is conceivable that breast binding could once again be introduced; however, there is little possibility that it would be so ubiquitously accepted. Tight corsets were the vogue in the late 19th century to produce the "wasp waist." The result of this bit of physical restraint was a high incidence of pulmonary pathology.

There is considerable evidence to suggest that in pre-Columbian culture, people with harelip, dwarfism, and spinal deformities (hunchback, etc.) were revered and even accorded special privileges. Some records show that spinal deformities were induced to enhance a fashionable concept of physical beauty (Waisman, (1967). Various deforming incisions were made in virtually every part of the body to enhance a popular concept of beauty in Africa, Asia, and the South Pacific, where such practices persist to this day.

Forming perforations of the nose, ears, cheeks, and lips through which various articles of adornment such as shells, wooden plugs and stakes, precious and semi-precious stones, and, more recently, metals of different types could be

1

worn is also an ancient and widespread custom. Even in higher cultures such as those of India and China, nose and ear perforation for the wearing of jewelry was a highly acceptable form of self-adornment.

The use of makeup was probably one of the first forms of self-decoration. Cosmetics, particularly facial, were highly developed and entirely socially acceptable among the upper classes in ancient Crete. It should therefore surprise no one that body painting has recently enjoyed a brief vogue.

Lest we forget our heritage and tend to look with disdain on our more "primitive" brothers, several examples of interesting forms of self-adornment (or is it self-mutilation?) have been selected as they are represented in different cultures. The author wishes to express his deep gratitude to the publishers and staff of the National Geographic Magazine and the American Museum of Natural History for their help and cooperation in making these reproductions available.

After viewing some of the methods of obtaining beauty on the following pages, it should seem apparent that modern cosmetic surgery is by all standards a mild form of torture to obtain the sought-after ends. This is not meant to infer, however, that there is any direct relationship between cosmetic surgery and what follows.

Vanity, it would seem, is shared by all members of the human race despite cultural differences imposed by genetics, religion, geography, or historical custom.

REFERENCES

Phillips, R. H., and Muzaffer, A.: Recurrent self-mutilation. Psychiatric Quart., 35:3, 1961.

Rees, T.D., and Daniller, A.: Self-mutilation: Some problems in reconstruction. Plast. Reconstr. Surg., 43:300, 1969.

Schedter, D.C.: Breast mutilation in the Amazones. Surgery, 51:554, 1962.

Waisman, A. I.: Ancient surgery of the Americas. Int. Surg., 47:129, 1967.

Nose, lip, or ear perforations, through which jewelry or ornamentation can be worn, are popular in many parts of the world, including New Guinea and much of Africa. The practice is almost ubiquitous among "stone age" New Guineans such as this man.

See illustration on the opposite page.

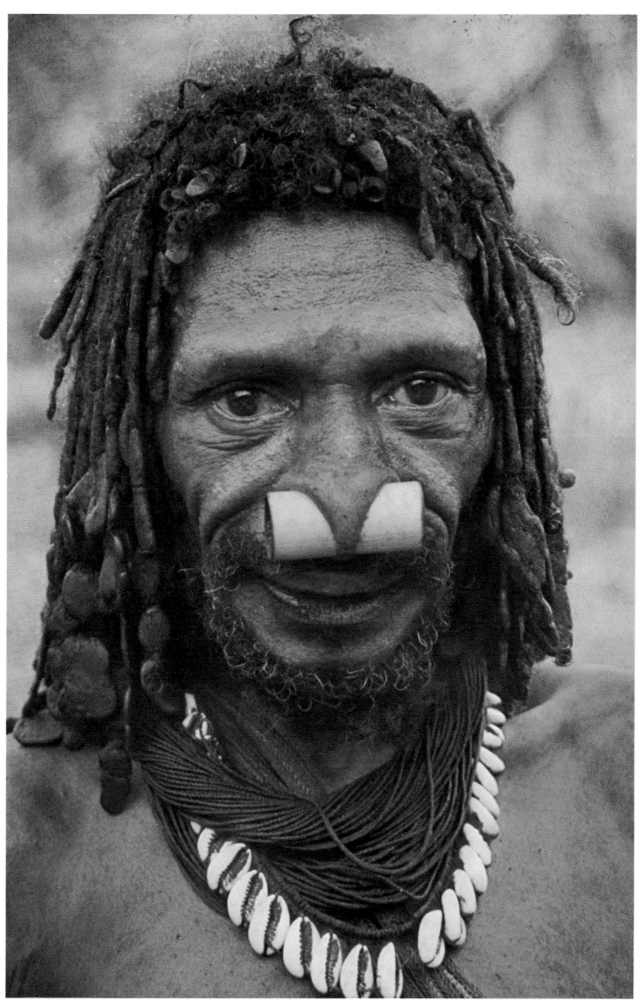

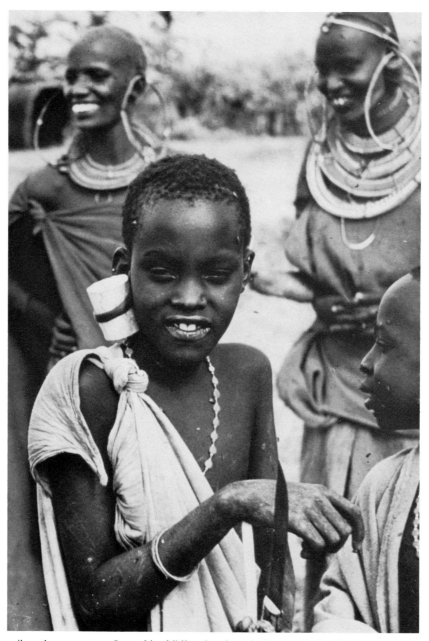

In many African tribes, the ears are perforated in childhood and gradually stretched to form great loops. These are considered decorative in themselves, but they also support various objects. Wooden plugs of graduated sizes are used to stretch the loops, as seen in this Masai boy.

Massive earrings of solid gold are seen in the ear loops of a Fulani maid, a resident of Mali in the sub-Sahara. Her permanent "lipstick" is an effect of tattooing. The mountain maid of Mandara wears in her ear a spent cartridge case left behind by the German rulers of the Cameroons before World War I.

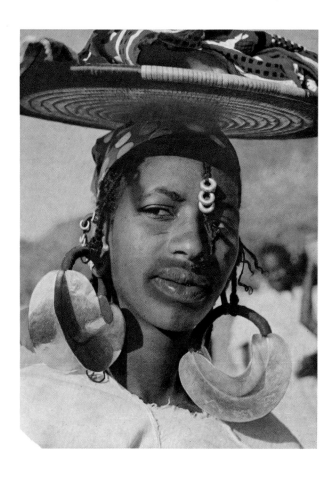

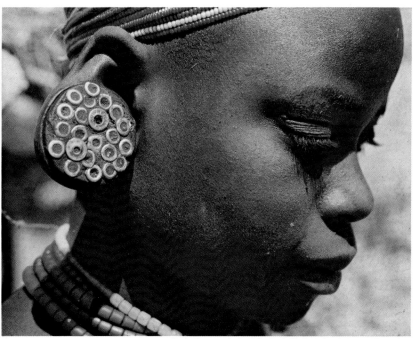

Both photographs by John Scofield, © National Geographic Society

5

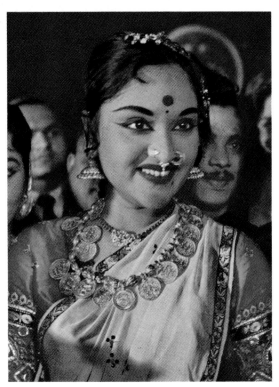

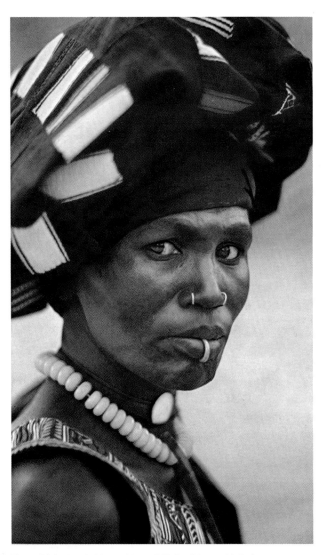

An Indian dancing girl wears precious stones in perforations of the alae of the nose as well as the columella. Tribesmen of the Bergen Country of Mali often adorn themselves with metal ornaments through perforations of the nose and lips.

If modern surgery to improve one's appearance seems like an ordeal, consider the filing of teeth as it is practiced in Micronesia, Indonesia, and elsewhere. The young man in this picture lives in Bali.

See illustration on the opposite page.

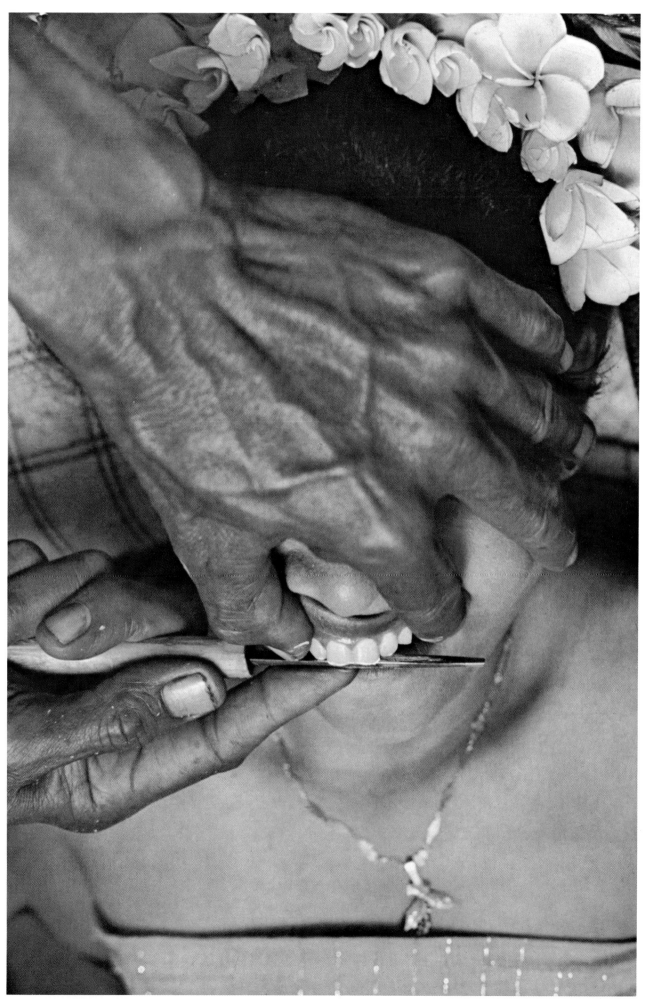

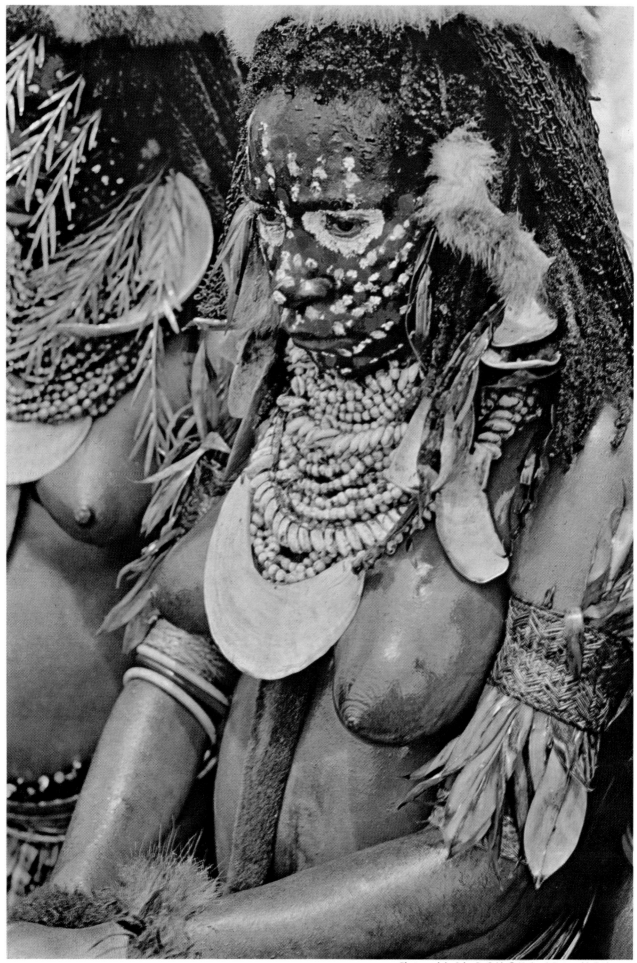

A lady of New Guinea in full ornamental regalia. Clearly most of these decorations have been fashioned from the local environment, with liberal use of shells, leaves, palm fronds, mud, and natural pigments. The arm bands probably came from traders.

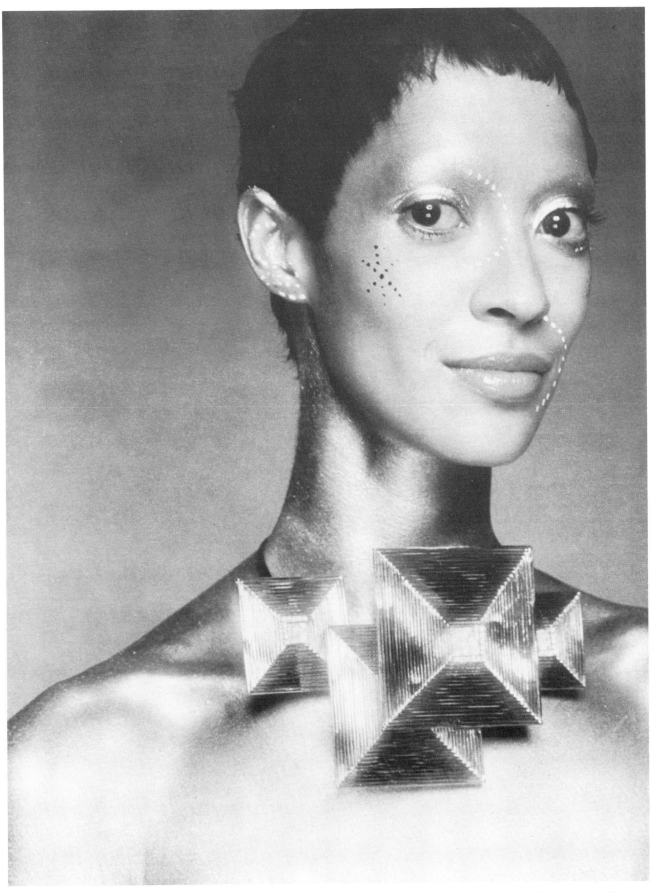

A modern civilized woman adorned with body paint, exotic make-up that is not entirely out of the realm of fashion possibilities these days.

This Kenyan has availed himself of ancient as well as modern techniques for self-adornment. The wearing of plugs or other objects in perforated and stretched ear lobes is a very old custom in Africa, as is painting of the face. Coral and glass beads worn on strings around the neck or head are of relatively recent origin, introduced by Arab and Indian traders. The sunglasses and a neck band made from a chrome-plated headlight rim are the most recent additions to the ensemble.

See illustration on the opposite page.

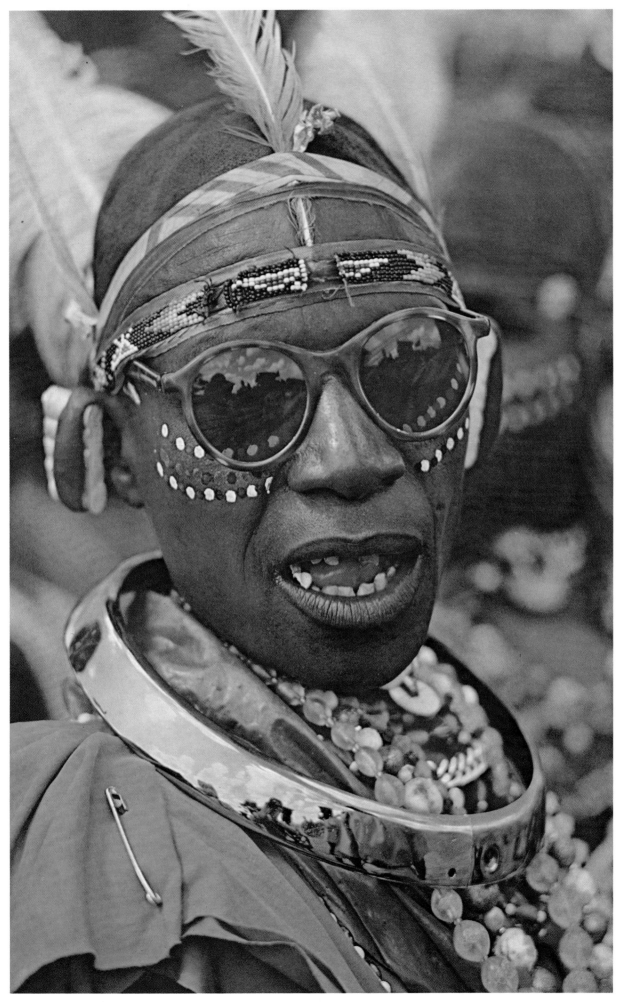

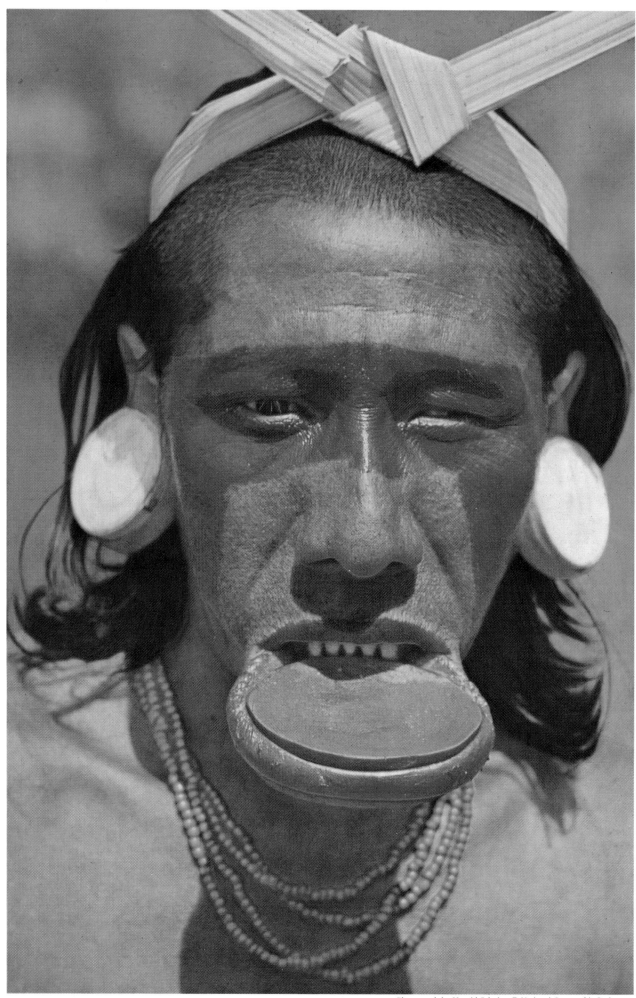

An African lady photographed during a transcontinental safari in 1938. Her lower lip measured 25 inches in circumference, and in this photograph it encircles a can that once contained 400 feet of motion picture film. The writer who visited her reported that her skin was so elastic that when pulled it snapped back "like a rubber band." This form of "mutilation" was probably begun centuries ago; tradition tells us that its original purpose was to make Ubangi women unattractive to slave traders. In the years since then the fashion has caught on, and these women are now considered appealing. Note the scarification marks on the forehead, and the scalloped ears.

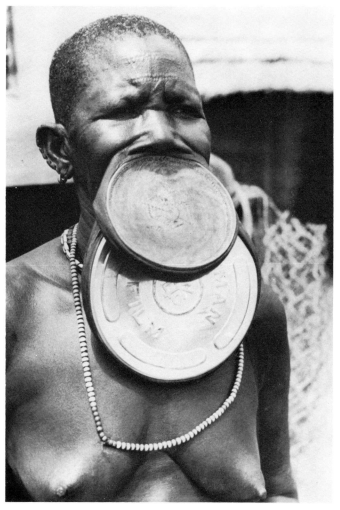

Stretching the lip is popular in both hemispheres, as the photos on these two pages suggest. The Brazilian gentleman on page 12, who belongs to the Suyá tribe, wears his lip disk in style, complete with red dye painting of the lip and face, earplugs of twisted palm leaves, a palm frond headband, and file-pointed teeth. He is a member of a vanishing tribe.

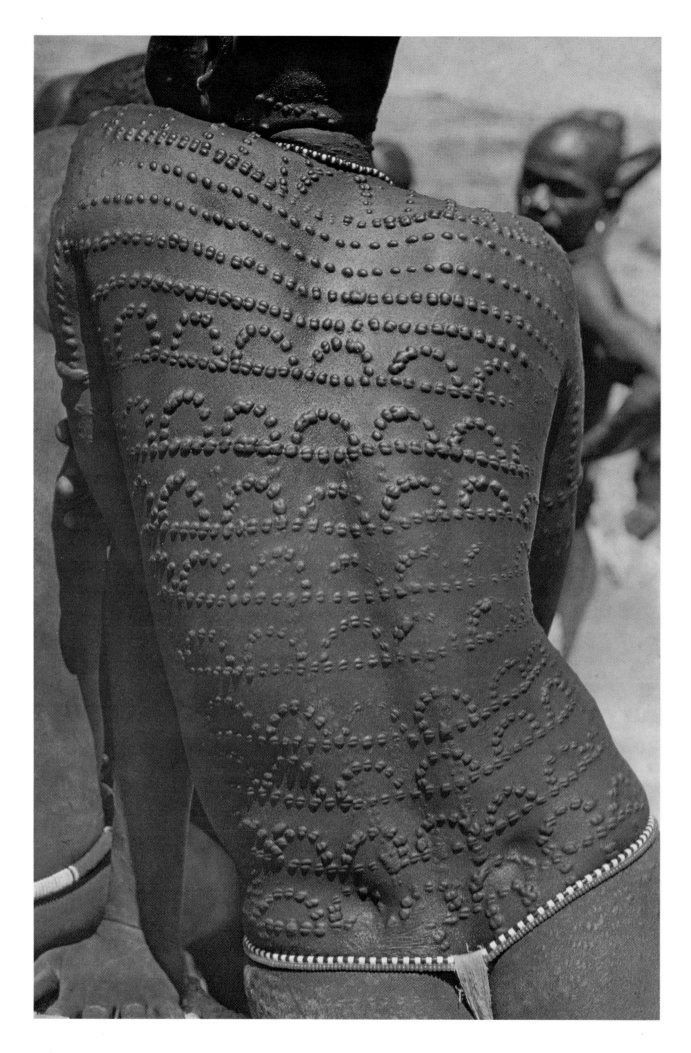

The people of the Masakin Qisar, a Nuba tribe, live in a remote part of the Sudan. Clothing is sparse or absent in the blistering sun of the region. For centuries these people have scarified the skin of their women as a method of beautification in the absence of the finery of clothes. Such scars, also found elsewhere in the world, often have significance. The three freshly cut rows of incisions across the left shoulder of the young girl pictured on this page are a particularly favored design because, lying over the heart, they are believed to make one's love life more favorable.

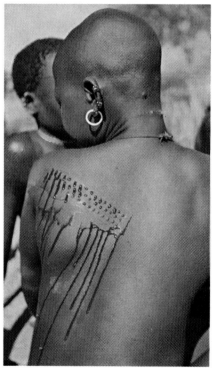

Both photographs by Oscar Luz, © National Geographic Society

Part 1

GENERAL
CONSIDERATIONS

Chapter 1

Selection of Patients

Thomas D. Rees, M.D., F.A.C.S.

Experience is the best teacher for most surgeons when it comes to patient selection for plastic surgery. This chapter is based on impressions gained by the author through many years of experience as a practicing surgeon. However, this is not a documented or disciplined study.

Chapter 2, written by Frances Macgregor, provides a complete and authoritative discussion of many aspects of patient evaluation and selection. Macgregor has had a long and rich experience investigating social and psychologic factors in plastic surgery patients. She has also worked closely with several plastic surgeons, and any surgeon seeking to enrich his understanding of this complex issue is advised to read Macgregor's chapter carefully.

CAN THE PATIENT BE SATISFIED?

The aim of cosmetic surgery is, after all, to make the patient happy. Generally, if the patient is happy, so is the surgeon. When a satisfactory result is not achieved, frustration and misunderstanding ensue and can lead to unpleasantness and, sometimes, litigation. Communication is the key to all human intercourse. For success, the total experience of a cosmetic surgical operation from consultation until the final follow-up visit depends upon a series of communications. It is distressing how rarely complete communication occurs.

Plastic surgeons have long sought a simple "A, B, C" guide that could characterize preoperatively the personality of a patient and therefore predict behavior patterns. Perhaps a battery of behavioral examinations could define a "personality profile" that would indicate those individuals apt to be pleased by physical improvment through surgery and those who would not; or maybe such a profile might indicate those with a realistic self-image. Such a quick and easy test has not been developed, probably because of the complicated natures of

humans. It is this very diversity that makes the study of personality so fascinating, yet so elusive.

CONSULTATIONS

There is no substitute for thorough personal interviewing and consultation prior to surgery. Primary aims of consultation are to establish meaningful communication between patient and surgeon at a personal level as well as to diagnose and plan treatment.

The first alarm that a patient may be unsuitable for cosmetic surgery is often signaled during the first telephone contact. The patient who is pushy, obnoxious, or rude is frequently egocentric, overdemanding, uncooperative, and difficult to communicate with. Patients who apply extraordinary pressure to obtain an early appointment and who are unwilling to accept an appointment at the normal allotted time almost certainly will expect "superservice" all along the way. Such patients are not only overdemanding but may well prove to be unrealistic about the results they expect from surgery. Concerted attempts to interfere with the normal office structure should always be viewed with caution and suspicion.

No surgeon likes to keep patients waiting; however, precise schedules in active day-to-day practice can rarely be maintained. The patient who shows extreme irritation at these minor vexations should be viewed by the surgeon and his staff as one who is more apt to be unduly irritated if some problems develop during or after the course of surgery. Everyone has the right to be impatient with delay, but excessive signs of impatience evidenced by the patient on the first visit may herald a difficult relationship and result in an unhappy patient.

It is a good practice to leave a new patient alone in the consulting room for a few moments before the actual consultation. Much can be
Text continued on page 23.

19

To   : My Patients
From : Thomas D. Rees, M.D.
Re   : Some Facts for Patients About Cosmetic Facial
       and Eyelid Surgery

You will do yourself a service if you read what follows carefully, for here you will find answers to many of the questions that are most often asked about plastic surgery of the face, neck and eyelids. Most of these questions are universally asked by patients interested in this type of surgical correction.

The purpose of cosmetic surgery is to make you look as good as it is possible for you to look. It cannot do more than that. If you are expecting a transforming miracle from surgery, you will unquestionably be disappointed. Plastic surgery is a combination of art and science. Surgery is altogether not an exact science, and because some of the factors involved in producing the final result (such as the healing process), are not entirely within the control of either the surgeon or patient, it is impossible to warranty or guarantee results. Surgical results from facial and eyelid plastic surgery, however, are more predictable in some patients than in others. This is determined by a number of factors such as the physical condition of the face, the thickness and condition of the skin, the presence or absence of facial fat, the relative "age" of the skin, the numbers and types of wrinkles present, the underlying bone structure, heredity and hormonal influences, and others.

It is not possible, by surgical operation, to make someone who is over 40 years old look as if he or she is 20 years old or younger! While this may seem obvious, I mention it because some patients through misconceptions or misinformation believe the clock can be turned back in this miraculous fashion. It cannot.

Surgery intended to improve sagging skin or wrinkles necessarily leaves scars. Despite what you may have heard, all surgical scars are permanent and cannot be erased. The job of the plastic surgeon is to place scars in natural lines of the face and eyelids, where they are least noticeable and are more easily camouflaged by make-up or hair styles. While such scars are permanent, they are rarely noticeable or cause any trouble.

Preconsultation Letter for Patients

Figure 1-1. *Legend continued on the opposite page.*

- 2 -

Now for some specific questions:

1.   How long will the surgical results last?

Plastic surgery of the face, neck and eyelids retards the aging process and actually slows it up. It "slows down the clock, but does not stop it." It is not a question of a sudden "falling down." How soon you will want, or require, another operation is highly individualized. I can only speak in averages. In general, the operation of facial and neck lift, which is for the improvement of the jowls along the jaw line and the loose skin of the neck, may need to be redone in about five to eight years. Some very few patients are encountered who, for one reason or another, age more rapidly so that another operation may be desired in a shorter period of time than five years. Of course there are some who never require it again. The operation to improve or correct "bags" of the eyelids usually lasts longer. In most instances, the pouches beneath the lower lids do not recur. As one grows older the skin becomes looser and redundant and a trim of loose skin may be necessary at a later time. In those patients in whom there is exceedingly marked aging and excessive skin of the neck, face and jaw, sometimes (but extremely rarely) it is necessary to perform a second operation within a year to achieve the maximum improvement possible. If this seems to be the situation in your case, I will so inform you in advance.

2.   Is facial surgery considered to be a major operation?

This type of surgery very rarely produces serious complications. It is, however, a surgical procedure and, as such, can be subject to unpredictables. Fortunately these are usually minor and amenable to treatment. These will be discussed with you in detail if you so desire.

3.   Why are preoperative photographs important?

Just as the chest surgeon cannot operate in an intelligent way without x-rays of the chest, the plastic surgeon cannot operate on the face or eyelids without medical photographs.

These photographs are not meant to flatter you. You probably will find it a harsh photograph unsuitable for framing. The photos will show your face in every detail. This aids greatly in the surgical performance of technical variations in the surgery.

4. What type of anesthesia is used during the operation?

Either local or general anesthesia can be used, according to preference. I prefer to use a combination of light general anesthesia and local anesthesia, which I find is more comfortable for the patient. This technique permits a light anesthesia. A high level of oxygen is maintained throughout the surgery, which promotes safety. Local anesthesia is preferred by some patients and is completely adequate for this purpose. General anesthesia requires the services of an expert anesthesiologist, who charges separately. His fee is explained in the preoperative instructions. Whether you have a local or general anesthesia, there will be no pain during the operation.

5. How long is the operation?

The actual surgical time will vary, depending on the amount of surgery necessary for each patient. A face lift usually requires about two hours and eyelid surgery one hour.

6. How long is the hospital stay?

The usual hospital stay is three days. Admission is usually one day prior to the operation at about 2 p.m. and discharge time is about 10 a.m. the second or third day after surgery. Admission to the hospital may seem unnecessarily early, but is necessary in order to perform the required laboratory work and examinations by the resident surgeon and anesthesiologist.

Although the room accommodations are booked well in advance of admission, it may not always be possible to have the accommodation you desire on admission to the hospital. Every attempt will be made on my part to handle this problem to your advantage.

Figure 1-1. *Continued. Illustration continued on the following page.*

7. Are bandages applied?

Bandages are applied to the head and neck after a face lift. These are removed 48 hours after surgery. Bandages may or may not be applied to the eyelids for a few hours. Following removal of the bandages, ice compresses are applied to the eyes for several hours. Although this will not prevent all bruising and swelling it will help to minimize it. After you leave the hospital these ice compresses may be continued at home from time to time if you find them comforting. Bandages are applied for several reasons, one being to keep the operated area as immobile as possible; therefore, it is also important that telephone calls and visitors should be kept to a minimum for the first 48 hours after the operation. Postoperative pain is rare, and whatever discomfort there may be is usually mild and short-lived and is easily handled with routine medication.

8. When are the stitches removed?

Most eyelid stitches will be removed on the second day after operation. The remainder are removed on the third or fourth day. Some stitches in front of the ears are removed on the sixth or seventh day after a face lift. In most instances, all remaining stitches are removed by the tenth day. Removing stitches is quick and uncomplicated. But you must remain in the New York area for a minimum of 10 days following facial surgery and one week following eyelid surgery so that the removal may be done.

9. When can make-up be applied?

Eye make-up may usually be applied three days following the removal of the last sutures. This includes mascara, eye shadow and artificial eyelashes. Facial make-up can usually be applied about the tenth day. At this time, you may have to use some type of covering cream if there are still bruises below the eyes. It is important to remove all make-up very thoroughly, using an upward motion, at the end of the day. Oiled eye pads are recommended for the removal of eye make-up. My office staff will provide detailed instructions on use of make-up during the postoperative period.

10. <u>When may I get my hair done?</u>

On the fourth day following surgery you may comb your hair out by using a solution of warm water and a large-tooth comb. Your first shampoo will not be possible until the eighth day following surgery. You may do this yourself or go to a hairdresser who is acquainted with the special procedure of the first hairset after plastic surgery. My office can recommend someone suitable. Rollers may be used, but loosely. A hair dryer may also be used but must be kept at the "comfort zone" (never hot), since at this time you may not have full sensation in the areas operated upon. Tinting and coloring usually may be done about three weeks following the operation.

11. <u>Is hair shaved in preparation for the operation?</u>

The hair is not shaved. At the time of surgery a small margin of hair behind the ears is trimmed where the incision will be. A similar area is trimmed inside the hairline above the ears. Neither area is visible once the hair is combed over the incision.

12. <u>Who takes care of me after surgery?</u>

Except over the weekends, you will be visited every day in the hospital by me. If for unforeseen reasons I am unable to visit you, you will be seen by one of my staff. There is an expert team of associates and assistants always in attendance, and they are continuously in touch with me. It is also not possible for me to visit you the night of admission to the hospital. Therefore, it is important that any unresolved questions be discussed prior to admission, if necessary, by a further visit to the office.

13. <u>Who actually performs the operation?</u>

I perform all surgery on my patients. I do have assistants who play an active role in your operation by assisting me just as the anesthetist and the nurse do. However, the actual operative procedure is performed by me.

Figure 1-1. *Continued.*

14. <u>What happens in the postoperative period?</u>

You must remember that before you see the improvement you are expecting you will go through a standard postoperative period in which you will look quite battered and bruised, followed by another temporary period of time when you may look "strange" to yourself. This varies considerably with each individual. When both facial and eyelid surgery are performed together you should set aside three weeks for recovery. At the end of this time most patients are able to appear in public, although the scars may need camouflaging with make-up. In some patients this time may be shortened by a few days and in others a slightly longer period is required. I think you should also bear in mind that in some patients undergoing facial and eyelid surgery there is a temporary period of slight emotional depression immediately following the surgery, during the period of time when you look your worst. This is quite normal and should not alarm you. It is not easy to look bruised and swollen, particularly when natural expectations are toward improvement of your appearance. Fortunately this period usually passes rather quickly.

15. <u>Are private nurses available?</u>

Although not a necessity, some patients feel happier knowing that someone will be with them following surgery. Some hospitals require the patient to book private nurses at the time of admission. At other hospitals we are able to arrange for nurses in advance. In spite of booking well in advance of surgery, because of the critical shortage of such help there is no guarantee that nurses will be available.

If you have any other questions be sure to get them answered in advance by me or my office staff. Many members of my office staff have been with me for years and are thoroughly informed, trained and able to answer questions that may occur to you. Well meaning friends are not a good source of information. Find out everything you want to know. A well informed patient is a happy one.

Thomas D. Rees, M.D., F.A.C.S.

learned from his or her behavior during this short period. Those who help themselves from the surgeon's bookshelves, desk drawers, or personal effects are literally putting up a red flag, signalling difficulties to come. Such incursions should be duly noted by the surgeon and, if the bounds of propriety are significantly overstepped, other parameters of the patient's behavior should be investigated.

I have found it useful throughout the past several years to address a personal letter to patients seeking cosmetic surgery that outlines in some detail what may and may not be expected from the operation. This is given to the patient for study prior to consultation. This form of communication has also proved helpful in answering many of the routine questions posed by most patients. It therefore not only serves to inform the patient but discusses in a general way that complications can and do occur and that the results of surgery are considerably less than perfect. A sample letter is shown in Figure 1–1.

PATIENT BEHAVIOR

Patients who are overly solicitous of the surgeon's attention or who demonstrate overt tendencies toward seductiveness are usually disturbed and insecure individuals for whom striking a "sexy" attitude is a cover-up for deep-seated insecurities and neurotic tendencies. The surgeon is well advised to be wary of such individuals and to insist on a preliminary psychiatric interview before making a surgical decision. In this context, it may be said that although the surgeon often sees patients who show many symptoms indicating neurosis or instability, it is not so easy or practical to obtain psychiatric evaluation. Clinics that have full-time psychiatric help are fortunate indeed; however, the average practicing surgeon does not have this type of specialized help at his beck and call, and he must often make many judgments on his own. Such decisions are often predicated on a sixth sense borne of long experience, but they can also be erroneous. The safest rule to apply is, when in doubt, do not operate until further information can be obtained. Psychiatrists are in short supply everywhere, and those with specialized knowledge applicable to plastic surgery are rare indeed. This is perhaps one of the most poorly understood areas in the field of cosmetic surgery, and one that deserves much attention. Current studies are limited to a very few medical centers in which psychiatrists interested in this subject are available.

Many patients harbor personality disorders that can be improved by cosmetic surgery. Nevertheless, the risks are significant, and the gamble should be undertaken only when an educated calculation indicates that the odds are favorable for satisfactory outcome.

Patients who are hospitalized often feel neglected in the absence of constant attention. It is therefore important that the surgeon try to make clear to the patient what can be expected in the hospital. It is also important to make sure that all arrangements for office visits and follow-up care are clarified to avoid misunderstanding.

Similarly, if the patient and the surgeon elect to proceed with the operation on an ambulatory basis, the patient should be informed in detail of the process and the plan of after-care. It is interesting that most patients who elect to undergo the surgery on an outpatient basis are easier to care for in every way than the average hospital patient. Generally, they communicate more easily, require less sedation and narcotics, follow instructions with less difficulty, and seem to recover more easily than hospitalized patients. It may well be that the patient who minimizes the threat of surgery and chooses outpatient facilities also minimizes life's problems in general. A study of outpatient personalities would be revealing in this regard. This experience is ubiquitous among doctors who perform a significant amount of ambulatory surgery. In the author's experience, it is often the parents or other family members who insist on hospitalization, rather than the patient.

PROBLEM PATIENTS

Patients who complain of a very minor superficial defect are particularly difficult to please. Such patients frequently have an unrealistic image of themselves. Any attempts at surgical correction of minor defects are almost certainly destined to failure. Fredricks further pointed out that the patient who speaks in a flat monotone may be harboring significant psychologic illness.

Generally, patients (especially women) who are in the age group to be candidates for rhytidectomy (40 and over) are in a period of life when the disappointments tend to outweigh the pleasant surprises. For most, the anticipation of new explorations and the joy of discovery are fading, and for some, they are already gone. Children, around whom their entire life may have revolved, have left home. The middle years have arrived, and with them the inevitable physical decline into old age and death. The sense of death becomes real to most people about this time. Before, it had been something that affected only others — the old or the infirm. In addition to this growing, distressing realization, especially in this second half of the 20th century, is the ever-growing emphasis on youth — its power and its desirability. Although physical health is better protected today so that most people actually "feel young" throughout middle age, they realize that youth has gone, never to be regained. Nevertheless, the pressure everywhere is to remain, and above all, to *look* young. It is not hard to understand, therefore, why facial rehabilitative surgery is undergoing an incredible boom.

On the other hand, most patients who seek rhinoplastic surgery are younger: in their teens or twenties. The defect is usually obvious and the desire for corrective surgery is clear. Unless the nose is a difficult, unpredictable one, or there is failure of proper communication between the surgeon and patient as to the aim of surgery, the surgical result is almost sure to be a success. The patient is usually pleased and the old nose is soon forgotten.

The situation is altogether different for the face-lift patient. The time of life, the motivations, the expectations, and the lifestyle are different. Much has been said about the older (over 35) rhinoplasty patient. Several years ago, it was unquestionably true that the general results of rhinoplasty in older patients (particularly males) was disappointing and often led to bitter problems for both patient and surgeon. With the growth of plastic surgery in recent years, and the change in attitude of many social and cultural groups toward altering appearance, our views of the older patient must be reevaluated. The patient today is well informed, knows his inner motivations, and is released from much of the guilt that used to accompany the desire for cosmetic surgery. Once again, only careful consultation and deeper investigation into the patient's desires and motives can provide the clues. It is the surgeon's job to listen and to learn before making a hasty decision.

Perhaps the hardest but the most important lesson for the young surgeon to learn is how to recognize which of the burgeoning number of patients seeking cosmetic surgery will become postoperative problems. He must learn to detect which patients will be unsatisfied or unhappy with the results, for these patients can and will make life miserable for everyone — themselves, their families, the surgeon, and the surgeon's staff. Experience is the greatest teacher in learning how to weed out the poor candidate for cosmetic surgery, but intuition plays an important role. The latter, unfortunately, cannot be taught, and some surgeons continue to have great difficulty developing the highly tuned psychic apparatus that makes it possible to pick up early danger signals.

Questionable candidates do not always present a cut and dried, black and white case. It is the group of patients in this "gray" area that causes most concern to the surgeon, and it is precisely in this group of patients that intuitiveness, experience, and a certain degree of luck are needed to achieve a happy result for all.

THE SELF-IMAGE

Much has been written on the subject, but only the surface has been scratched in our understanding of the psychologic nuances involved in evaluating the prospective cosmetic patient. Probably we will never have a clear-cut evaluative technique that is thorough enough to prevent postoperative problems from arising, for cosmetic surgery deals with the very core of human behavior and that most delicate of all human perceptions, the self-image. Despite all that has been published about the self-image, our knowledge of it is exceedingly superficial. It is often astonishing to the young surgeon to find out just how people visualize themselves, and how far removed this self-visualization can be from the interviewer's or surgeon's evaluation. There is no doubt that we all distort our self-image somewhat, so this should be expected to some degree in any patient. The line of demarcation between the normal range of distortion and the bizarre, however, is an important one in plastic surgery, because any cosmetic operation results in a certain change in self-image. When such a change is beneficial as far as the patient is concerned, all is well. When the change is viewed as a negative one by the patient, despite the fact that the surgeon and even other observers may feel differently, the result can be disastrous for both patient and surgeon. Sometimes the result can even be a tragedy.

How can the surgeon who is not a trained psychiatrist, and who does not have the services of a trained psychiatrist or psychologist instantly available, effectively evaluate the emotional status of the patient requesting a change of physical appearance? The problem arises almost every day for most plastic surgeons, and it consumes a considerable portion of their time and interest. It also has, of course, a direct economic bearing on the surgeon's life, as there is no doubt that most lawsuits in the field of aesthetic surgery arise from a misunderstanding between patient and surgeon on this all-important question of the patient's self-image. Most settlements to patients who have had cosmetic surgery are made not on the basis of malpractice or negligence but more on what is termed "breach of contract" — i.e., the doctor did not produce the result that the patient expected or liked. Clearly the surgeon and the patient were miles apart in understanding and interpreting what was to have been done. Such settlements have driven the insurance premium rates for malpractice sky high, and in some cases, insurance policies covering plastic surgery have been cancelled altogether. With the threat of litigation constantly hanging over the surgeon's head, it behooves him to develop his techniques of patient evaluation to the highest degree possible.

A patient can become very unhappy if the results of the surgery are criticized by family or close friends in the immediate postoperative period. It is not rare to see a patient soon after surgery who is ecstatic on one visit and deeply depressed on the next. An unkind or thoughtless word from someone close can turn the tide, arouse the guilt, and possibly reinforce a deep-seated doubt. A long-standing conflict with a spouse or a friend provides a typical setting in which cutting remarks are made after cosmetic surgery. Such conflicts cannot be resolved by the surgeon, but he should be patient and investigate further when a pleased patient becomes a depressed one. A few kind words or gentle probing as to what the problem really is can change a situation from one of potential hostility and lasting displeasure to one of closer communication and support during the trying postoperative period.

For the same reason, the surgeon should watch for signs of trouble between the patient and the family during consultation. Telltale symptoms of conflict can often be sensed between husbands and wives or adolescents, and parents during the consultation. Such signs should alert the surgeon that further investigation is warranted. Does the husband really object to the operation? Are the small derogatory jokes about the proposed surgery meant in jest, or are they sincere? Does the young lady really want the rhinoplasty, or was she dragged into the office by one or both parents who want the surgery for their own purposes? Is the father [or spouse] really so against the operation that he does not plan to pay the bill [therefore forcing the patient to pay]? These are only a few of the questions that bear investigation. They are warnings of problems to come and certainly should not be ignored. Often, innuendoes are detected by experienced staff in the office and then passed on to the surgeon. To ignore these small situations is to court problems.

PSYCHOSOCIAL EVALUATION

In the author's view, the ability to evaluate cosmetic patients on the basis of the flimsy and superficial knowledge gathered during one or two rather short interviews unfortunately is more a matter of intuitiveness than of behavioral science. Perhaps this is why some surgeons are constantly facing problems in their selection of patients whereas others seem to have little difficulty. The ability to penetrate the mask of human behavior and to sense deep-seated disturbance is a gift that many doctors do not have. Such doctors might be better off in another field of medicine than in plastic surgery, where this sense is vital in day-to-day practice. Some surgeons who have little native ability in this area are able to learn and to train their intuitive abilities so that they make fewer and fewer misjudgments. Eventually, with experience, some of these surgeons become quite skilled in this regard.

A great deal of intensive research is needed in the area of psychosocial evaluation of the plastic surgery patient. As more and more patients seek cosmetic reconstruction, the demand for this knowledge increases. Currently, very few centers have even a semblance of such research programs. Some of the problems retarding research in this area are the limited manpower available and the chronic lack of funds. It is surprising that more psychiatrists and psychologists have not realized the opportunities for study in patients seeking cosmetic surgery. Such patients are often quite eager and cooperative about psychiatric probing. Frequently, they are aware that there is a relationship between their self-image and their desire to change their appearance, and they are often willing to explore the relationship.

Assuming a lack of scientific criteria and a dearth of psychiatric aid, what are the more superficial indications that can guide the young surgeon in his patient selection? Some of these have been described by various authorities. Certain syndromes, such as that of the "insatiable cosmetic patient," exist and are not hard to recognize. As mentioned previously, it is the patient with more subtle problems who causes difficulty.

The first interview with the patient is the best time to detect potential problems, carried out under certain rather rigid circumstances in a controlled environment. This is of great importance, since the initial consultation sets the tone of the relationship between surgeon and patient. The consultation should be conducted in a private room without the presence of nurses, assistants, or others. The room should be comfortably decorated and aesthetically pleasing so that the patient can feel relaxed.

It is preferable that the first interview be conducted without interruptions. A cut-off switch should be placed on the telephone. The secretary should hold all calls, if possible, enabling the surgeon to devote his entire attention to the patient. Some surgeons prefer to see new patients at specific times that do not conflict with follow-up practice or day-to-day office routine. Although this may not be necessary, every effort should be made to provide peace and tranquility in this first interview, which rarely needs to exceed 20 or 30 minutes. Interviews lasting longer than 30 minutes or those in which the patient demands more time should arouse some suspicion in the surgeon that all is not quite right. If more time is required, the surgeon should arrange a second interview or consultation, particularly for those patients about whom he is unsure. Often, a second interview can be arranged after photographs have been taken or after other indicated studies such as x-rays, urine tests, blood work, and consultation with other specialists have been finished. This hiatus between consultations can be of great value for both surgeon and patient. The interval allows seeds of suggestions and questions planted at the first interview to germinate and sometimes brings forth valuable information at the second interview.

To avoid problems of communication, it is important for the surgeon to get a clear idea as to exactly what physical problem is disturbing the patient. It is fascinating to find that what might be considered an obvious deformity to the surgeon or his staff is not what is disturbing the patient. Markedly protruding ears, for example, are ignored by some.

Before the surgeon makes a fool of himself by suggesting a corrective operation for the wrong deformity, he should *listen* to the patient. It is best to begin an interview by asking the patient what it is that brought him to the surgeon, or to say, as my friend Dr. John Williams does, "What do you want to talk about?" Such an approach gives the patient the opportunity to speak about his problem. The complaint may be astonishing to the surgeon. Sometimes it is clearly unreal, but it is always revealing. The surgeon can then take the clue, and the remainder of the consultation proceeds along the lines indicated.

I have often found it helpful to pass a hand mirror to the patient and ask him to describe the particular physical problem that bothers him. In this way, particularly in rhinoplasty, the surgeon can gain a more defined picture of the patient's problem, and he can evaluate more accurately what he may be able to accomplish with surgery.

Several situations tend to contraindicate, temporarily at least, face-lifting procedures in men or women. These include severe emotional crises such as marital problems, divorce, or the death of a loved one, and those of late middle age — e.g., a sudden change in job status. If the emotional status of the patient becomes stabilized, however, he may benefit greatly, psychologically as well as physically, from the operation.

There are certain other signs that will indicate a disturbed or unsatisfactory cosmetic surgery patient. These signs admittedly are generalities and may be subject to severe criticism by psychiatric colleagues. Nevertheless, many have been proven by the test of time and experience. The following are presented here only as the opinion (or bias) of the author.

Perhaps the most commonly observed psychologic contraindication to surgery is in the patient who brings to the surgeon photographs of celebrities he or she would like to resemble. Most people who admire the appearance of others in this way are attractive in their own right, but they have the unrealistic attitude that choosing a face is like choosing a hair style.

The patient who is disheveled and unkempt, or who appears in inappropriate or sloppy dress with uncombed hair or signs of poor personal hygiene, should be viewed with slight suspicion. Although many patients assume a drastically different view of themselves following successful cosmetic surgery and take an increased interest in clothes, makeup, and hair styling, it does not necessarily follow that a sloppy and disorganized-appearing individual will benefit from such surgery. There is no guarantee that he will take a fresh interest in grooming when he had little such interest preoperatively. Furthermore, total disinterest in self-grooming or appearance may be symptomatic of a serious underlying mental disorder. Borderline psychotics frequently are disorganized in this way. The dishevelment of the withdrawn psychotic is even more apparent. However, it must be noted that everyone who is poorly groomed is not psychotic or even potentially so. The surgeon's personal biases in reference to what is a neat appearance must also be reckoned with. Many people dress casually in a studied sloppiness and do not consider themselves disheveled in any way, and their self-images are well developed.

The patient who seeks consultation at the insistence of a friend or relative and does not seem convincingly self-motivated is a questionable candidate. Every effort should be made to establish that the patient truly wants the operation. The surgeon should be wary of patients who present with statements such as, "I don't really want to be here or have this operation, but my boyfriend thinks I should." If the patient even implies that the surgery is being done solely to please someone else, the surgeon is well advised to refuse to operate.

The patient who tends to ask repeated questions but apparently does not listen to the surgeon's answers is also a potential problem. Conflicts will undoubtedly arise with such patients in the area of advised consent; they are best avoided.

One of the most telling signals on the basis of which to reject a patient for surgery can be detected within the first seconds of the interview. This is when the patient, almost immediately, begins to deprecate another surgeon, or surgeons, or doctors in general. Many such patients have severe conflicts with authority, and physicians represent the ultimate authority in their minds. They are almost never satisfied with surgery, either primary or secondary. It is often very tempting for the young surgeon to accept such a patient, particularly when a facial deformity seems obviously amenable to surgical correction. The temptation increases when such patients often warmly infer that all other doctors are incapable except the surgeon with whom they are consulting. This is both flattering and ego-building to the unwary. Such patients, however, are destructive and usually neurotic. Even if the surgery is successful, the relationship will be an unpleasant and exasperating one.

The perfectionist presents a separate problem that is difficult to resolve. Perfectionist patients are often recognized by their immaculate dress, highly detailed and probing questions, desire to know every detail, and above all, very detailed description of exactly what they would like to have done — sometimes complete with drawings, tracings, and photographs. These patients are very apt to be disappointed in the minor details of the surgical correction, but often in the end they are pleased with the overall result. Superperfectionists cannot be pleased. Expectations of such patients cannot be fulfilled, and they should be informed of this quite directly and turned away. Perfectionists of a lesser degree require more time and attention from the surgeon, including more than one interview to emphasize and to explain everything in great detail, especially the inadequacies, drawbacks, defects, and shortcomings of the operative procedure and the expected results.

If the surgeon decides to operate on a perfectionist patient, he must accept a certain risk that the patient may not be happy or may arrive at some measure of acceptance only after many weeks and a good deal of annoyance and irritation to the surgeon and his staff. On the other side of the ledger, however, is the astonishing fact that in some rare instances, pefectionists become the most devoted patients a surgeon can have. Suffice it to say that prior to surgery, the relationship between such a patient and the surgeon must be firmly established, and every detail must be explored to the utmost.

Another patient to avoid in most instances is the one who is rude, arrogant, difficult, insulting, or otherwise unpleasant to the secretary or receptionist. Often, such patients are the epitome of politeness and attention to the surgeon. When a secretary informs the surgeon of such rude behavior, he should be on guard and should make a very careful evaluation of the situation before accepting the patient.

In my view, a valid reason for deciding against surgery of a given patient can only be described as "negative vibrations." Such nebulous feelings between two individuals are recognized by us all, and they should not be denied. Aesthetic surgery demands a more intimate involvement between surgeon and patient (transference) than do other surgical specialties. If the "vibes" are not right, there is a good possibility that the final results, both surgical and psychologic, will not be satisfactory for either patient or surgeon. Certainly, any minor conflicts that arise will be magnified out of proportion by such poor compatability. Usually, this disturbance of communication is felt by both. When sensed, it is best discussed with the patient.

The patient who seems to ignore preoperative instructions as to medication, photographs, and other details may also prove to be a problem. Some such patients are simply a bit absent-minded, but others may be severely neurotic. Losing instructions or making repeated phone calls to the office staff to inquire about the same points is a fairly reliable tip-off to the surgeon that he had better make sure that he has investigated all aspects of his relationship with the patient before surgery is undertaken. It is such patients who are required by many surgeons to sign an informed consent form, although the legality of such forms is open to question. Usually, this type of patient is also the one who leaves personal belongings in the office or misses appointments one or more times. Sometimes, they do not even show up at the hospital at the appointed time, offering some lame excuse. Such patients may not be real trouble, but they can generate more than their share of minor irritation, including their failure to pay their fee either before or after surgery.

Although much has been written about evaluation of the patient, one aspect that is rarely considered is the surgeon's evaluation of himself and his reaction to the patient. Surgeons tend to be egotists, and their ego tends to grow and feed upon itself as experience is gained and success increases. Egotists have difficult understanding why they run into trouble with patient relationships.

Understanding should increase, given a little time for introspection, but the immediate reaction of most surgeons to a challenge by a patient is one of annoyance or even rage. Ask any surgeon what he feels when challenged by a potential lawsuit, for example, and if he is honest, he will admit to feelings of rage and depression as well as hostility directed at the patient. Actually, what these feelings represent is an unspoken, "How can they do this to me when I did such a great job?" When anger and ego take over in such a situation, reason disappears and communication breaks down. The loss of communication between surgeon and patient has been shown over and over again to be the prime cause of final litigation. Often, litigation can be aborted in the early stages if solid communication exists. This is not to say that a highly developed ego is not a positive attribute for a surgeon, but an overly developed sense of self-importance can certainly become a handicap if the surgeon has a poor understanding of himself and his reaction to his patients.

Such an ego can also push the surgeon into accepting patients that he would otherwise reject. Patients who massage the surgeon's ego are often accepted as surgical candidates, even by experienced surgeons, when all other evidence suggests that the patients should be turned down.

Surgeon, know thyself and be aware of thine own ego.

There are many other patient types that could be discussed. However, the interested reader is now invited to delve more deeply into the literature on the subject. The foregoing rather superficial discussion is meant more as an aid to the surgeon beginning in the field of cosmetic surgery than to the "old hands," although it is clear that these lessons have to be learned several times by most before they really sink in.

(For references, see page 47.)

Chapter 2

Social and Psychologic Considerations in Aesthetic Plastic Surgery: Old Trends and New

Frances C. Macgregor, M.A.

Aesthetic plastic surgery, a beginning specialty 40 years ago, has come to full maturity. Once regarded as slightly suspect and discounted because it dealt with what were considered "frivolous" rather than lifesaving matters, it has now assumed a stature within the medical profession as an important therapeutic specialty whose essential function is to improve the quality of life. No longer is it regarded as an indulgence to be sought furtively by wealthy women, vain and aging celebrities, and "neurotics," but it is seen rather as a social, psychologic, and economic necessity.

In the past decade, we have seen a dramatic growth both in the number of plastic surgeons and in the demand for their services. In addition to requests for rhinoplasties, face lifts, and the removal of eye bags — with which aesthetic surgery has been primarily associated — there is a growing demand for modifications and corrections of areas of the entire body, which new techniques and tools now make possible.

There are several reasons for what is being referred to today as "the boom in plastic surgery." One obvious one is the amount of publicity it is receiving. In the proliferation of books, magazine articles, and television programs, attention is focused upon the dramatic facial and bodily alterations that can be achieved, with discussions in simplistic terms of the surgical procedures, costs,

and psychologic benefits. Of special interest are the public testimonies of well known personalities who unabashedly discuss in detail not only their operations but also the emotional and social rewards derived from them. Having plastic surgery to enhance one's appearance is no longer a matter to be embarrassed about or to be hidden from one's best friends. Instead, it is a topic of conversation at health spas, cocktail parties, and beauty parlors. Both men and women freely talk about their surgery, recommend it to friends and acquaintances, and exchange information about surgeons and their competence.

From a sociologic perspective, the popularity of aesthetic surgery is a reflection of and a response to a variety of social pressures and changing values. In our youth-oriented culture, aging has become a dreaded prospect. It is not just those over 65 who are suddenly viewed as incompetent and often treated as social rejects; those in or approaching middle age are also beset by realistic fears. In the crowded and fiercely competitive marketplace, obsolescence comes early, and such aging signs as bald heads, double chins, and wrinkles are real impediments. Today, a job lost at age 35 or 40 may be the last job.

The sexual revolution, the preoccupation with eroticism, and the permissiveness about public exposure of the body are also reflected in the motiva-

29

tions and broad spectrum of requests for plastic surgery. For example, more and more women are undergoing surgery for augmentation or reduction of their breasts and for the removal of abdominal stretch marks, redundant skin from buttocks and thighs,and other bodily imperfections. In their wish to change their sexual identities, male transsexuals and transvestites, who once would have sought anonymity for such surgery in a foreign country or else taken no action at all, are in increasing numbers seeking a range of external alterations that will make them look more feminine. As for male homosexuals, a youthful appearance is highly valued within their community. Motivated by a fear of looking old, more and more individuals are to be found in the plastic surgery patient population.

A final impetus to the practice of aesthetic surgery is economic. The wide coverage of insurance plans and the expanding number of plastic surgery clinics throughout the country now make it possible for people from most socioeconomic levels to seek and to receive treatment for facial or bodily imperfections that cause them distress.

In the light of these converging developments, the motivations of patients appear to be far less complex psychologically than they were found to be in the majority of studies made prior to the 1960's and 1970's. For example, in a psychiatric evaluation of male patients seeking cosmetic surgery, Jacobson and his associates (1960) found that every patient warranted a psychiatric diagnosis. In a study of women seeking rhinoplasties, Meyer et al. (1960) concluded that preconscious and unconscious factors played a significant role in patients' motivations such as conflicts in sexual identification, the symbolic (sexual) meaning of the nose and the wish for surgery, and ambivalence in patients' identification with parents. In reports of mammoplasty and rhytidectomy patients, the incidence of pathology was also found to be high. For example, Knorr, Hoopes, and Edgerton (1968) found that many adolescent and adult females requesting breast augmentation exhibited hysterical character traits and were prone to frequent depressive episodes. Meerloo (1956), reporting on psychiatric patients who had had rhytidectomies, claimed that following surgery, an initially hidden depression emerged. Moreover, he observed that "a masochistic strategy was fortified by the operation, and the road to self-acceptance was blocked by a real loss, more difficult than the previous state to heal by psychotherapy."

The implied caveats in these and similar reports were such that many surgeons, fearful of postoperative reactions, held operations in abeyance until questionable patients received psychiatric clearance. Were these studies to be replicated today, the probability is that quantitatively, the findings would be different. This is not to suggest that the earlier ones were invalid or that the fears of the surgeons were entirely unjustified. To account for the extent of pathology found in these studies, one must judge them within the time context in which they were made, as well as their strong psychiatric orientation. Appropriate and inappropriate behavior are socially and culturally defined, and behavior is defined as pathologic when it veers too far from the norms of society. In the years when these investigations were made, shoulder-length hair and beads worn by men, unisex clothes, and overt proclamations of homosexual preferences would also have been considered manifestations of pathologic disorders. As we have seen in the last few years, however, there have been radical alterations in our social and sexual mores, with resulting changes in definitions of "normal" and "abnormal" behavior.

But these changes, coupled with the fact that requests today for aesthetic surgery are perceived as rational responses to realistic needs and situations, do not mean that in the selection of patients, caution is not mandatory, or that surgeons need no longer be concerned with patients' motivations for and expectations of an operation. Indeed, as the scope and range of surgical accomplishments widen, the potential hazards increase.

Although the major consideration of the surgeon is whether or not surgery is in the patient's best interest, the matter of litigation is also one of concern. As the public is becoming increasingly informed about medical care, competence, and legal aspects, dissatisfied patients are more inclined to speak out and, if necessary, to seek legal aid. With the current excessively high insurance rates for malpractice and the overeagerness of some attorneys to help in the courts, the plastic surgeon is particularly vulnerable. In many instances, however, such difficulties are not necessarily related to the surgeon's technical skill but lie in the area of human relations and communications. For the protection of both surgeon and patient, careful screening and selection of candidates are necessary.

Unfortunately, no "personality profile" or statistical chart exists, as some plastic surgeons have been heard to long for, by which one can learn in seconds whether a patient will be a psychologic risk: What is his real motivation for surgery, what are his subjective expectations, will he cooperate or be a management problem, will he be punitive or litigious if things go wrong? At best, a personality profile is a concept that rests on normative assumptions, and although statistical frequency may be interpreted as statistically normal, it does not follow that the patient is normal in a mental health sense. Even if one had a chart covering all types of personalities with mathematic weighting of characteristics that, when submitted to statistical analysis, would indicate or contraindicate surgery, other variables (social class and ethnicity, for example) would still make such an instrument one of dubious value.

Because of the nature and complexity of human relationships, the possibility of mistakes cannot be eliminated, but the more aware the surgeon is of factors that affect his decisions or color his judgments, the greater the potential reduction in unhappy surprises or outcomes for himself and the patient.

WHAT CAN GO WRONG AND WHY

Since lack of relevant information is one of the major causes not only of errors in evaluation but also of misunderstandings in the management of soundly selected patients, the importance of knowing the individual cannot be overemphasized, To know him well enough even to decide judiciously whether to operate often takes more interviewing time than many surgeons feel is either possible or essential. Though some doctors supplement their direct patient contact with chart reading and consultations with colleagues, these too may receive insufficient attention because of daily pressures and priorities. Neglect is not implied, but unawareness of certain pertinent facts is often apparent.

For instance, it is generally assumed that when a cosmetic defect about which a patient complains is evident and operable, it is both unnecessary and unprofitable to investigate or to discuss with him his problems, motives, and expectations. This assumption is erroneous. In contrast to the conspicuously disfigured patient, whose needs are obvious, the one who presents a "minor" defect requires particular attention. The former's complaints are situationally real, whereas with the latter, one cannot be sure. He poses special problems.

SPECIAL PROBLEMS IN AESTHETIC SURGERY

As evidenced by research (Macgregor et al., 1953), patients with slight defects tend to assess them as more conspicuous than they are, and they are also apt to be the most demanding patients. Additionally, the smaller the defect that troubles the patient, the more likely he is to focus on minute details and to magnify any residual imperfections following the surgery.

Cursory consultations with such patients seldom expose their underlying motives. Given reasons such as wanting to look better or to get or hold a job or a spouse are so highly sanctioned today as to obviate questioning. In many instances, the stated reasons may be the real ones. But in as many others, they can be oversimplifications or lesser elements in the motivation for the request. For example, one investigation of rhinoplasty patients showed that, although not verbalized to the surgeons, a dominant factor in the requests of approximately half the 89 people interviewed was the desire to reduce or eradicate ethnic visibility (Macgregor, 1967).

Besides the person who presents a single complaint, it is not uncommon to meet in one's practice a patient obsessed with real or imagined defects who shifts attention from one body part to another and who moves from one surgeon to another seeking relief but often finding none and ending in disaster. The following case underscores the importance of careful interviewing prior to acceptance of patients.

Miss G., aged 30, was convinced that her slightly large nose was the source of all her troubles. The surgeon accepted her request for rhinoplasty without attempting to review her history or to learn what she expected of surgery. Though he considered his results good, she did not, and she demanded a second operation and then a third. When he refused her a fourth procedure, she sought other surgeons. Two told her that further surgery was not advisable. Another, recognizing her disturbed state, suggested psychotherapy, but Miss G. argued that her first doctor hadn't thought she was "crazy," since he had agreed with her and operated three times. When seen at still another surgeon's office, she believed her nose to be actually disfigured and was highly agitated. To the social scientist who interviewed Miss G., it was apparent that she needed immediate psychiatric care. She resisted this idea but a few days later was committed to an institution because she had become violent and threatened suicide.

Had Miss G.'s first surgeon taken time to talk with her, he would have found strong evidence that her complaints were symptomatic of emotional illness and that psychiatry, not surgery, was indicated. In adolescence, she had been obsessed with what she considered her "ugly" complexion (acne). She spent hours in front of the mirror and aggravated the condition with heavy makeup. Because of this preoccupation and her refusal to go out socially, she was a problem to her family. When the acne finally subsided, she became absorbed with the size of her breasts. Though they were not abnormally large, she underwent reduction mammoplasty. She next focused upon her nose, blaming it for her unhappiness and difficulties with others. By accepting her for rhinoplasty, the surgeon unwittingly validated her complaint, with results that eventuated in a complete breakdown.

BREAST SURGERY

Demands for surgical alterations of the body in order to conform to prevailing trends and fashions require special attention. This is particularly important in the case of breast augmentation. Many women who would never before have considered mammoplasty now feel pressured by what has become almost a fetish in our culture. Slight imperfections in size or symmetry, for instance, once a private matter and easily concealed, are suddenly perceived as aesthetic deficiencies in today's climate with its insistent and intrusive exposure of women whose "ideal" physical attributes are so widely exploited.

Of the hazards inherent in breast alterations for aesthetic purposes, one is related to the decision to undergo this particular procedure. The given motivation of patients — to look or to feel more feminine and sexually attractive — is for most plastic surgeons a rationale that requires no elaboration or justification. Yet, more often than is generally recognized, the precipitating factor in the visit to the surgeon's office is not a long-felt need on the part of the patient but, as exemplified in the following cases, a wish to please a man.

Patient #1, aged 22, had been married just a little over a year. Because of her husband, a professional photographer, she had asked to have breast augmentation. "The size of my breasts doesn't make that much difference to me. But my husband — he's a breast man, and he just likes women's bosoms —like he'll see Raquel Welch on the TV and go 'M-m-m!' He said he had never dated any girl under a 36D until he met and fell in love with me. And gee, I'm only a 32A, and I think I ought to do something about it." After reading a magazine article about breast augmentation, with pictures of a woman who resembled the patient, the couple decided that "since it wouldn't hurt," an operation "would be a good idea." Although the patient admitted to wishing at times that her breats were larger, like many other young women she had worn padded bras and had given the matter little thought. But now she wanted to please her husband because, she said, "I am his woman."

Patient #2, a divorcee aged 35, had had a breast augmentation five years before. Three years later, complications had arisen, and because the implants were too large, they were replaced with smaller ones. On this occasion, the patient had just undergone surgery on the left breast, which was larger than the right. She was angry at herself and the doctors. Asked if she had told the latter about her feelings, she replied, "What's the use of saying anything? Doctors seem to lose their feelings about people. They're not interested in *you* — only in the operation. Anyway, I don't feel I have the right to complain, since what I've done is not a necessity."

To make matters worse, the patient said that her boyfriend, for whom she had surgery in the first place, now told her that he wished she had never had anything done. "He said he wished I was the way I was before. I hadn't noticed until he mentioned it, but my breasts are cooler than the rest of my body, and he doesn't like these 'bumps.' (She described her breasts as feeling like "two bricks.") He said, 'What good are they? *You* can't feel anything, so it doesn't do anything for me either.'"

Patient #3, a young, attractive model, had been married one year to an airline pilot. Her reason for requesting breast augmentation was that her husband wanted her to have large bosoms. "He said that when we are sitting around swimming pools he wants other men to envy him."

Patient #4, a young woman married one year, was frankly reluctant to request surgery but was doing so at the insistence of her husband. He objected to the fact that her breasts were asymmetrical. Passing displays in shop windows, he continually pointed out to her the symmetry of "normal women's breasts." His badgering had reached a point where she felt that her marriage actually depended upon her acquiescence to his demand.

Interestingly enough, none of the above women had revealed these facts during consultations with their surgeons. They would have been, they said, too embarrassed to divulge the real reasons behind their requests.

Since breast surgery is by no means a minor procedure, it would seem to be incumbent upon the physician to probe more deeply into what has brought the patient to his office. Perhaps, as the above cases suggest, he should turn his attention to the motivations of the men whose discontent with their wives and girlfriends develops "when the honeymoon is over." Marriages or relationships that depend on the size of the woman's breasts are not likely to be sound and lasting, and such faultfinding will most likely spread to other "imperfections." What is essential in such instances is to protect the patient from undergoing surgery for the wrong reasons, which later can turn into feelings of deep resentment and self-devaluation.

Many requests for mammoplasty have their origin in prospects for jobs. Naive young women are sometimes persuaded, directly or by innuendo, that they could have a position if they had larger bosoms. For example, 28-year-old M.G., who believed she looked like Marilyn Monroe, was told by a modeling agent that she would be acceptable for modeling bras provided she had a size 36C or D cup. But the offer was not firm. "Get the big ones," the agent had told her. "Then come and see me."

SECONDARY SCARS

Another potential problem, and one that has received practically no attention, is the effect upon patients of secondary scars. As used here, "secondary" refers to scars that have been surgically induced in adjacent or distal body areas by removal of skin, cartilage, or bone. Such sequelae can be troubling for patient and surgeon alike. In seeking correction of an aesthetic defect, the

average person is either unaware of or has not considered the possibility of residual scars. Despite the terms "incision," "skin grafts," and "donor sites," the notion exists that surgical scars are invisible or, if not, that they can later be eradicated.

For some patients, the distress caused by scarring may equal if not surpass that generated by the original defect. Although the surgeon considers the primary correction on which he has concentrated to be satisfactory — an opinion that may well be shared by the patient — the effect of unexpected but unavoidable scars on other parts of the body may undermine the psychologic benefits that were achieved by the initial procedure.

In our culture, negative reactions to unsightly body scars are universal, and today, with the fading taboos about nudity, such imperfections take on added significance. This is particularly true for adolescents and young adults. Normally preoccupied as they are with appearance, sexual attractiveness, and self image, they are especially sensitive to that which is aesthetically offensive. For patients in these age groups, unsightly scars may, as the following case shows, have serious social and psychologic consequences.

Before undergoing surgery for his malformed ear, Henry at 13 had been exceedingly proud of his "good-looking" body, especially his "manly" chest and his athletic ability. In the course of several operations, however, he had acquired scars on his chest, neck and leg. Angry and ashamed about "these obnoxious body blemishes," which to him were violations of his body and worse than having an imperfect ear, he had withdrawn from both athletic and social activities. By the time he was 16, Henry's parents were seeking psychologic help for him. He had not only grown alarmingly depressed but also refused a final procedure for his ear on the grounds that "it is a shame to fix one part of the body and ruin the rest of it."

Some patients who are not satisfied with the aesthetic outcome of the initial correction view a scondary imperfection as an extension of their original problem, and other view it as substituting one blemish for another. Patients who seek surgery because of attributed difficulties that are more imagined than real may transfer their preoccupation from the original defect to the secondary "mutilation" or use it as an additional cause of unhappiness. Regardless of age or sex, negative reactions are more likely to be pronounced in those individuals who are perfectionists or have narcissistic tendencies. For such patients, a scar that is hardly perceptible can become a source of inordinate concern.

Patients' resentment about surgical sequelae is usually aggravated by but more often has its origin in the fact that they are unexpected. Even if patients are forewarned by the surgeon, they may not be prepared for the extent or the appearance of the defect. Well documented is the fact that patients frequently fail to hear what the doctor tells them, and that ambiguous or nonspecific statements such as "there may be some residual scarring" make no impression at the time they are said. When unpleasantly surprised postoperatively, patients tend to feel misled, and they direct their anger at the surgeon. His assurance that the scar isn't very big or doesn't show under one's clothes is often cold comfort to the one who has it. In my research, I have found that the ability to accept unavoidable scarring is highly correlated with the degree to which the patient has been realistically and psychologically prepared. To avoid or mitigate untoward reactions, the surgeon should explain in careful detail his procedures and, insofar as he can anticipate, what may be expected. For some individuals, a scar may be more objectionable than the imperfection for which they originally sought relief. Information from the surgeon beforehand will give these patients an opportunity to weigh the alternatives.

CRITERIA FOR REJECTING CANDIDATES

Most plastic surgeons have rules of thumb for deciding if a person is a risky candidate psychologically. Strict adherence to these, however, can preclude objective judgment, thereby depriving some people of the attention they deserve.

HISTORY OF PSYCHIATRIC TREATMENT

Because symptom removal has long been regarded by psychiatry with suspicion, a common caveat is a history of psychiatric treatment. As already indicated, there is good reason to examine each potential patient's emotional status. But not all forms of neurosis result from basic personality disturbances. Many are realistic responses to external situations. Yet for most surgeons, the fact that a person has a record of emotional instability makes him immediately suspect, even when his complaint is valid. There is doubt whether surgery will satisfy him, whether he will become a management problem, or, worse still, whether surgery will precipitate a psychologic breakdown. His chances of being accepted are even weaker if he has the reputation of being hostile or a "personality problem."

J.B., aged 22, was such a person. When first seen by plastic surgeons in a Veterans Administration Hospital, to which he had been admitted for a complaint diagnosed as "psychosomatic," he was arrogant, defensive, and had untenable relationships with both personnel and patients. The surgeons described him as a "pain in the neck."

To a psychiatrist, J.B. had disclosed his feelings about his face and how it interfered with his relationships. He had what has been called the "FLK syndrome" (funny-looking kid). His large ears stood out from the sides of his rather small head. His upper jaw protruded, making the teeth so prominent that he could not bring his lips together. In contrast, the lower jaw receded.

An otoplasty was permitted, but two surgeons discouraged additional surgery and orthodontic treatment lest these trigger a psychotic episode. In any event, they regarded J.B. as "too difficult" and predicted he would be " a lot of trouble." "I wouldn't touch him," said one. "He's a kook," said another. The psychiatrist didn't consider J.B.'s appearance significant in the etiology of his personality disorder and was skeptical about the psychologic effectiveness of surgery. One resident surgeon, however, was inclined to operate. Because of conflicting opinions, the patient was referred to the social scientist on the rehabilitation team.

A review of J.B.'s life history revealed that his emotional problems had stemmed in large measure from ridicule and social rejection. At school, his peculiar face on his small, thin body provoked the nicknames "Long-legged Spider," "Elephant Ears," and "Buck Teeth" — epithets that he ruefully admitted were "appropriate, but this makes an impression. I always looked odd, and therefore I was considered odd."

Frequent family moves and new schools compounded his difficulties. Though bright, J.B. dropped out before finishing eighth grade. "You can't go to school if you're not accepted by the kids, and you can't learn something if everyone around you is making faces at you and you have arguments every morning. Kids are naturally going to pick on you. If you don't look right, you're singled out as the bad guy."

When he became interested in girls, his frustration continued. "I used to go up to a girl at a dance, but I was always rejected. When I was young, everyone else went out with girls — I didn't.

Convinced that he would have to go through life looking "odd," his efforts to cope with a hostile environment took the following forms: He developed " a very short, sharp tongue." He rationalized leaving school on the grounds that he was "creative" and so musically gifted that he didn't need formal training; that since he was "talented" his looks weren't "the most important." To cover his real feelings of inferiority and insecurity, he became arrogant and "put on an air of superiority and super-security." His isolation from others, he convinced himself, was self-imposed, since he had "superior intelligence and most other people were boring and unintelligent." Though his evaluation of his appearance was realistic, the defenses and stratagems he used to cope with his situation only led to further social rejection, withdrawal, and severe maladjustment.

J.B.'s growing intolerance of others multiplied his problems when he was drafted into the Army. Because he hated it, he developed psychosomatic symptoms and was unable to perform routine physical activities. Following hospitalization for bronchitis and pneumonia, he refused to return to duty. He was eventually given a psychiatric discharge, after having been placed in a mental hospital.

His behavior at the V.A. hospital in which he had undergone otoplasty tended to substantiate the surgeons' impressions of J.B.'s instability. His neurosis, however, was situational, and his days were fraught with unmitigated humiliation. Surgery could not be expected to heal his psychic wounds, but correction

of his appearance would remove a stigmatic barrier to his relations with other and help him to gain some self-esteem. For these reasons, the social scientist endorsed surgery.

Postoperatively, there was a striking change in J.B.'s face. Striking also was his dress: "mod" clothes, square gold-rimmed glasses, and ornate rings. He was delighted with the surgical results. He had begun to date and for the first time spoke hopefully of marriage. Although his improved appearance gave him an almost immediate sense of well being and more confidence when meeting people, he had sufficient insight to realize that he lacked the skills of normal social interaction. "It will take a lot more time being with people to change from the way I was before. Because I kept to myself, I have to learn how to act around people. It's not that I'm not fairly well mannered and so on, but I can't carry on a conversation. There seem to be certain intricacies in human relationships that you have to learn before you can actually get along."

J.B. got a job as assistant nurse in a department of physical medicine. He found the patients interesting and enjoyed his work. Within a few months, his former hostility and arrogance had almost vanished.

POSSIBILITY OF LITIGATION

Another criterion for rejecting candidates is the possibility of punitive action by those who may find fault with their postoperative results, even though these may be satisfactory from the surgeon's point of view. In a specialty that has one of the highest records for malpractice suits, surgeons are perforce wary of accepting any patient who they suspect may retaliate if his expectations are not fulfilled. Patients who have had cosmetic surgery elsewhere but wish additional operations tend to be viewed with caution. Derogatory remarks about the original doctor and vindictive attitudes are seen as red flags; any hint of legal action is so threatening that most surgeons close the door on further consideration of the patient's needs. This fear, realistic and justifiable as it may be in some cases, is so generalized that some patients who merit help are denied it. Caught in the rigid system of medical values and the stigma attached to those who seek any form of retribution, such patients are left to work out their problems alone. Even experienced specialists may make injudicious decisions when biases have priority and positions are taken without an effort to ascertain the facts.

A case in point is that of S.F., in whose infancy a skin infection on her nose had left conspicuous pitting about which she became exceedingly self-conscious. At age 24, she consulted a plastic surgeon who performed dermabrasion and rhinoplasty that unfortunately resulted in further scarring and also notched alae. Four years later, she requested evaluation at a plastic surgery clinic and was accepted for another dermabrasion. Dubious about this procedure because of its previous failure to eradicate the pitting, she asked instead for a skin overgraft. Although advised of the risk involved (possible scarring and a differentiation in skin color), she chose to take the chance, preferring this possible outcome to the pitting. Moreover, she volunteered to sign any document exonerating the surgeons should the operation fail.

While awaiting arrangement of her surgical appointment, S.F. mentioned to another patient that she had sued her first surgeon. The recipient of this information, an "old patient," told the head nurse. The surgeons' immediate reaction was to cancel the operation.

The story about the lawsuit was correct, but S.F. had not instigated it. The surgeon had also been disappointed with the surgical results. Several days before operating, he had broken his leg. According to S.F., he was in great pain and therefore hadn't done "as good a job as he might have. I felt sorry for him and I didn't blame him for what happened. He even offered to perform another operation." At the time, S.F. was a secretary in a law firm. It was her employers who instituted procedures on her behalf, on the grounds that the surgery had been "botched up." She described the trial as "a terrible ordeal. I would never want to go through anything like it again." She still felt sorry for surgeon and held no grudge. Her employers, however, had persisted and won the suit.

When the details of this case were reported to the surgeons who had refused to operate, S.F. was brought to the clinic for reevaluation. Several members of the group favored surgery, but others who were more skeptical and worried about legal action vetoed the idea. The patient, whose hopes had been raised, left the clinic in tears.

SURGEONS' MOTIVATIONS

Although the plastic surgeon may sometimes be overly cautious in selection, he may also err on the side of suggesting surgery. For instance, his high sensitivity to the slightest deviation or asymmetry and his zeal to make "beautiful people" may tempt him to propose unnecessary aesthetic improvements. This enthusiasm to make alterations, referred to as the "Pygmalion complex," is a potential pitfall and can obscure the difference between "desire to cure and the need to cure" (Meyer, 1977). Surgeons' suggestions may also be motivated by professional self-interest such as eagerness to obtain operating experience or to recruit patients — phenomena not uncommon in resident training programs of teaching hospitals or in building up a practice.

In some instances, correction can safely be initiated and should be. However, the surgeon needs to be conscious of his motives. To suggest that an individual's appearance can be improved is to point up a deficiency, and this is a responsibility that must be carefully weighed. If the person is nonreceptive, he will only be disconcerted. On the other hand, he may be more than ready to comply; but if he is dissatisfied with the outcome, the doctor may have to bear the full onus.

Such a consequence was aborted in the case of R.L., aged 39, who said she had come to the clinic because the previous week, while she was being treated in the ENT clinic for a sinus infection, a plastic surgery resident observed that rhinoplasty would make her look better. She asserted she had never thought of having an operation, but "since the doctor thought it would be a good idea" she was "willing" to have it.

Interviewing disclosed that R.L. actually had long desired to have her nose altered but had refrained for fear the results would fall short of her standards of perfection. In the event of an imperfect result, she would have only herself to blame, a situation that she seemed unable to handle psychologically. Discussion of her work experience and social relationships revealed a vindictive need to hold others responsible whenever she failed. Fortuitously, in this instance, the resident's casual suggestion of a rhinoplasty had provided a solution to her dilemma. Should the operation fail to fulfill her hopes, he could be a convenient scapegoat. Considering the psychologic hazard involved, it was decided not to operate.

CONFLICTING CONCEPTS OF "SUCCESS"

Another source of problems in aesthetic surgery is the dichotomy between the surgeon's concept of a satisfactory result and the patient's expectations. Since the surgeon's training is necessarily concerned with reconstruction or correction that approximates in form and contour the anatomic "ideal," he assumes that the patient has the same objective. That there are cultural variations in concepts of the "ideal" may be forgotten. Confident in his judgment of what can and should be done, the surgeon is dismayed and puzzled when a patient views technically successful results as disappointing.

Arbitrary ascription of physicians' standards in the controversial area of aesthetic surgery, where patients' subjective responses are so often the criteria for success, is to invite complications, as shown in the following case.

Tired of being called "Ski Snoot" and teased about her "Bob Hope" nose, 29-year-old N.H. requested correction of its retroussé tip. The surgeon achieved what he considered an excellent result, but N.H. first wept hysterically, then became depressed. Though the modified tip pleased her, she had not expected the elimination of a slight dorsal concavity. To her, this was a calamity because she was Irish and extremely proud of her heritage. Equating Irishness with a turned-up nose, she had tacitly valued the dorsal curvature. The surgeon's perception and creation of the "best" esthetic effect — in this instance, a straight dorsum — destroyed what the patient prized, her Irish identity.

As already indicated, preoperative consensus could forestall such deleterious outcomes. Of central importance to satisfactory results, along with good doctor-patient relationships, is a clear understanding of the patient's perception of his defect, what it means to him, its symbolic significance, and what he expects surgery to achieve both aesthetically and subjectively. The surgeon should insist on as much specificity as possible from patients about what they do or do not want done and why, and in turn he should explain as definitively as he can what alterations he has in mind.

RELIANCE ON OTHER PROFESSIONALS

Because of the exigencies of treatment, it is important for plastic surgeons to have other professionals on whom they can rely in making judgments in the patients' best interests. Most medical centers have psychiatrists, clinical psychologists, and psychiatric social workers available for referral and consultation, and it has become customary to turn to these specialists when questions arise regarding psychologic diagnosis and management. They are also the ones most often included as participants in rehabilitation and research programs. Their use of such methods as interviews, psychologic tests, and projective techniques often provides helpful adjunctive information and insights.

In depending on these disciplines for psychosocial evaluations and solutions to behavioral problems, the plastic surgeon should also be cognizant of certain limitations. The traditional training of psychiatrists, psychologists, and social workers is rooted in Freudian theory and individual psychology, and as such it has focused on personality development, the unconscious, and the intrapsychic processes of people who manifest some form of psychopathology or behavior considered abnormal. This orientation, aimed at understanding the individual, is concerned primarily with such idiosyncratic features as his emotional life, personality structure, and primary sexual identification. Interpretations of behavior considered deviant (which implies the existence of norms) tend to be couched in negative terms: repression, guilt, hostility, fixation, neurosis, and so on. Such interpretations fail to consider the person in the context of his social, cultural, and religious background; the influence of the social world in which he lives; and the impact of these factors on his attitudes and behavior.

Today, the narrowness and shortcomings of the individual psychologic approach to behavior are recognized, and increasing attention is given to broader perspectives that include those of sociology and anthropology. According to the noted psychiatrist Jurgen Reusch, emphasis must "shift away from man as an isolated entity and towards consideration of man in his environment" (1966). Man's social needs and his interdependence with his environment — including his interaction with his surroundings — must be considered. In a similar vein, Murphy stated, "The conception of personality as a self-contained . . . whole . . . goes badly with the world of reality (1968).

For the person with a visible physical defect, the "world of reality" has unique import and must be taken into account. A facial flaw in particular can have profound consequences for personal adjustment and social interaction. More often than not, his problems are sociogenic rather than psychogenic (Macgregor, 1974). Referral to the psychiatrically oriented, therefore, for diagnosis and solution of patients' problems, is not always the answer. Consider the following two cases.

C.A., a young mother of three, had incurred a slight facial scar in a car accident. In view of her low socioeconomic level and her established role as a housewife, her intense anxiety about her appearance seemed to the surgeons disproportionate and thus symptomatic of emotional disturbance. It was suggested that she needed a psychiatrist more than she did surgery. C.A. happened to be Puerto Rican, and interviewing by a social science researcher revealed that indeed she had reason to be disturbed. In her sociocultural milieu, a scar on a woman's face is a sign that one has been branded for unfaithfulness. She was distressed more for her husband, whom she loved, than she was about herself, since his acquaintances were assuming he had slashed her cheek because she had committed adultery. The stigma that Puerto Ricans attach to such scars was the sole reason both for her visit to the clinic and for what the surgeons had perceived as an overreaction. Fortunately, in this instance, a serious diagnostic mistake was averted.

Sarah was a 14-year-old girl whose lack of psychologic readiness for facial surgery was the subject of a clinic conference. The surgeon suggested that the excessive anxiety of the mother was a factor in the child's resistance to a minor opera-

tion. The psychiatrist to whom Sarah was referred declared that in his opinion, the mother was not so much anxious as outright hostile toward her daughter. What kind of mother was it, he asked, who would slap her child's face on learning that the child's menses had begun? This fact he had learned from Sarah herself while questioning her about the menarche. For him, this was evidence of the mother's hostility, even cruelty. What he failed to take into consideration was the possibility that there might be some other explanation for the mother's behavior.

Both Sarah and her mother were Orthodox Jews from East Europe, among whom it is the custom for the mother to slap her daughter's face at the time of the menarche "to bring the roses to the cheeks," or to bring good luck. By assessing behavior in terms of his own cultural standards of what is normal or abnormal, the psychiatrist was led to a false interpretation. The mother's behavior in this situation was not aberrant. As a custom of her culture, it had no deeper meaning for the child than the ritualistic and facetious spanking given an American child on his birthday (Macgregor, 1960).

In using the services of other professionals, plastic surgeons should have a knowledge of and weigh the former's special orientations and biases. Indiscriminate and unquestioning reliance on any single discipline for interpretations of behavior can make for judgmental errors. On the other hand, appreciation of the training, value orientation, role, and function of each specialist enables the surgeon to make optimal use of those he may wish to consult.

SUMMARY

As current demands for aesthetic surgery increase, so too do the possibilities of postoperative problems for surgeons and patients alike. To avoid these, special care must be taken in the selection of patients.

In assessing the validity of the request for surgery, the patient's presenting complaint must be considered in the context of his emotional state, sociocultural background, motives, and expectations. Because people with "minor" imperfections may pose special problems, careful screening is essential. Vital too is the surgeon's awareness of his personal biases and examination of his criteria and motives for accepting or rejecting patients. Although mutual satisfaction cannot be guaranteed, preoperative consensus based on understanding what the patient perceives and wants, and what the surgeon can recommend as technically feasible, helps to minimize their possibly conflicting concepts of success.

Knowledge of the orientations and limitations of other professionals can enable the plastic surgeon to use their services judiciously in making psychosocial evaluations and in managing behavioral problems. Traditional reliance on disciplines that stress Freudian theory and individual psychology needs to be augmented by broader perspectives, including those of sociology and anthropology.

(For references, see page 47.)

Chapter 3

Anesthesia

Seamus Lynch, M.D.

Be gentle with me, ... Treat me tenderly, I need the gentle touch, ... They've been so many who didn't understand. . . . but give it gently. Please.

Rod McKuen, *Two*
"Listen to the Warm"

Gentleness is an art when inducing and sustaining a pain-free unconscious state. Administering an anesthetic means applying a measured physiologic insult to a patient under precise pharmacologic control. Unnecessary fluctuations of blood pressure and pulse, irregularity of respiratory depth and rate, bucking and coughing (on the endotracheal tube), increased bleeding in the wound, straining and moving during application of the surgical dressing, and bulky and obtrusive endotracheal equipment are all signs of the crude, casual, and careless approach to anesthesia so frequently encountered in the operating room. Problems that are considered of little consequence in general surgery are of major importance to the patient undergoing cosmetic surgery, probably because postoperative pain is minimal, particularly in facial or eyelid plasty. The loss of a capped incisor or a broken bridge, the ecchymoses produced by an intravenous needle poorly placed in the dorsum of the hand, or hours of retching and vomiting can only tarnish the image of both the surgeon and the anesthesiologist. Such problems can be virtually eliminated by a gentle, knowledgeable, and sympathetic approach to anesthesia and by the concept of the "esthetic anesthetic."

Preoperative Evaluation

It is essential that the anesthesiologist visit and examine the patient undergoing cosmetic plastic surgery the day before the operation in order to gain the confidence of the patient and to relieve any fears and anxieties. The choice of premedication and anesthetic agents is made at this time. Halothane certainly will not be administered to the patient with a history of jaundice, just as methoxyflurane (Penthrane) would not be considered for the patient with a history of chronic kidney disease. Because of the increased risk involved, elective surgery should not be attempted following a myocardial infarction unless a minimum of six months has passed since the cardiac injury. The patient who is accustomed to a daily alcohol intake, who uses tranquilizers, or who routinely takes sedatives for insomnia will require heavier premedication and, most likely, higher concentrations of anesthetic agents to produce a satisfactory anesthetic state. A detailed oral examination is mandatory because of the many delicate dental restorations commonly observed today. Most potential errors in the management of anesthesia can be avoided by careful preoperative evaluation and planning.

Premedication

The patient who has been properly premedicated arrives in the operating room in a drowsy, amnesic, and cooperative state, with no circulatory or respiratory depression. This optimal condition usually is achieved by a combination of drugs. Because of its pharmacologic activity, each drug plays an important role in the final result. Drugs used for premedication include barbiturates, belladonna alkaloids, tranquilizers, and narcotics.

Barbiturates. Short-acting barbiturates such as secobarbital (Seconal) or Pentobarbital (Nembutal) are rarely used today. The combination of postoperative pain and barbiturates produces restlessness.

Tranquilizers. The addition of a phenothiazine such as prochlorperazine (Compazine), 10 to

40

20 mg, or perphenazine (Trilafon), 5 to 10 mg, enhances the hypnotic effects of the barbiturates and the narcotics without producing significant hypotension. As shown by Bellville, Bross, and Howland (1960), the particular value of tranquilizers is in their potent antiemetic properties, since reduction in postoperative nausea and vomiting is best for both patient and surgeon. The patient has a smooth and pleasant emergence from the anesthetic, and the surgeon need not contend with vomitus-soaked dressings.

Valium. Valium is a benzodiazepine derivative. It is an excellent tranquilizer in a 10 to 20 mg oral dose. It should never be injected intramuscularly, as it is painful and ineffective. Given intravenously, it produces a significant degree of amnesia. Its main drawback is that there is a small incidence of phlebitis.

Narcotics. Morphine sulfate, 8 to 10 mg, and meperidine (Demerol), 50 to 100 mg, are the commonly used narcotics. They enhance the sedative effect of the tranquilizer and, because of their analgesic action, reduce the amount of anesthetic agent necessary during the operative procedure.

Belladonna Alkaloids. Atropine sulfate and scopolamine hydrobromide, 0.4 to 0.6 mg, are important in proper preoperative medication. Their primary value is in drying secretions in the airway. They also diminish the reflex activity of the pharynx, the larynx, and the heart. Because it is an excellent drying agent and has an important specific amnesic effect on the patient, scopolamine is preferred. Atropine sulfate, however, effects greater control on the reflex activity of the myocardium. The narcotic and belladonna drugs are miscible and are administered by intramuscular injection one hour prior to surgery.

Innovar. Innovar is the combination, in a 50:1 ratio, of a tranquilizer and a short-acting narcotic analgesic. Droperidol (Inapsine) is the tranquilizer and neuroleptic agent and sublimaze (Fentanyl) is the narcotic. Each cubic centimeter contains Fentanyl 0.05 mg and Inapsine 2.5 mg. Innovar can be used intramuscularly as premedication or intravenously during surgery to produce the state of neuroleptanalgesia (Fox and Fox, 1966). The neuroleptic state is characterized by (1) mental withdrawal, (2) hypomotility, a disinclination to move, (3) homeostatic stabilization by blockade of the adrenergic receptors, and (4) potent antiemesis.

Pentazocine (Talwin). Talwin is a potent analgesic. In a dose of 30 mg, it is usually equivalent in effect to morphine, 10 mg, or meperidine, 75 to 100 mg. Analgesia occurs within 15 to 20 minutes after intramuscular injection and should last three hours. The usual narcotic antagonists such as nalorphine are not effective to reverse the respiratory depression caused by Talwin. Although it is not under narcotic control, dependency can occur.

Propranolol (Inderal). Propranolol is a β-adrenergic blocking agent that is used in the treatment of various supraventricular cardiac arrhythmias such as atrial fibrillation, flutter, and paroxysmal tachycardia since it prolongs the A-V nodal refractory period. Inderal is of interest to the anesthesiologist because of its use for the aftercare of the patient who has had a myocardial infarction and for those patients with angina pectoris, since propranolol blocks the catecholamine ability to increase myocardial work and oxygen consumption. Propranolol causes a depression of A-V conduction and direct myocardial depression, so caution is warranted when anesthetizing patients who are being treated with this drug. However, such patients should be maintained on their usual propranolol therapy, as acute withdrawal may induce serious sequelae. Propranolol is dispensed as 10 to 40 mg tablets. The daily maintenance dose is 20 to 80 mg. It is available also in ampule form for intravenous use, 1 mg per cc. The dose here is 0.5 cc to a maximum of 4 cc.

PRINCIPLES OF SAFE LOCAL ANALGESIA

The safe administration of local analgesia depends upon (1) reasonable premedication, (2) the application or injection of the proper dose and concentration of the selected agent, (3) avoidance of intravenous injections of solutions, (4) use of vasoconstrictor drugs, and (5) preparedness at all times to treat adverse reactions.

Reasonable Premedication

The desire to avoid patient discomfort during local anesthesia leads the surgeon to attempt to produce the state of general anesthesia by ordering heavy premedication. The induction of varying degrees of stupor and coma is unwise and unsafe and is best left in the hands of the anesthesiologist, who has the knowledge to sustain and to resuscitate a patient so deeply anesthetized. Premedication is designed merely to produce a state of calm relaxation while unusual or uncomfortable situations occur. The patient should sustain all vital functions, including responsiveness.

Snoring is a sign of respiratory obstruction and, therefore, of hypoxia and hypocarbia. It is much safer to undermedicate than to risk the complications of iatrogenic coma. Valium, 10 mg

TABLE 3–1

Drug	Maximum Dose	Topical	Infiltration
Procaine (Novocain)	1 gm	Has no topical action	200 cc of 0.5% = 1 gm 100 cc of 1% = 1 gm 50 cc of 2% = 1 gm
Lidocaine (Xylocaine)	0.5 gm	10 cc of 2% = 200 mg 5 cc of 4% = 200 mg	100 cc of 0.5% = 0.5 gm 50 cc of 1% = 0.5 gm 25 cc of 2% = 0.5 gm
Hexylcaine (Cyclaine)	0.5 gm	10 cc of 5% = 0.5 gm	100 cc of 0.5% = 0.5 gm 50 cc of 1% = 0.5 gm 25 cc of 2% = 0.5 gm
Cocaine	200 mg	4 cc of 5% = 200 mg 2 cc of 10% = 200 mg	Not used; too toxic
Tetracaine (Pontocaine)	200 mg	4 cc of 2% = 80 mg 8 cc of 1% = 80 mg	80 cc of 0.25% = 200 mg

orally, or compazine, 10 mg intramuscularly, and Demerol 50 to 100 mg given one hour prior to surgery should be more than adequate for most patients. If on arrival in the operating room the patient should still be apprehensive, nervousness is controlled by starting an intravenous infusion and adding small amounts of narcotic or tranquilizer as required. Intermittent intravenous injections of 10 to 25 mg of meperidine and 5 to 10 mg of Valium should control any restless patient. The surgeon must remember that it is almost impossible to predetermine the exact amount of premedication that will be effective on each patient. Continuous titration of small doses intravenously will invariably produce the required precise degree of control.

Dose Concentration

Exceeding the toxic dose of an agent is a common error. All anesthetic agents have well established maximum dose levels, as indicated in Table 3–1.

Inadvertent Intravenous Injection

When a drug is injected intravenously, a high blood level results and may lead to cardiovascular and respiratory collapse. It behooves the surgeon, when injecting local anesthetic solutions, to aspirate — that is, to pull back on the plunger — before injecting the local anesthetic, unless the needle is moving. Secondly, when injecting in a known vascular area, it is necessary to reduce both the volume and the concentration of the drug.

Use of Vasoconstrictor Agents

These agents, by causing local vasoconstriction (chemical tourniquet effect), reduce the rate of absorption of the local anesthetic agent and so reduce the incidence of adverse reactions. They also prolong the duration of the anesthetic. The dangers of these agents, particularly epinephrine (which is the best), is in the use of unnecessarily high concentrations. Solutions of 1:100,000 will produce the maximal degree of vasoconstriction. Stronger solutions will not increase the vasoconstrictor effect and will only invite the complications of epinephrine intoxication — which are nervousness, cold sweats, hypertension, and tachycardia — and severe arrhythmias. Errors in the preparation of local analgesic agents containing epinephrine should be avoided. Table 3–2 outlines the proper concentrations.

Adverse Reactions

Toxic effects of local agents are usually due to high blood levels of the anesthetic agents. There are many classifications available (Bonica, 1953; Moore, 1957). It is important that the surgeon

TABLE 3–2

Anesthetic Volume	Epinephrine (1:1000 Solution)	Dilution	Recommended For:
100 ml	2 ml	1:50,000	Rhinoplasty
100 ml	1 ml	1:100,000	Blepharoplasty
100 ml	0.5 ml	1:200,000	Facial plasty (large volumes of solution are required)

recognize the seriousness of the situation at the earliest possible moment. If a patient who has been loquacious or restless suddenly settles down and becomes quiet, the surgeon should immediately examine the patient and check his respiration, pulse, and blood pressure, since tachycardia, tachypnea, and hypotension are the adverse signs most frequently encountered. A patient under local anesthesia should never be left unattended; means of monitoring the patient's vital signs must be available. Such essential monitoring can be done by trained technicians or by electronic devices, many of which are available on the market.

The treatment of adverse reactions is symptomatic. Reactions to toxicity exhibit themselves by symptoms referable to the central nervous system, the respiratory system, and the cardiovascular system. Actually, these symptoms are manifested by muscular twitching, tremors, and convulsions, hypopnea or apnea, and severe hypotension. They are the result of the depressing effects that local anesthetic agents have on the medulla and the myocardium and their dilatation effects on the vasculature. Treatment is urgent but symptomatic. Oxygen should be given immediately. Should convulsions occur, Valium, 5 to 20 mg intravenously, is most effective. If apnea occurs, artificial respiration by positive pressure on the rebreathing bag and endotracheal intubation are necessary. Circulatory depression, as indicated by hypotension and a weak pulse, requires an intravenous or intramuscular injection of a vasopressor such as ephedrine hydrochloride, 50 mg. Cardiac arrest should be treated by current methods.

ANESTHETIC AGENTS

Thiopental Sodium.   Thiopental sodium (Pentothal) is a very versatile agent for use in plastic surgery, with few contraindications to its use. Contrary to popular belief, it is not a true anesthetic. Although it belongs to the barbiturate family of drugs, thiopental sodium has no analgesic effect within its clinical range. When combined with a low-potency, nonflammable agent such as nitrous oxide, it can produce excellent anesthesia for a wide range of plastic cosmetic surgical procedures. Such a combination allows the free use of electrocoagulation. Neither Pentothal nor nitrous oxide sensitizes the heart to the arrhythmic effects of epinephrine; indeed, Pentothal affords protection against such effects. It is apparent that this combination of agents allows the surgeon wide latitude in surgical technique and provides the patient with a safe and smooth anesthetic.

Cyclopropane.   Cyclopropane is of little value in plastic cosmetic surgery. It is highly flammable, and the use of epinephrine is contraindicated during its administration because of the frequent occurrence of severe ventricular arrhythmias. McLoughlin (1954) demonstrated that cyclopropane increases the amount of bleeding in the wound. Its use should be reserved for the patient in shock from hemorrhage; then, cyclopropane is the agent of choice.

Halothane.   Halothane is the most valuable anesthetic agent available today. It is nonflammable — thus it allows free use of electrocoagulation. It obtunds the pharyngeal, laryngeal, and tracheal reflexes in light planes of anesthesia, so that coughing and straining are rarely encountered. Despite its proven value, its use is reserved for children owing to medicolegal implications because of its alleged responsibility in producing postoperative hepatitis.

Enflurane (Ethrane).   Also a halogenated ether, enflurane is nonflammable and nonexplosive. Although induction is slower with this drug than with halothane, enflurane provides excellent working conditions for the surgeon. Controlled hypotension is readily achieved when required to produce a relatively bloodless surgical field. Enflurane decreases cardiac output and peripheral vascular resistance. It produces enough vasodilation to prevent any increase in right atrial pressure. However, if the depth of anesthesia is excessive, especially when associated with hyperventilation and respiratory alkalosis, motor activity may be encountered, consisting of twitching or "jerking" of various muscle groups. This complication is self-limiting and can easily be terminated by lowering the anesthetic concentration. Enflurane can be used more freely in the presence of epinephrine. Squeezed-out, epinephrine-soaked pledgets may be used for wound packing; also, injected epinephrine mixed with a local anesthetic or saline in concentrations of 1:100,000 is well tolerated.

Sodium Methohexital.   Sodium methohexital (Brevital) is a rapid, ultra short-acting barbiturate. It differs chemically from the established barbiturate anesthetics in that it contains no sulfur. It is used in a 1 percent solution. The usual induction dose of 5 to 12 ml (50 to 100 mg) produces anesthesia for five to seven minutes.

Methoxyflurane.   Methoxyflurane (Penthrane) is a halogenated ethyl methyl ether that is nonflammable and nonexplosive. It is a valuable agent but its odor is usually considered unpleasant by the operating room personnel. Induction is much slower than with halothane. Because of the occasional occurrence of high-output kidney failure (Crandell et al., 1966), it should not be used for operations on the elderly or when prolonged surgery is anticipated.

Succinylcholine Chloride. Succinylcholine chloride is a short-acting muscle relaxant whose primary value is to relax the patient's jaw, pharynx, and larynx to facilitate atraumatic intubation of the trachea. Since its action is not selective for those muscles, the patient is totally paralyzed for the duration of its effect. Prior to intubation and immediately following, the anesthesiologist must breathe artificially for the patient until spontaneous respirations return, usually after a period of five to ten minutes.

Ketamine Hydrochloride. Ketamine hydrochloride is an intravenous or intramuscular anesthetic that produces a profound dissociated sleep. Muscle tone of the tongue and pharyngeal muscles remains as in the awake state, and the respiration is not depressed, so that the endotracheal tube and controlled respiration are rarely needed. It would seem to be the ideal anesthetic for cosmetic surgery. Unfortunately, blood pressure and pulse rates are elevated with ketamine and there is increased bleeding in the wound. Its main drawback is its high incidence of delirium, nightmares, delusions, and schizoid reactions during the awakening period. It seems to distort the perception of time. Such bad trips may last only a few seconds, but to the patient they seem to go on for hours. This "nightmare" anesthetic has no place in cosmetic surgery.

ATTENTION TO DETAIL

Airway Management

By its very nature, any surgical procedure on the head or neck usually demands the use of an endotracheal tube. It provides a free and unobstructed airway, even in the presence of blood in the pharynx, and it enables the anesthesiologist to be at a considerable distance from the surgical site. If resuscitation should be necessary during the course of surgery, it can be instituted immediately, thereby avoiding dangerous delays while efforts at intubation are attempted under conditions other than ideal. In expert hands, complications from the use of an endotracheal tube are rare and of minor significance. The simple technique of oral intubation is performed quickly and atraumatically while the patient is totally relaxed by succinylcholine. It is important to use an adequate dose of this drug (60 to 100 mg). A smaller dose will not produce complete relaxation, and pressure from the laryngoscope blade can damage the incisors or produce tears of the soft tissue in the hypopharynx. Its duration of action is directly related to the dose level, and recovery from a small dose is quite rapid. Such quick return of muscle activity following intubation does not allow sufficient time for the previously applied topical anesthetic agent to attain its peak effect and results in coughing and straining with the endotracheal tube in place. At the end of the operation, the tube must not be removed from the trachea while the patient is in a light plane of anesthesia, as this causes coughing and bucking. It is much better practice to maintain the level of anesthesia that was obtained during the operative procedure until the dressing has been applied and the surgeon is ready to leave the operating room. At this time, the tube is removed rapidly during the expiratory phase of the respiratory cycle. This technique will almost always avoid coughing and bucking on the tube.

Reduction in Bulk of Equipment

The presence of large, bulky equipment that encroaches on the operative field is a most annoying problem to the cosmetic plastic surgeon. To keep bulk at a minimum, the author prefers the use of a soft rubber Magill endotracheal tube with a curved metal adapter at its proximal end. The tube is cut to exact length so that following insertion, only this metal piece, resting on the patient's lower lip, is visible. The metal piece, in turn, is attached to a small cylindrical malleable connecting piece, and then to hoses leading to the machine. These hoses are extra long, allowing the anesthesiologist to sit below the level of the knee, in the case of oral intubation. Thus, there is no equipment in the way, and the whole field is open to the surgeon. A minimal number of short adhesive strips may be used to secure the tube. If distortion of the face is a problem, adhesive strips are not used, since distortion is virtually eliminated when the tube lies freely. If the operation requires the tube to be moved from side to side, as in the case of full-face dermabrasion, it can easily be moved by the anesthesiologist.

Carbon Dioxide Retention

Depressed respiration produces an elevated blood carbon dioxide level. Because of its vasodilating effect, this in turn increases the amount of oozing in the surgical field. The cosmetic plastic surgeon wants a bloodless field, if possible, as bleeding under a flap or graft prolongs the patient's convalescence. It is therefore most important that the patient's ventilation be augmented at all times by the technique of assisted or controlled respiration.

Airway Obstruction

The fact that the patient has been intubated successfully does not guarantee that the airway will remain patent for the duration of the anesthesia. Under certain conditions, the tube may become kinked by hyperextension or hyperflexion of the neck, or the lumen may be partially or completely occluded by a blood clot or inspissated mucus within or by the pressure of retractors or pharyngeal packs from without. When total obstruction occurs, it is readily diagnosed because breathing ceases. However, obstruction is easily and quickly remedied.

Unfortunately, when obstruction is not complete and a partial airway remains, it may go unnoticed. Partial obstruction can be recognized by the "rocking-boat" action of the patient's abdomen and chest, similar to that of asthmatic breathing. When such partial obstruction is uncorrected, the patient must exert considerable effort to overcome the resistance to breathing, and this results in annoying oozing of blood in the surgical field. This increased bleeding results from the elevation of the venous and the arterial blood pressures and the increase of carbon dioxide in the blood. If the surgeon notices any sudden change in the amount of bleeding in the wound, he must immediately ask the anesthesiologist to inspect the airway. Also, any change in the breathing pattern of the patient warrants an immediate check of the system. A kinked tube or a malfunctioning valve may be the cause of the obstruction.

Coughing

Coughing and straining with the endotracheal tube in place produce an elevation in the blood pressure and a rise in the peripheral venous pressure which undoubtedly increase the amount of bleeding. They can even cause a recurrence of bleeding in areas under hemostatic control. It is essential that the anesthesiologist institute adequate topical anesthesia. On the other hand, the surgeon should be aware that an otherwise smooth anesthesia can be marred by abrupt motions of the head and neck. These actions move the tube in the trachea and invariably lead to coughing and straining by the patient. The surgeon must warn the anesthesiologist of his intentions so that the anesthesiologist can either deepen the level of anesthesia or administer small amounts of short-acting muscle relaxant, after which the move can be made with no fear of causing annoying disturbances.

Premature Recovery

In cosmetic surgery, premature recovery of the patient is undesirable. The patient must not be allowed to awaken until the procedure is completely finished and the dressings have been applied. The anesthesiologist should realize that the application of the dressing is of great importance to the success of the surgical procedure. It is impossible to apply a dressing properly if the patient is coughing, vomiting, or resisting vigorously. It must be remembered that this straining may cause bleeding under a skin graft or flap. To maintain a quiescent patient until the end of the procedure, either an adequate depth of anesthesia must be maintained to the completion of the dressing or a small amount of succinylcholine must be administered.

Recovery Period

In the recovery room, the patient is closely watched by the anesthesia and the recovery room staffs for signs of airway impairment, particularly if pressure dressings on the face and neck compromise the airway. If there are signs of delirious emergence from the anesthesia, it may be controlled by the intravenous injection of a mixture containing Demerol, 10 mg, and Trilafon, 1 mg, in each cubic centimeter. One cubic centimeter of solution is given every five minutes until the desired effect is realized. If the restlessness is obviously not due to pain, Valium in 5 to 10 mg doses intramuscularly is excellent for tranquilizing the patient. This allows a quiet, relaxed awakening, which is greatly appreciated by the surgeon, the patient, and the nursing staff.

Often, the surgeon believes that tight dressings will stop the bleeding. However, heavy packs and tight dressings may cause soft tissue obstruction of the pharynx and thus interfere with the patient's breathing. Once the endotracheal tube is removed, the anesthesiologist should be prepared to cut away the dressings if there should be any indication of impaired breathing.

Induced Hypotension

The desire of the surgeon for a bloodless field in which to operate is as old as the specialty itself. Throughout the years, great effort has been expended in order to produce a dry, bloodless field in the anesthetized patient. The most dramatic approach is the application of induced hypotension to general anesthesia as fostered by Enderby (1958) in England.

Hypotension is induced by drugs that cause generalized peripheral vasodilation. Combined with posture, such as the head-up position for operations on the head and neck, hypotension allows pooling of blood in the dependent areas away from the surgical site. The venous return to the heart is reduced and the cardiac output falls, vastly reducing the amount of bleeding in the surgical wound. Such vasodilation is produced by drugs that block the automatic ganglia. Those commonly used are hexamethonium (Vegolysen), pentolinium tartrate (Ansolysen), trimethaphan camphorsulfonate (Arfonad), homatropinium (Trophenium), and sodium nitroprusside (Nipride).

An important part of the technique advocated by Enderby is controlled respiration. Positive pressure applied to the airway by intermittent manual pressure on the rebreathing bag can, by raising the intrapleural pressure, further reduce the venous return to the right heart. This has a very marked hypotension effect when used in combination with the ganglion-blocking agents.

On the other hand, it is such an exacting and demanding technique with so little margin for error that it cannot be recommended for general use. In expert hands, this technique can be applied safely with no significant increase of risk to the patient (Enderby, 1961; Linacre, 1961).

SPECIAL TECHNIQUES

Rhinoplasty

The discomfort of injections in and around the nose is a major fear of the patient undergoing rhinoplasty. This can be eliminated by a very simple technique that satisfies both the patient and the surgeon in that it produces the conditions that each desires. Such a patient welcomes the opportunity to be unconscious during that short critical period when the surgeon establishes the local anesthesia of the nose, as there is complete avoidance of the fears and apprehensions of discomfort that the patient associates with these injections.

Methohexital (Brevital), the ultra short-acting oxybarbiturate, is ideally suited to induce such a short period of sleep. The surgeon packs the nasal passages and inserts the pledgets of topical anesthetic and vasoconstrictor and then retires to scrub. During this interval, the anesthesiologist injects a solution of 1 percent Brevital in 1 ml increments, to a total of 4 to 6 ml, the endpoint being reached when the patient can no longer communicate with the anesthesiologist. The patient sleeps while the surgeon establishes the local anesthetic. During this period, there may be some motions or phonations on the part of the patient, but there is never any recollection of the injection. Once the local anesthetic is established, no additional Brevital is given. Within three to five minutes, the patient can respond to questions, and the procedure continues in the usual manner.

Chemabrasion

Full-face chemabrasion is not tolerated well by the patient unless he is placed under very heavy narcosis, with an ensuing prolonged arousal time. Pentothal sodium seems to be ideally suited for this short operation. The patient is premedicated in the usual manner. On his arrival in the operating room, a dilute solution of thiopental, 0.2 percent, is administered by continuous intravenous infusion. As soon as the eyelid reflex is obtunded, chemabrasion is begun. Very fine control of the depth of anesthesia is maintained, so that the patient is awake following the application of the adhesive strips. A recovery room stay is rarely necessary.

Neuroleptanalgesia

Neuroleptanalgesia is a euphemistic term that describes the condition of induced narcosis that produces profound analgesia and psychomotor sedation, while allegedly leaving the cortical and cardiovascular functions intact. The principal application of neuroleptanalgesia in cosmetic surgery is as a supplement to local anesthesia. Although the combination of any narcotic and tranquilizer may produce the condition of neuroleptanalgesia, the drug Innovar has become almost synonymous with this state of induced psychic indifference. It is of interest that when Innovar is properly administered, the patient can cooperate and respond to questions, yet when not stimulated by conversation, the neuroleptic state of calm detachment returns. Operations such as blepharoplasty, facial plasty, and scar revision lend themselves to this technique, since regional anesthesia is so readily established by the surgeon.

The patient is premedicated in the usual manner. On his arrival in the operating room, an intravenous infusion is started and Innovar is injected in increments of 1 ml through the infusion tubing until the patient is in the neuroleptic state. At this time, should there be any signs of respiratory obstruction, a soft nasal airway is inserted and the head is adjusted for optimal breathing. Also at this time, the surgeon administers the local anesthetic and operates. If the patient shows signs of awareness or movement, additional 1 ml increments of Innovar are given. For example, in blepharoplasty, the tugging during extirpation of the herniated fat usually elicits a pain response. At this phase of the procedure, the anesthesiologist should anticipate this pain response and should administer an additional 1 ml of Innovar. It must be stressed that Innovar is composed of a potent narcotic and a tranquilizer and should be used only when the patient's vital signs are constantly monitored by an anesthesiologist who is prepared, at a moment's notice, to institute endotracheal intubation, controlled respiration, and cardiovascular resuscitation.

Innovar can be used also for the establishment of the total anesthetic state should endotracheal intubation be required for the safe conduct of the operation. Here, the induction is by thiopental and succinylcholine, as previously described. The anesthesia is maintained with nitrous oxide by inhalation and with intermittent injections of Innovar in increments of 0.5 to 1.0 ml. This technique is of special value in the patient for whom halothane may be contraindicated — for example, a patient with a history of previous liver disease (Bunker et al., 1969). However, unlike anesthesia with enflurane, it behooves the surgeon, if there by any need to move the patient's head, to alert the anesthesiologist to this fact, so that a deeper plane of anesthesia can be established before this movement is made. If this is not done, bucking will surely occur, resulting in increased bleeding in the wound. It should be stressed that with enflurane, the surgeon is virtually guaranteed that the patient will not cough or buck. Such a guarantee cannot be made with Innovar. This unnecessary complication is much more likely to occur when Innovar is the nucleus of the anesthetic technique. A very satisfactory alternative to Innovar is the supplementation of local analgesia with a combination of diazepam (Valium) and sublimaze (Fentanyl) 0.05 mg. Valium, 10 mg, is injected intravenously as soon as the intravenous infusion is established. Sublimaze is then given to the patient in 0.05 mg increments until the appropriate neuroleptic state is achieved.

Postoperative Hematoma

It is unfortunate that, despite great care on the part of the surgeon to achieve hemostasis during the facial plastic operation, a small proportion of these patients must return to the operating room in the immediate postoperative period because of hematoma. This frequently requires removing most of the sutures to find the source of bleeding. It is not only difficult but indeed hazardous to attempt local anesthesia for this purpose. A more prudent course is to induce general anesthesia, thereby establishing a clear airway, eliminating the risk of toxic reaction to the local anesthetic agent because of the vascularity of the area, and, lastly, allowing the surgeon to effect hemostasis in an orderly manner.

EPILOGUE

The physician who undertakes the administration of potent drugs in order to render a patient semiconscious or unconscious assumes a great responsibility that cannot be undertaken in a capricious manner. Such degrees of insensibility can be produced only by prescribing potent sedatives, hypnotics, tranquilizers, and narcotics. The pharmacologic effects of these drugs on the patient can never be predicted accurately. It would seem prudent that the surgeon relieve himself of this unnecessary responsibility in order that he may direct his attention entirely to his surgical endeavors.

REFERENCES

Selection of Patients

Fredricks, S.: Personal communication, 1970.
Knorr, N. J., Hoopes, J. E., and Edgerton, M. T.: Psychiatric surgical approach to adolescent disturbance in self image. Plast. Reconstr. Surg. 41:248–253, 1968.
Macgregor, F. C., Abel, T. M., Bryt, A., Lauer, E., and Weissmann, S.: Facial Deformities and Plastic Surgery: A Psychosocial Study. Springfield, Ill., Charles C Thomas, 1953.
Macgregor, F. C., and Schaffner, B.: Screening patients for nasal plastic operations: some sociologic and psychiatric considerations. Psychosom. Med. 12:277–291, 1950.

Social and Psychologic Considerations

Jacobson, W. E., Edgerton, M. T., Meyer, E., Canter, A., and Slaughter, R.: Psychiatric evaluation of male patients seeking cosmetic surgery. Plast. Reconstr. Surg. 26:356–372, 1960.
Knorr, N. J., Hoopes, J. E., and Edgerton, M. T.: Psychiatric-surgical approach to adolescent disturbance in self image. Plast. Reconstr. Surg. 41:248–253, 1968.
Macgregor, F. C.: Social and cultural components in the motivations of persons seeking plastic surgery of the nose. J. Health Soc. Behav. 8:125–135, 1967.
Macgregor, F. C.: Social Science in Nursing: Applications for the Improvement of Patient Care. New York, Russell Sage Foundation, 1960.
Macgregor, F. C.: Transformation and Identity: The Face and Plastic Surgery. New York, Quadrangle/The New York Times Book Company, 1974.
Macgregor, F. C., Abel, T. M., Bryt, A., Lauer, E., and Weissmann, S.: Facial Deformities and Plastic Surgery: A Psychosocial Study. Springfield, Ill., Charles C Thomas, 1953.
Meerloo, J. A.: The fate of one's face. Psychiatr. Quart. 30:31–43, 1956.
Meyer, E.: Psychiatric aspects of plastic surgery. In Converse, J. M., ed.: Reconstructive Plastic Surgery, Volume I, General Principles, 2nd ed. Philadelphia, W. B. Saunders Company, 1977.
Meyer, E., Jacobson, W. E., Edgerton, M. T., and Canter, A.: Motivational patterns in patients seeking elective plastic surgery. I, Women who seek rhinoplasty. Psychosom. Med. 22:193–201, 1960.
Murphy, G.: Cited in Norbeck, E., Price-Williams, D., and McCord, W. M., eds.: The Study of Personality: An Interdisciplinary Appraisal. New York, Holt, Rinehart and Winston, 1968.
Ruesch, J.: The future of psychologically oriented psychiatry. In Masserman, J. H., ed.: Sexuality of Women. New York, Grune & Stratton, 1966.

Anesthesia

Bellville, J. W., Bross, D. D. J., and Howland, W. S.: Postoperative nausea and vomiting. Clin. Pharmacol. Ther., 1:590, 1960.
Bonica, J. J.: The Management of Pain. Philadelphia, Lea & Febiger, 1953.
Bunker, J. P., Forrest, W. H., Jr., Mosteller, F., and Vandam, L. D. (eds): National Halothane Study: The study of the possible association between halothane anesthesia and postoperative hepatic necrosis. Bethesda, Md., National Institutes of Health and of General Medical Sciences, 1969.

Crandell, W. B., Pappas, S. G., and Macdonald, A.: Nephrotoxicity associated with methoxyflurane anesthesia. Anesthesiology, 27:591, 1966.

Enderby, G. E. H.: The advantages of controlled hypotension in surgery. Brit. Bull., 14:1, 1958.

Enderby, G. E. H.: Halothane and hypotension. Anesthesia, 15:25, 1960.

Enderby, G. E. H.: A report on the mortality and morbidity following 9,106 hypotensive anesthetics. Brit. J. Anaesth., 33:109, 1961.

Fox, J. W. C., and Fox, E.: Neuroleptanalgesia: a review. N. Carolina Med. J., 27:471, 1966.

Katz, R. M., Matteo, R. S., and Papper, E. M.: Injection of epinephrine during general anesthesia with halogenated hydrocarbons and by cyclopropane in man. Anesthesiology, 23:597, 1962.

Linacre, J. L.: Induced hypotension in gynecological surgery. Brit. J. Anaesth., 33:45, 1961.

McLoughlin, G.: Bleeding from cut skin and subcutaneous tissue surfaces during cyclopropane anesthesia. Brit. J. Anaesth., 26:84, 1954.

Moore, D. C.: Regional Block. Springfield, Ill., Charles C Thomas, 1957.

Part 2

RHINOPLASTY

Chapter 4

History

Thomas D. Rees, M.D., F.A.C.S.

There is evidence that plastic surgical operations directed at the nose were performed in India and Egypt as early as 600 B.C. Denecke and Meyer (1967) cite Egyptian hieroglyphics and ancient Indian writings in their review and quote the Edwin Smith surgical papyrus hieroglyphics description of the first recorded use of pressure dressings applied to the nose.

Amputation of the nose was a frequent form of punishment in ancient India, dealt out primarily for adultery but also used for other crimes. The use of the forehead flap for reconstruction of the missing organ was described by Susruta Samhita in his work, *Ayur-Veda*. Other contributions to reconstruction of the partially or totally missing nose were made by the Brancas about 1450 A.D., who further developed the median forehead flap method of reconstruction. Antonio Branca began using a pedicle flap from the upper arm for nasal reconstruction. This method was described by Gaspare Tagliacozzi in 1597 and is generally ascribed to him. Because of its development in Italy, it became popularized as the Italian method. Tagliacozzi's efforts to repair the human form were considered heresy at the time, since deformities were considered to be the will of God. He was persecuted considerably for his efforts, and his teachings were lost for many years, only to be rediscovered from time to time by other surgeons of Europe such as Cortesi of Mesina and Graffon of Lucerne.

Other attempts were described in the *Madras Gazette* in 1793, in which a nasal reconstruction was performed on an Indian bullock driver by a surgeon of Poona, India, by the name of Maharatta. He also used the forehead flap method. Joseph Carpue, an English surgeon, used the same technique to reconstruct the nose of an English officer in 1814, apparently with success. Many of the great surgeons of Europe such as Dupuytren, Delpech, Syme, Beck, Zeis, and Warren were stimulated by

these previous reports to develop further methods of reconstruction of the nose as well as of the lips and cheeks. The modern age of corrective rhinoplasty, however, did not begin, according to Rogers (1976), until the work of John Orlando Roe in 1887. An otolaryngologist from Rochester, New York, Roe described an operation performed within the nose but confined to the tip. The name of this work was "The Deformity Termed Pug Nose and Its Correction by a Simple Operation." Subsequently, in 1891, in another paper entitled "The Correction of Angular Deformities of the Nose by Subcutaneous Operation," Roe described corrective rhinoplasty of the entire nose. Reduction of the bony and cartilaginous hump and profile was described in this paper.

In 1845, Dieffenbach was probably the first to record an attempt to reduce a large nose. Dieffenbach's efforts were directed primarily at reducing the soft tissue of the nose, and he made extensive use of external incisions to accomplish this end. Apparently, the concept of an intranasal approach did not occur to him. In addition to his soft tissue work, he did, however, describe attempts to correct deviated noses by chiseling the septum loose from the palate and fracturing the nasal bone. It is interesting that it was not until almost four decades later that the intranasal approach to rhinoplasty was described by Roe. Roe's initial account in 1887 was followed by the detailed accounts of reduction rhinoplasty by Joseph, the famous German surgeon, in 1898. Joseph has been generally recognized as the father of modern nasal corrective surgery. His techniques were described in *Nasenplastik und Sonstige Gesichtsplastik Nebst Mammaplastik* (1931).

Weir was another important contributor to the history of corrective rhinoplasty. In 1892, he described utilizing intranasal incisions to stabilize fractured nasal bones in a medial position with the use of steel needles that were inserted transversely

51

to the entire nose and held in place by lateral clamps.

It is impossible to credit all the many pioneers who made meaningful contributions to the technique of corrective rhinoplasty since its inception. This surgery has caught the imagination of surgeons the world over and has produced voluminous literature, some of which is sound and constructive and some of which is but interesting conjecture. Surgeons of various disciplines have become fascinated by rhinoplasty; most of the contributions to technique, however, have come from general plastic surgeons and rhinologists. The scope of this book does not permit a detailed chronology of the development of rhinoplasty, nor does it allow for proper credit to be given to each surgeon who has devoted his time and effort to this interesting subject.

In the development of corrective surgery of the nose since the early work of Roe and Joseph, certain pioneer names should be mentioned. These include Gustave Aufricht and Joseph Safian, both students of Joseph who developed their craft in America.

An excellent detailed history of the development of corrective rhinoplasty was provided by Blair O. Rogers in 1976, and a comprehensive reference work on nasal surgery is available in *Surgery of the Nose* (Denecke and Meyer, 1967).

THE TECHNIQUE

The rhinoplasty operation has undergone definitive changes in concept and approach since the time of Joseph. The key emphasis today is on subtlety. To accomplish this, many surgeons have abandoned the time-honored technical steps used in the operation of Joseph and his students. For example, the tip is frequently corrected early in the operation, followed by reduction of the dorsal hump and finally by infracture. The alar cartilages are treated in a much more conservative manner. Maintenance of as much natural architecture as possible is stressed. Similarly, the nose is usually shortened only slightly.

This conservative swing in attitude toward the operation evolved after study and observation of many patients who underwent nasal plastic surgery many years ago. Long-term observation indicated the necessity of conservation of all tissue and established the guidelines of modern surgery. The children and offspring of the first and second rhinoplasty generation patients wish to avoid the "operated look" at all costs. This recent emphasis in teaching on a more conservative and subtle rhinoplastic technique (Peck, 1976; Sheen, 1976; Rees, 1977; and others) has unquestionably improved results everywhere.

(For references, see pages 450 to 453.)

Chapter 5

Anatomy

Thomas D. Rees, M.D., F.A.C.S.

From a surgical point of view, it is well to consider the nose as an osteocartilaginous vault divided into two chambers by the median septum, lined on the inside by mucous membranes and various appendages (turbinates) and covered externally by skin. The osteocartilaginous vault may appropriately be compared to the structural framework of a tent and the skin may be compared to the covering. Adjustments of the framework will be effective only insofar as the covering conforms to the new contour changes in skeleton. Other structures that must be considered include the muscles, vessels, nerves, and lymphatics.

Appreciation of the external landmarks of the nose is important, since a grasp of their relationship is vital to understanding operations designed to change them (Figure 5–1). Landmarks and immediately adjacent structures of importance to the surgeon include the glabella, nasion, nasofrontal angle, dorsum of the nose, lower (mobile) nose, (which includes the tip), nostrils, columella, nasolabial angle, alae, and alar grooves. On examination of sagittal sections of the nose, it becomes apparent that a considerable portion, if not most, of the "hump" of the nose consists of cartilage rather than bone. Appreciation of this fact has been partly responsible for a change in the technique of hump removal whereby the saw has been discarded in favor of the sharp rasp or finely honed osteotome.

THE SOFT TISSUES OF THE NOSE

The skin plays a critical role in the final appearance of the nose after surgery. Although it is closely adherent to the underlying alar cartilages, the skin is loosely attached and mobile over the upper lateral cartilages and nasal bones. Of particular importance to the final results is the quality of skin of the nasal tip and lobule, since a lack of delicacy and pliability militates against achieving fine definition. Normally, the tip skin contains many sebaceous glands, which diminish in number over the lateral cartilages. The skin can be either thin or thick, or it may be padded with a considerable layer of subcutaneous fat. The abundant sebaceous glands, in addition to large amounts of subcutaneous fat, make the skin unpliable, and it is therefore unlikely to "drape" well over the adjusted cartilaginous framework beneath. In the aging individual, the skin usually becomes thinner, and in some cases, overactivity of the glandular structures can produce a rhinophymatous condition.

Pitanguy (1965) identified a subcutaneous "ligament" closely identified with the dorsal skin in the supratip region, particularly in noses of mixed or noncaucasian origin. This ligament may be important in anatomic and surgical thinning of the soft tissue of the nasal tip structures.

Arterial, venous, and neural supplies to the skin lie quite superficially in the soft tissues. Accordingly, the dissection plane of the skin from the underlying bony and cartilaginous skeletons should lie immediately adjacent to these structures, maintaining the integrity of the skin and subcutaneous tissues insofar as possible to avoid injury to the blood supply.

THE NASAL BONY FRAMEWORK

The framework of the pyramidal external structure of the nose is formed by the paired nasal bones, which project from the nasal process of the frontal bone superiorly and from the nasal (frontal) processes of the maxilla laterally. The paired nasal bones are rarely symmetrical, and in general terms they constitute a smaller portion of the nasal hump than is generally thought. Nasal bones are quadrangular, and they are thicker above than below; the usual location of a nasal bone fracture is at the junction between the thicker and thinner portions. Inadvertent fractures during surgery tend to occur at this location and sometimes cause troublesome small spurs, which must be corrected with either a fine osteotome or a rasp.

The septum serves as the central support for the nasal bone at the midline. The perpendicular plate of the ethmoid is the osseous support of the septum, ending at its junction with the septal cartilage at precisely the terminal point of the inferior portion of the nasal bone. During traumatic or purposeful fractures of the nasal bones and septum, disruption of the septum most often occurs at this point.

The superior suture line of the nasal bone lies at its junction with the hard and thick bone of the glabella. The depression of the profile here is known as the nasofrontal angle, commonly re-

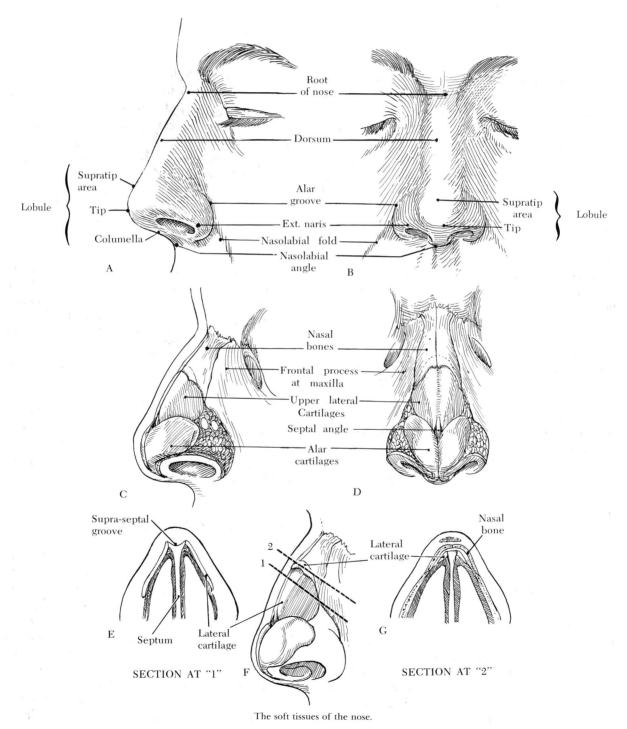

The soft tissues of the nose.

Figure 5–1.

ferred to as the nasion. There is no visible depression in many patients. Surgical reconstruction of this depression may be exceedingly difficult owing to an absence of normal "bossing" of the glabellar area and because it is difficult to shape the excessively thick bone of the glabella by chisel or to gouge enough to register on the profile.

The combination of the joined nasal bones and frontal processes of the maxilla forms the pyriform aperture in the anterior aspect of the skull. The posterolateral border of the frontal process of the maxilla, along with the corresponding groove along the lacrimal bone, forms the lacrimal groove, which contains the lacrimal duct. A lateral osteotomy must not violate the groove because of the important structure it contains. In practice, it is exceedingly difficult to cut the bone at such a level during the usual surgical approach unless the osteotome is angled in an extremely posterior direction.

It is important to remember that true fusion of the internasal, nasal-maxillary, and nasal-frontal sutures is rare. Fractures of these structures commonly occur in the thinner portions of the bones and heal by fibrous union and sparse ossification of the callous. Fractures made during surgery by purposeful osteotomies are therefore frequently associated with comminution along old fracture lines.

CARTILAGES OF THE NOSE

Septal Cartilage. The septal cartilage (also known as the quadrangular cartilage) borders superiorly and posteriorly on the perpendicular plate of the ethmoid and inferiorly and posteriorly on the vomer, and in combination with the bony nasal septum, it divides the nasal cavity into two chambers (Fig. 5–2). The septal cartilage protrudes in front of the pyriform aperture. The anterior-superior projection of the septal cartilage is known as the septal angle. It is of considerable importance at operation and is a key element in altering the profile.

The major portion of the septal cartilage is firmly adherent to the vomer along the floor, the perichondrium of the cartilage being perceived as continuous with the periosteum of the vomer (Fig. 5–3). Insertion of these fibers is from front to back. Therefore, elevation of a mucoperichondrial flap along this junction is best accomplished from back to front with a sharp elevator. At best, this maneuver is difficult; it frequently tears through the flap because of the peculiar anatomic junction of the cartilage with the bone and the arrangement of the perichondrium and periosteal fibrous interconnections.

The caudal border of the septal cartilage extends over the smooth surface of the nasal spine. The septum is mobile in this area with considerable side to side motion, probably because of the flexibility of the cartilage and the instability of the cartilaginous-osseous joint.

Studying the septal cartilage in a sagittal section once again confirms that most nasal humps are formed by the dorsal border of the septal cartilage in combination with its junction with the upper lateral cartilages and the nasal bones. Cur-

Figure 5–2.

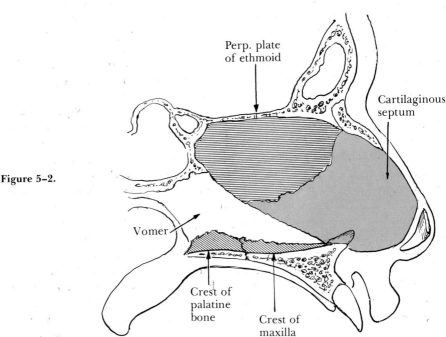

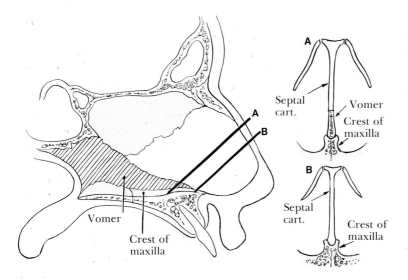

Septal cart.

Vomer
Crest of maxilla

Septal cart.

Crest of maxilla

Figure 5–3.

rent practice is to remove more cartilage and less bone than previously. The free margin of the septal cartilage at its caudal end is separated from the columella containing the medial crura of the alar cartilages by the membranous septum. This was formerly sacrificed in most rhinoplasties, but it should be preserved whenever possible to permit normal mobility of the lower nose.

The Nasal Cartilages. The nasal cartilages constitute the largest part of the external nasal structure. The cartilaginous external nose is anterior to the pyriform aperture and is constantly moved by the musculature of the nose. Such constant motion plays an important role in regulating airflow through the nostrils. Consequently, the shape of the nasal cartilages is important in nasal physiology. They are derived embryologically from a portion of the chondrocranium — the cartilaginous nasal capsule — which is a paired structure. In fact, the only structure of importance in the nose that is not paired is the nasal septum.

The paired lateral cartilages (upper lateral cartilages) are essentially a caudal continuation of the nasal bones, although they are not anatomically fused to these bones (see Figure 5–1). They are roughly triangular, are attached to the medial portion of the frontal process of the maxilla and the medial aspect of the nasal bones, and lie in very close proximity (although not fused) to the septal cartilage in the midline. The lateral cartilages are overlapped in their inferior (caudal) margins by the upper (cephalic) borders of the alar cartilages, which override the lateral cartilages on their external surfaces (see Figure 5–1). A groove (the limen nasi) is thereby created, which serves as a landmark for incisions just above the vestibule. The two cartilages are joined at this point by connective tissue.

The outer margin of the cartilage is separated from the rim of the pyriform aperture by dense fibroareolar connective tissue. Overlapping of the upper end of the lateral cartilages by the nasal bone is established during embryologic growth (see Figure 5–1, *G*). The nasal bones develop from a membrane on the surface of the cartilaginous nasal capsule, thus explaining the upward extension of the lateral cartilage on the inner surface of the nasal bones. This overlapping may extend from 2 or 3 mm to as much as 10 mm. Fusion of the perichondrium of the upper lateral cartilages to the periosteum of the nasal bone produces a firm adherence between these structures, so that any motion of the nasal bones, either purposeful (as in surgery) or accidental (as in unexpected trauma), moves the entire unit as a continuous plate. The membranous development of the nasal bones may explain their excellent behavior as implants. Absorption of free implants of nasal bone or cartilage is unusual, in contradistinction to the significant dissolution of cancellous bone grafts from the iliac crest.

The Septum and Lateral Cartilages. The septal cartilage extends up under the nasal bones for a distance approximating that of the extension of the lateral cartilages. The septal cartilage has a fairly sharp edge in the regions of the septal angle and adjacent portion of its dorsal border, but it becomes thicker at its junction with the perpendicular plate of the ethmoid. This increased width is most evident where the cartilage becomes identified with the nasal bones to form the typical "hump." In some individuals, the widened septum may be accentuated by a midline groove that may be palpable but usually is not visible. A perceptible diastasis of the nasal bones can occur, with the septum sandwiched between the bones.

Although there is an intimate relationship between the lateral and septal cartilages near the nasal bones, the cartilages are not fused histologically (see Figure 5–1, *E*, *F*, and *G*). Continuity of the perichondrium is not rare. Caudal to the nasal bones, the septal and lateral cartilages are separated by a narrow cleft, which becomes more obvious near the septal angle. Dense connective tissue adherence in this region prevents medial and lateral motion of the lateral cartilages. The narrow angle formed by this close relationship of the lateral cartilages and the septum is critical during respiration. In the internal nose, it is of importance for the eddying currents of airflow. Obstruction of this angle from scar tissue or trauma results in a loss of the sensation of air flow and the symptom of nasal obstruction, which will be discussed more fully in the section on physiology. The inferior margins of the lateral cartilages, where they lie in close association with the alar cartilages, are also important in the breathing mechanism, since this region is under control of the nasal musculature and acts similarly to a valve. From a surgical point of view, the lateral cartilages are clearly of utmost importance not only in achieving aesthetic results but in maintaining proper nasal physiology. Conservatism is important during trimming of the alar cartilages, particularly at their inferior extremities. After hump removal, the dorsal borders of the lateral cartilages are trimmed flush with the septal dorsum so that the anatomic relationships of the triangle are carefully reestablished.

The Alar Cartilages. The tip and columella (lobule) is supported primarily by the paired major alar cartilages also known as the lower lateral cartilages (Fig. 5–4). When viewed end on, these structures are roughly c-shaped with a medial component — the medial crus — which provides most of the structural framework for the columella, and a lateral component — the lateral crus — which provides the framework that, along with the skin, determines the shape of the tip. The point at which the medial and lateral crura meet might best be referred to as the transition area. The arrangement resembles a wishbone. Although the transition area can constitute the dome in some patients, the true dome usually is formed by the lateral crus, where it arches immediately superior and lateral to its junction with the medial crus. Maximal projection of the tip occurs at different points in different patients, but it is usually at the transition (junction).

Many illustrations of the alar cartilages are erroneous. There are several variations in the size and shape of the alar cartilages of both the lateral and medial crura (Figs. 5–5 and 5–6). It behooves the student of rhinoplasty to study the size and shape of the alar cartilages preoperatively. Only by understanding the anatomy of the alar cartilages can the astute surgeon design an appropriate operative procedure to improve the tip.

The paired cartilages are separated by varying amounts of fibroareolar tissue. The medial crura can be in close proximity to each other, or they can be significantly separated in a diastasis that can readily be seen from external examination (the medial crura curve downward into the columella, where they provide the principal support for this structure). Variations in the anatomy of the medial crura include excessive curvature of the inferior (caudal) margins, producing a rounded or hanging columella, and divergence of the bases (feet) of the medial crura, producing a widened base of the columella, which can constitute an obstruction to airflow at the entrance vestibule. The medial crura are attached to each other by fibroareolar connective tissue.

The lateral crura of the alar cartilages require the most attention during surgery because of the many variations that can exist. They extend from their junction with the medial crura in a posterolateral direction, a fact not always understood by young surgeons who tend to associate the lateral crura with the nostril rim. The nostril rim, in fact, is composed of soft tissue and not cartilage throughout most of its length. A "soft triangle" is formed by soft tissue at the apex of the nose between the junction of the columella and the alae. Where the skin and lining are very thin, the soft triangle should not be surgically violated, since postoperative deformities such as notching are difficult or impossible to repair. The inferior margins of the alar cartilages can be identified by retracting the nostril rim with a two-pronged retractor and exerting downward pressure on the lateral crus. A small ridge is readily seen.

The lateral crura of the alar cartilages diverge in the supratip area, leaving a triangular area between them that contains the septal angle. The dorsum of the nose in this immediate supratip area is supported only by the septal angle of the septal cartilage and the thickness of the overlying skin and subcutaneous tissue. The lateral crus of the alar cartilage forms only slightly more than half the nostril rim. The remainder is composed of dense collagenous fibers arranged longitudinally.

The Columella. The nasolabial angle is the angle formed between the lip and the base of the columella. The shape of the columella is determined largely by the configuration of the caudal margin of the septum in combination with the medial crura of the alar cartilages. The width of the

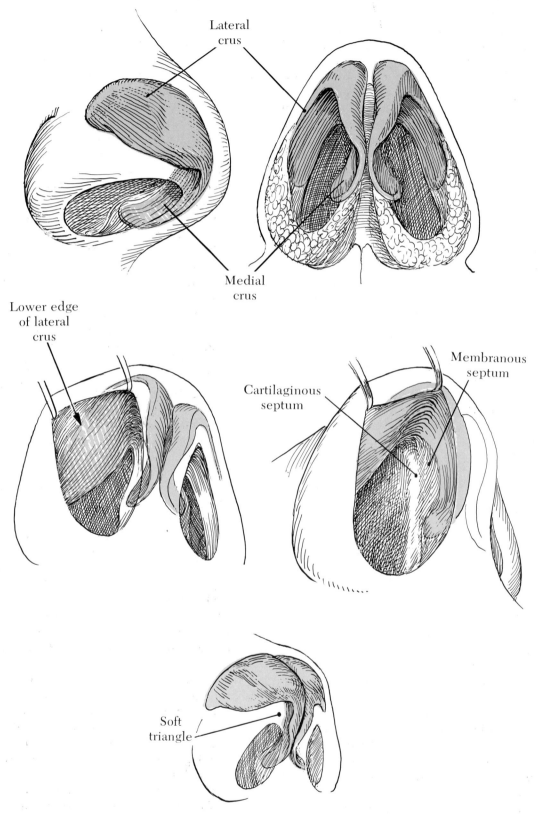

Figure 5-4.   The alar cartilages.

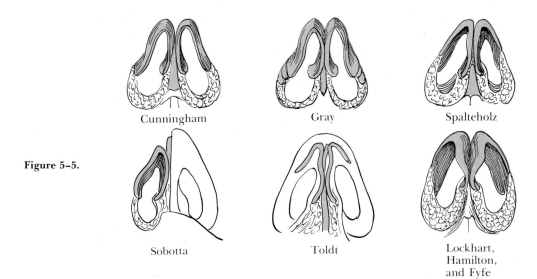

Figure 5–5.

Cunningham   Gray   Spalteholz

Sobotta   Toldt   Lockhart, Hamilton, and Fyfe

columella is determined by the distance between the feet of the medial crura and their divergence. The columella is often amenable to surgical reshaping of the medial crura. Total or subtotal loss of the columella is exceedingly difficult to reconstruct. The retracted columella, so common after "radical" submucuous resection, is also a very difficult surgical problem.

The Membranous Septum. The membranous septum joins the columella with the caudal border of the septal cartilage. It consists of two layers of skin separated by loose areolar tissue. The membranous septum is an important structure, providing flexibility and resiliency of the lobule. It is subject to the dynamic action of the depressor septi nasi, which extends through the columella, traverses the membranous septum, and inserts over the caudal septum. The action of this muscle on the membranous septum is important during nasal ventilation. During deep inspiration, the orbicu-

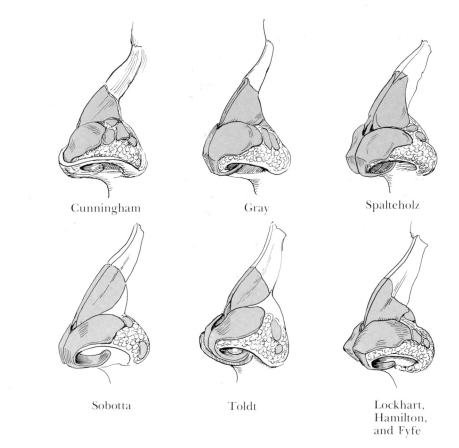

Cunningham   Gray   Spalteholz

Figure 5–6.

Sobotta   Toldt   Lockhart, Hamilton, and Fyfe

laris oris muscle contracts the lips, and the depressor septi nasi muscle (in combination with the zygomaticus) acts to tense the membranous septum and the columella. By this action, the internal nares are narrowed, and a negative intranasal pressure rises around the tense columella and membranous septum. The internal nares then dilate, allowing air to flow into the nasal fossa. This same combined muscular action results in an unsightly plunging of the nose — an animation in those patients with a strong hump and septal angle. This is the main complaint of many patients. It was common practice in the past to resect the membranous septum in the mistaken belief that it would fix the nasal tip and thus minimize postoperative dropping. In certain deformities, of course, the membranous septum must be sacrificed. However, it is generally desirable to maintain as much of this structure as possible to insure mobility of the lobule.

The Vestibule. The vestibule lies immediately inside the nostril rims and slightly above them. It can be considered as a cavity that is lined with skin containing numerous hair follicles (vibrissae) and sebaceous glands. The vestibule forms the anterior or inferior part of the nose, depending on one's orientation, and it becomes continuous with the internal nose. Transition between skin and mucosa occurs at the level of the sulcus between the upper border of the alar cartilage, where they overlap the inferior borders of the lateral nasal cartilages. The vestibule of the nose forms the entrance port to the airflow, and it begins the filtering, warming, and moistening process where the epithelial transition area begins. The motion of the upper lateral cartilages in relationship to the septum plays an important role in regulating the amount of airflow that passes through the internal nares.

The Internal Nose. Past the transition nose or the limen nasi, the lateral wall of the nasal cavity is lined with pseudostratified filiated columellar epithelium. Physiologically this functions as respiratory epithelium by filtering, moistening, and regulating the various eddies and currents of the airflow. The three tuberances on the lateral walls — the superior, middle, and inferior turbinates (also known as concha) — are sensitive to disturbances in the internal nose. The mucous membrane overlying these structures is highly vascularized with many venous networks that are erectile in action. The inferior turbinate is of particular importance in rhinoplasty, since this structure often hypertrophies to compensate for anatomic derangements of the septum. Many surgeons outfracture the inferior turbinate, which theoretically provides air space. Turbinectomy is out of vogue and rarely performed today; however, steroid injections are common. These techniques will be discussed in the section on physiology.

MUSCLES OF THE NOSE

The muscles of the nose are arranged in two layers that partially overlap (Fig. 5–7). The frontalis muscle of the forehead extends as a continuation known as the procerus, which shortens the nose. The lower portion of the levator labi superioris is known as the caput angular muscle, which acts to shorten the nose and dilate the nostrils. The pars alaris musculi nasalis and the depressor septi nasi depress and lengthen the nose as well as dilate the nostrils. The zygomaticus exerts a pulling effect on the orbicularis oris, which activates many of the muscles of the lower nose, adding an external but direct influence on nasal motion (Figure 5–8). The pars transversalis musculi nasalis compresses, lengthens, and contracts the nose. When the face is not animated, the nostrils and internal nares usually remain open, chiefly as a result of the stability of the upper lateral cartilages abutting with the wishbone-like support provided by the alar cartilages.

All muscles of the nose are innervated by the seventh cranial nerve. During nasal surgery, it is important that dissection be carried out in the subperichondrial and subperiosteal planes to prevent damage to the nasal framework. Surgical interruption of the musculature is sometimes purposefully done in order to modify plunging of the nasal tip during animation and in an attempt to prevent unnatural or exaggerated dilatation of the nostrils.

NERVE SUPPLY (Figure 5–9)

Sensory innervation of the external nose is derived from the fifth cranial nerve, and the motor nerve supply to the muscles of facial expression is derived from the seventh cranial nerve. Sensation to the dorsum and tip of the nose is supplied by the external nasal ramus from the ophthalmic nerve, which, early in its course, passes deep to the nasal bones and becomes superficial between the nasal bones and the lateral nasal cartilages. The infraorbital nerve is a branch of the maxillary division of the trigeminal nerve (fifth nerve). It supplies sensation to the lateral nasal and alar wall. These two nerve branches are easily blocked by small deposits of local anesthesia injected as a field block at the base of the nostrils over the dorsum of

Text continued on page 64.

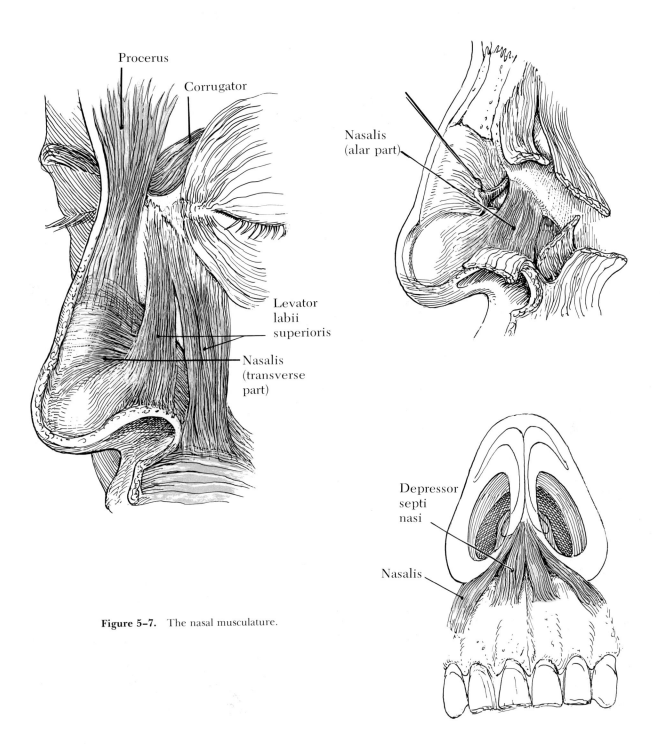

Procerus

Corrugator

Nasalis
(alar part)

Levator
labii
superioris

Nasalis
(transverse
part)

Depressor
septi
nasi

Nasalis

Figure 5–7. The nasal musculature.

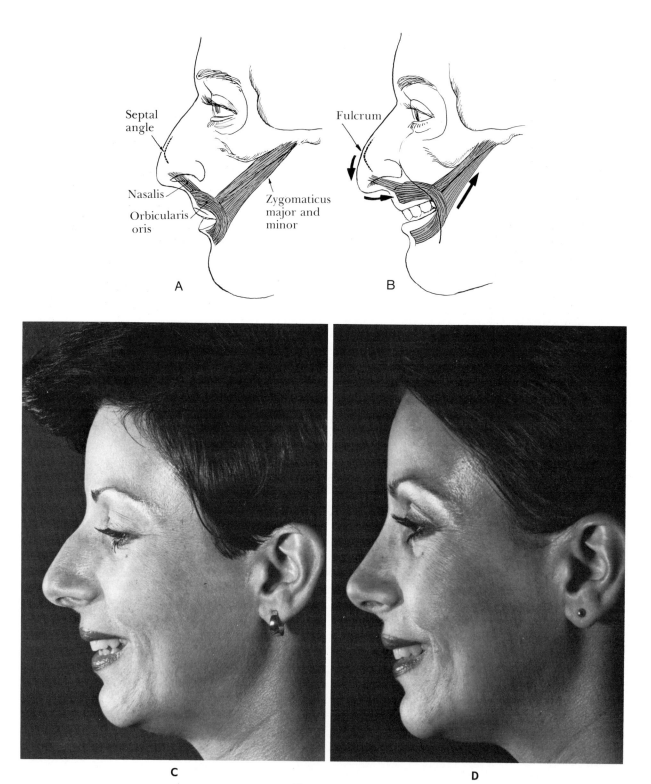

Figure 5–8.

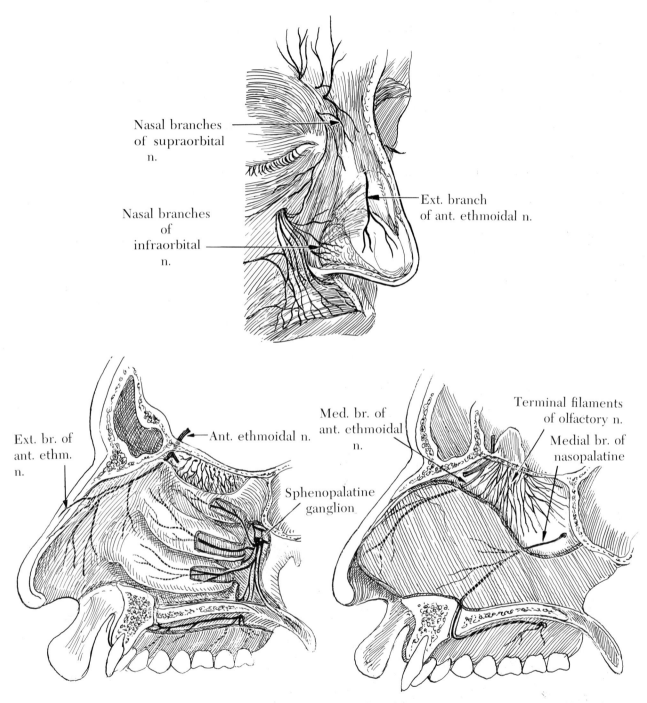

Nasal branches of supraorbital n.

Ext. branch of ant. ethmoidal n.

Nasal branches of infraorbital n.

Ext. br. of ant. ethm. n.

Ant. ethmoidal n.

Med. br. of ant. ethmoidal n.

Terminal filaments of olfactory n.

Medial br. of nasopalatine

Sphenopalatine ganglion

Figure 5–9. The nerve supply to the nose.

the nose, in conjunction with topical anesthesia administered high in the triangle formed by the nasal bones and lateral cartilages to the septum. It is this area that causes most anesthetic problems for the new surgeon and that is responsible for pain during surgery. Care should be taken to apply the topical anesthesia in a high and dorsal position in the internal nose in order to block the external nasal ramus.

The sphenopalatine ganglion supplies sensory fibers from the maxillary division of the fifth nerve and parasympathetic fibers from a great superficial petrosal nerve from the geniculate ganglion of the seventh nerve, as well as sympathetic fibers from the deep petrosal nerve (Vidian nerve). It supplies the inferoposterior mucosa of the nasal walls septum. This ganglion lies near the sphenopalatine foramen and is easily accessible to topical anesthetics. The sphenopalatine foramen is just behind and above the posterior end of the middle turbinate. The mucosa of the nasal sinuses are supplied by sensory fibers from the nasal wall of the cavity. Other nerve supplies to the internal nose come from the internal branches of the anterior ethmoidal nerve.

BLOOD SUPPLY (Figures 5–10 and 5–11)

The blood supply to the external nose comes from the external carotid artery via the external and internal maxillary arteries and the ophthalmic artery, which is a branch of the internal carotid. The facial artery, also known as the external maxillary, probably provides the major blood supply through its several branches. The internal maxillary artery, also known as the infraorbital artery, sends small branches that communicate with the external maxillary arteries supplying the lateral walls and the dorsum of the nose. A small branch of the ophthalmic artery, the supraorbital, contributes to the blood supply of the root of the nose.

Branches from the superior labial artery supply much of the ala and lower septum, where they anastomose with nasal branches of the ophthalmic artery (from the internal carotid system). The rich arterial supply to the soft tissues of the nose is well demonstrated by the copious bleeding that occurs during alar base resection.

The sphenopalatine artery and the descending palatine artery supply most of the blood to the internal nose (Figure 5–11). The descending pala-

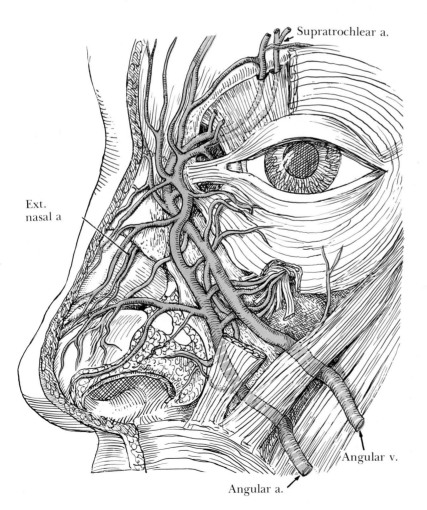

Supratrochlear a.

Ext. nasal a

Angular a.

Angular v.

Figure 5–10.

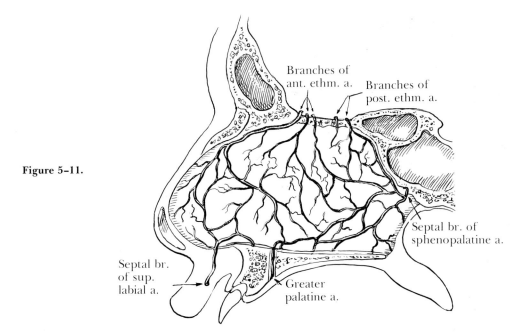

Figure 5–11.

Branches of ant. ethm. a.

Branches of post. ethm. a.

Septal br. of sphenopalatine a.

Septal br. of sup. labial a.

Greater palatine a.

tine artery is also known as the major palatine artery, and it travels through the nasal-palatine foramen. The nasal palatine branch is the terminal portion of this artery, where it leaves the submucosal region of the hard palate and ascends to the nasal cavity through the incisive canal. Here, it has a high anastomosis with the septal branches of the sphenopalatine artery. This artery supplies a large part of the nasal cavity and is the last of the terminal branches of the maxillary arteries.

The sphenopalatine artery sends many branches to the nose, particularly the nasal septum. The lateral wall is supplied by the osterolateral nasal arterial branch of the sphenopalatine artery. Many smaller branches supply the mucosa of the sinuses. The posterior portion of the nasal septum is supplied by the posterior septal artery, which travels over the roof of the nasal cavity and then descends to supply the septum. This artery also has a rich anastomosis with the nasopalatine branch of the major palatine artery.

The venous and lymphatic drainage of the nose generally parallels the arterial supply. It is well to remember that part of the venous drainage of the nose occurs via the ophthalmic veins to the cavernous sinus of the anterior fossa of the skull. Ascending infection and thrombosis of the cavernous sinus is a dreaded complication, but it is fortunately very rare. Likewise, the ethmoid vein drains into the superior sagittal sinus. These rich venous communications between the intracranial and intranasal cavities provide a menacing communication to the spread of intranasal infection.

THE LOBULE OF THE NOSE

The lobule of the nose is an anatomic unit that includes the tip, ala, columella, and membranous septum, as well as the internal structures they surround and envelope (including the alar cartilages and the minor cartilages). The entire unit (lobule) is moveable because there is no fixed cartilaginous or bony continuity. The septum and lateral nasal cartilages are connected only by connective tissue.

The skin of the lobule is important in rhinoplasty. It is thicker than the upper two thirds of the nasal skin and contains considerably more appendages. The structure of the dense connective tissue that forms the soft tissue and support of much of the lobule of the nose also may provide obstacles to the result in rhinoplasty, since much of it cannot be sculpted as can the cartilaginous structures. Trimming of the skin and subcutaneous tissue results inevitably in scars that may cause secondary deformities such as notching and depressions.

(For references, see pages 450 to 455.)

Chapter 6

Physiology

Daniel C. Baker, M.D.

The patient requesting rhinoplasty is usually motivated by a desire for cosmetic improvement and, not infrequently, more comfort in breathing. A successful rhinoplasty should not only be aesthetically pleasing to the patient and surgeon but should also maintain or restore normal physiologic nasal function. Any surgeon performing rhinoplasty must be familiar with nasal physiology and the intimate relationship of nasal function to nasal form, both in its internal and external variations.

The stuffy nose is a common complaint in a sizeable proportion of patients. Unfortunately, nasal obstruction is one of the least understood and most frequently mismanaged and inadequately treated conditions associated with rhinoplastic surgery. Too often, the emphasis has been on structural deformities that must be corrected surgically, leading to the attitude of "when in doubt, do a submucous resection." However, many preoperative and postoperative nasal obstructive problems are physiologic rather than structural, and they can be treated with patience and medical care (Baker and Strauss, 1977).

Most disorders of nasal breathing are the result of turbinate dysfunction (Goode, 1977), yet there is no acceptable, simple diagnostic standard or test for the common nasal pathologies. The variety of medical and surgical treatments available bears testimony to their frequent ineffectiveness and the frustration of the physician or surgeon caring for these patients.

This chapter will provide the surgeon performing rhinoplasty with a basis for understanding nasal physiology and pathophysiology. It should enable him to make a rational evaluation and intelligent treatment plan for the patient with nasal obstruction, and to obtain a satisfactory result in the normal, functioning nose without unfavorably altering physiology.

HISTORY

It is generally considered that Galen, 2000 years ago, was the first scientist to perceive the key functions of the nose and accurately describe its anatomy (Cinelli, 1971). However, it was not until the 19th century that significant physiologic investigations of nasal function were performed, and it is only in the past 50 years that major progress has been made in our understanding of nasal physiology (Proctor, 1977).

In 1876, Braune and Clausen made classical observations on nasal air currents and pressures under various conditions, and their findings are still valid today (Proetz, 1941). Until the latter part of the 19th century, physiologists believed that air currents took a straight course through the nose; Paulsen (1882) refuted this concept by studying the streaming of air in cadavers. His studies were confirmed by experiments of Zwaardemaker and Franke, which demonstrated that the air currents entering the nose during inspiration follow a parabolic curve (Cinelli, 1971; Wright, 1914). This was further confirmed by studies of Tonndorf (1939), Proetz (1941), and Konno (1973). Konno's studies were based on measurements and observations of the pattern and velocity of airflow through a nasal model made from a silicone cast of the human nasal cavity.

In 1884, Zuckerkandl published a classic work on the anatomy of the nose, including a description of the vasculature of the turbinates. Wright (1885) studied the vascular mucous membrane and its vasomotor reaction to irritation of the mucosa. This has recently been elaborated by Ritter (1970) and Taylor (1973). The presence of a normal cycle of congestion and decongestion of the cavernous tissues of the nasal conchae was first described by Kayser in 1895, and he termed this the "nasal cycle." His observations have been corroborated by the studies of Heetderks (1927), Stoksted (1952, 1953), and Hasegawa and Kern (1977).

The earliest surgical attempts to overcome nasal obstruction were directed at correction of septal deformities. Total or partial removal of the cartilaginous septum had been advocated by Langenbeck (1843), Dieffenbach (1845), and Chassaginac (1851). Adams (1895) proposed straightening the deviated septum by moving it into the midline either by fracturing or crushing (Cinelli, 1971; Wright, 1914). Although the basis of the submucous operation was already in the medical literature based on the work of Ash, Burghardt, and Krieg, it was the publications of Freer (1902) and Killian (1904) that described the submucous septal operation that was to become the standard procedure for several decades and that is still used today to correct certain deformities (Walter, 1973). Since then, the various techniques of septal surgery have been thoroughly examined. Today, septal plasty, septal reconstruction, and septal repositioning are preferred over submucous resection when they can be accomplished.

In more recent studies in nasal physiology, Cottle (1960), Negus (1948), Williams (1954), Bridger (1970), Proetz (1941), Ogura (1966, 1968), and others have corroborated and elucidated the physiologic principles and theories of the 19th century. Although numerous methods have been devised to measure nasal pressure-flow relationships and nasal resistance, there is still no effective standard.

The surgeon needs a simple test for an objective evaluation of nasal obstruction that can be adapted to the clinical situation to determine what surgical procedure is indicated. Although nasal surgery to improve physiologic function is extensively practiced, there is a scarcity of objective preoperative and postoperative studies and statistics on the results obtained. Evaluation relies primarily on the patient's subjective opinion and the surgeon's view through the nasal speculum.

FUNCTIONS OF THE NOSE

The nose is an active organ with numerous functions. Most notably, the nose acts as a complex air conditioning apparatus and an airway to the lower respiratory tract. The nasal mucosa probably receives more exposure to the environment than any other part of the body, and although most nasal functions are taken for granted, significant impairment is soon noted by the patient and manifested by various nasal symptoms.

Respiration. The most important function of the nose is to provide a route for adequate airflow to the lungs. The physiologic superiority of nasal breathing over mouth breathing has been demonstrated, although nasal breathing nearly doubles the total respiratory resistance to airflow (Proctor, 1977). Mouth breathing is felt to be unphysiologic and inefficient, requiring an increased expenditure of energy for a given alveolar ventilation as well as causing excessive water loss. Studies suggest that the nose has an important respiratory control function that cannot be completely compensated for by mouth breathing (Williams, 1973).

Filtration. Filtration and cleansing of the inspired air occurs in two ways. The vibrissae in the anterior nares filter out very coarse foreign material such as soot, leaves, and insects. Smaller particles such as dust, pollens, powders, and bacteria are projected against the mucous blanket on the nasal walls, where they are caught and retained to be conveyed to the pharynx and swallowed (Proetz, 1941). This latter process is made more effective by electrostatic charges that are constantly maintained on the body surface; when the nose and dust particles bear opposite charges, adsorption occurs.

Humidification. The nose regulates the moisture of the inspired air as it passes over the turbinates. It is estimated that inspired air becomes humidified to approximately 90 percent before reaching the lungs and, in performing this function, approximately one liter of water is emitted by the nose every 24 hours (Proetz, 1941). The normal nose is able to saturate inspired air with water under nearly all conditions of humidity. To accomplish this function, the average nose has about 158 square cm of mucous membrane and an airstream width along the turbinates of about 1 mm (Goode, 1977). Absence of this function is demonstrated by the devastating effects of pharyngitis or laryngitis sicca such as inspissated secretions, crusts, and swallowing difficulty (Taylor, 1974).

Heating. Of equal importance with humidification of inspired air is heating, which is also controlled by the turbinates. The dense arrangement of blood vessels in these structures permits a rapid accommodation of a large blood volume that can circulate and radiate heat.

Air entering the nasal cavity is brought to a temperature of 31° to 37° C, although inspired air can vary in temperature from −5° to 55° C and may be dry or saturated (Konno, 1973). Approximately 70 kilocalories of energy are required to perform the functions of humidification and heating. According to Cole (1953), almost one third of the heat and moisture supplied by the nose is recovered during expiration and transferred to the inspiratory cycle.

Protection and Self-Cleansing. The nose delivers inspired air to the lungs under relatively constant conditions for effective respiration. The filtration system is also self-cleansing by action of the cilia and mucous glands. Approximately one liter of mucus is produced every 24 hours by the goblet cells and mucous glands, and it is composed predominantly of water with about 3 percent mucin and 1 percent salts (Goode, 1977). Nasal mucus also contains antibodies that are active against viruses and bacteria (Remington, Vosti, Lietze et al., 1964). Particles are trapped on the sticky surface, and the constant action of the cilia moves the mucous blanket posteriorly toward the pharynx at a speed of about 1 cm per minute as they beat at rates estimated at from 160 to 1500 beats per minute (Proetz, 1941; Goode, 1977). Although the cilia are hardy structures that quickly regenerate, removal of the mucous blanket and drying may incapacitate the cilia in a matter of minutes. The surgeon must therefore be careful about incisions and scars so as to avoid producing nonciliated areas in locations that could interfere with the normal cleansing action of the nose. During acute viral rhinitis, ciliary paralysis is a common occurrence.

Olfaction. Smell is certainly an important function of the nose, but in man, this sense is relatively feeble in comparison with olfaction in lower animals (Negus, 1958). Man has developed the senses of sight and hearing, which protect him more quickly against dangers. In man, the olfactory membrane occupies a position high in the nasal cavity, out of the mainstream of airflow.

Secondary Sexual Organ. The nose also serves as a secondary sexual organ. Most wild animals react acutely to animal odors and find them pleasant; a male dog with anosmia becomes quite philosophical about his sex life (Brown, 1951). Because the sense of smell in man is relatively undeveloped, a woman tries to improve upon nature by using elaborate perfumes and aromas usually made from oils extracted from animals. Besides the intimate connection of the olfactory sense with sexual reflexes, certain nasal disorders may be related to sexual irritation — e.g., honeymoon rhinitis, menstrual and prepubertal epistaxis, and rhinitis of pregnancy. The anatomic similarity of the engorged turbinates to the erect penis is a well-studied fact (MacKenzie, 1884).

Phonation. The nasal cavities exert a profound influence upon vocalization by acting as an additional resonating chamber for certain consonants. Any pathologic or anatomic condition that blocks the nasal passages will change the tone and timber of the human voice. If the nose is obstructed, a nasal tone known as rhinolalia is given to the voice.

AIRFLOW IN THE NASAL CAVITY

There are diverse opinions on the pathway of air through the normal nose, and much of this disagreement is due to the various models used in experiments as well as to the varying widths of the nasal cavities (Konno, 1973). Most rhinologists agree that the air currents follow a parabolic course rather than a straight course from nostril to choanae (Figure 6–1).

The majority of experiments on nasal air currents have been done on human cadaver skulls, casts, or latex models of the nasal cavities in which the septum has been replaced by glass. With these, the air currents can be visualized using smoke or acid fumes contacting pieces of litmus paper distributed throughout the model. Therefore, the basic airflow determined by these means can only be considered an approximation (Abramson and Harker, 1973), as these models may differ in size, shape, contour, and texture from the nose *in vivo*.

From 1.5 to 2.5 cm beyond the anterior nares, the airstream converges to pass through the small cross section of the ostium internum. It then bends in a parabolic curve of 60 to 130 degrees from its initial direction to pass mainly through the middle meatus over the inferior turbinates; a lesser stream travels through the inferior meatus and along the nasal floor. The least airflow is through the narrower superior aspect of the nasal cavity (Proctor, 1977; Abramson and Harker, 1973). Following the bend in the nasopharynx, the airflow moves in a more or less straight direction through the pharynx and larynx into the trachea.

On expiration, the pathway is essentially reversed with air entering the choanae uniformly, passing upward and taking a parabolic curve to exit through the nostrils. One difference is that the resistance at the nasal vestibule causes some secondary air currents and eddies to form so that air is recirculated to the roof of the nose (Abramson and Harker, 1973).

Airflow in the nose may be of two types: laminar or turbulent. Laminar flow is one in which the direction and speed is constant and uniform. Circling motions can be part of laminar flow if they are reasonably constant in speed and direction. Turbulent flow consists of currents that vary constantly according to time and direction and are

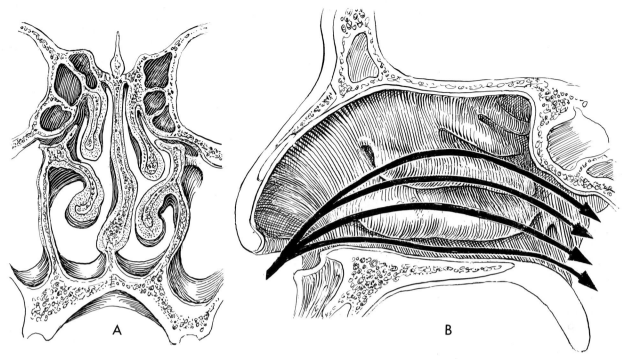

Figure 6–1.   *A*, Coronal section through the midnose showing available airspaces in the "normal" nose. Slight septal deflections must be considered the norm. *B*, The passage of air through the meatus in the presence of normal mucosa. The main air current takes a parabolic curve to pass through the middle meatus over the inferior turbinate; a lesser stream travels through the inferior meatus and along the nasal floor; the least airflow is through the narrower superior aspect of the nasal cavity.

irregular, resulting in decreased airflow efficiency and increased resistance.

Airflow is dependent upon the minimal cross-sectional diameter of the nose and the pressure differential produced by the lungs between the anterior and posterior nares. As air flows through the nose, laminar resistance increases in inverse proportion to the fourth power of the diameter (Poiseuille's law). Thus, as the effective diameter of the nasal cavity decreases by half, laminar resistance may increase by as much as 16 times (Abramson and Harker, 1973). In order to perform its many functions — especially warming, humidification, and cleansing — in the presence of varying environmental conditions, the nose possesses a wide range of control over the erectile and contractile tissues of the nasal mucosa — airway space can be rapidly reduced or enlarged at any given moment.

During quiet respiration when the velocity of air is slow, airflow is primarily laminar and streamlined. However, any decrease in the cross-sectional area of the nose or increase in respiratory rate allows eddies to form and favors turbulent flow. In such a complex structure as the nose, airflow is both laminar and turbulent. According to Goode (1977), in the ideal nose there is a narrow laminar flow of air passing over as much mucosa as possible at a velocity slow enough to enable the mucosa to humidify, warm, and cleanse the air, yet fast

enough so nasal dyspnea does not occur. On expiration, a certain amount of turbulence is normal and improves olfactory sense.

What may increase turbulence of the air flow is a deformity such as a septal spur or scar contracture of the internal nasal valve area. Constrictions of the inside cross section of the nose caused by septal spurs or ridges whose maximal extension is parallel to the direction of airflow have little effect on the air current. However, obstructions placed at right angles to the direction of airflow may change the type and velocity of flow considerably, since the volume of air passing through the nose is proportional to the narrowest cross section that normally corresponds to the internal valve. In anatomic causes of nasal obstruction, the narrowest cross section may be nearer the vestibule or inside the main nasal cavity (Naumann, 1972). The most marked turbulence is seen in the nasal cavity of a patient with atrophic rhinitis where the narrow, streamlined width of the nose is lost.

NASAL AIRWAY RESISTANCE AND NASAL OBSTRUCTION

Some rhinoplastic surgeons regard the nose as a passive conduit for airflow from the external environment to the lungs. In patients with complaints of nasal obstruction, they make the erroneous interpretation that the passage must be enlarged to accommodate a maximal inspiratory airflow. On the contrary, the nose acts as a variable resistor to airflow, and the various air conditioning functions of the nose depend on the interaction between the air and the nasal surface. In order to perform these functions efficiently the normal nose is constructed to have a narrow width and wide surface area with a smooth contour and convolutions. A certain degree of nasal resistance seems to be normal for comfort and health, and although nasal surgery is performed to improve airflow, there is little data to determine the ideal endpoint for any given patient (Abramson and Harker, 1973).

The nasal cavity does not have a constant diameter, and therefore the total nasal resistance is a summation of the resistances of the varying effective diameters of the cavity (Konno, 1973). This resistance also varies with each individual in relation to changes in posture, exercise, vascular congestion, and disease.

Nasal obstruction is a subjective feeling and sensation caused by an increase in nasal airway resistance. In most cases, the sensation of nasal obstruction is consistent with the objective measurement of nasal airway resistance, although there is a wide individual variation among patients because or natural or acquired patterns of respiration. Most importantly, there is a difference of threshold and adaptation of sensation of nasal obstruction (Konno, 1973). An increase of nasal airway resistance may be caused not only by anatomic changes in the nasal cavity or external nose but also by a reversible rapid change of the turbinate size.

When a patient's complaints do not correspond to the objective findings, it may be necessary to repeat the rhinoscopy examination at another time. In certain cases, the sensation of nasal obstruction may not be caused by an increase of nasal airway resistance, but by other abnormal sensations of the nose or by physiologic factors that cause the patient to be constantly aware of nasal respiration.

THE NASAL CYCLE

At any given moment, most individuals have unilateral nasal obstruction, although they are usually unaware of it. This obstruction is due to a normal physiologic phenomenon of a cyclic, rhythmic variation between congestion and decongestion of the turbinates. It may be so complete that the major nasal airflow may be almost entirely through the patent side. This phenomenon was first observed and studied by Kayser in 1895 and has been termed "nasal cycle." Despite the alternating congestion and decongestion of each side, the normal person does not complain of the subjective sensation of nasal obstruction because the total airway resistance remains relatively constant (Hasegawa and Kern, 1977). As one nasal airway is opening and its turbinates are shrinking and giving off secretions of serous fluid and mucus, the opposite nasal airway is closing.

This cycle has been demonstrated in about 80 percent of normal individuals and has been reported to occur over periods of 30 minutes to 5 hours (Stoksted, 1952, 1953; Williams, 1973). Usually, a damp and cold atmosphere brings about the greatest engorgement of the turbinates. The cycle has also been reported to be more active during adolescence, presumably on the basis of increased hormonal activity. The exact function of the nasal cycle has not been adequately explained, although it is conceivable that such a rhythmic shift of nasal airflow might provide an opportunity for recovery from ambient air-related injury (Proctor, 1977). For the rhinoplasty surgeon, it is important to recognize the cycle as a normal physiologic response and to differentiate it from true causes of nasal obstruction.

EFFECT OF NASAL STRUCTURES ON AIRFLOW

NOSTRILS AND VESTIBULE

The position, shape, and direction of the nostrils play an important role in directing nasal airflow and affecting nasal resistance. The ventral boundary of the nostrils is the nasal tip, and the normal contour is formed by a graceful rounding of the angles of the lower lateral cartilages. Excessively narrow tips can cause slit-like nostrils, which impair inspiratory airflow. A twisted tip caused by dislocation of the caudal septum or hypertrophy or buckling of the lower lateral cartilage can create nostril asymmetry; pendulous tips, retroussé tips, and recessed tips all may affect airflow, since the direction of flow into the vestibule is controlled by the nasolabial angle and shape of the nostrils (Proetz, 1941) (Figure 6–2). The anterior nares directs inspired air upward to the internal valve area. In the long nose with a plunging tip and acute nasolabial angle, the main air current will be directed relatively high in the nasal cavity; conversely, in the patient with a retroussé tip and large nasolabial angle or saddle deformity, the main air current is lowered (Konno, 1973).

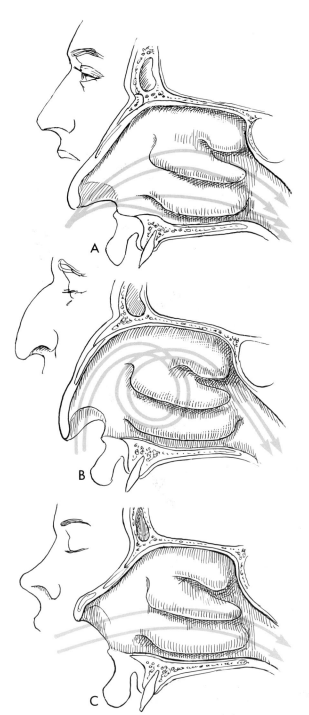

Figure 6–2. Inspiratory current: *A,* Normal nose, parabolic curve.

B, Dependent tip with impingement of the inspiratory current on the dorsum and formation of eddies.

C, Excessively elevated tip with flattening of the air current and more direct course. (After Fomon and associates, 1948.)

The lateral boundaries of the nostrils are the alae, whose shape is largely determined by the lateral crura of the lower lateral cartilages and soft tissue covering (Figure 6–3). The cartilages may be thick and rigid or thin and frail allowing easy collapse; they may be abnormally long producing vo-

luminous nostrils or very short in small nostrils. Their position may be elevated or depressed due to heredity or to trauma or surgery. The alae may be so thick as to encroach upon the nares, or they may be thin, allowing a wide opening. Concavity may produce narrow or pinched nostrils; flaring is typical of the noses of blacks (Fomon, Silver, Gilbert, and Syracuse, 1948).

The medial boundary of the nostril is formed by the columella, the contour of which is largely determined by the flare of the medial crura and soft tissue. The columella may be excessively wide, producing narrow nostrils; too short, creating small horizontal nostrils; or too long, giving rise to slit-like nostrils. Retraction of the columella can lead to collapse of the nostrils following excessive shortening of the nose in rhinoplasty.

The nostril is a dynamic structure subject to constant motion and modified during respiration by the action of the nasalis muscles. If a horse is observed while it is galloping, it will be noticed that the nostrils dilate on inspiration and contract on expiration. This opening of the nostrils allows for a free inlet of air and corresponds to the demands of respiration. In fast-running species of animals, the movements of the alae nasi are marked; man, with less strenuous needs of respiration, still demonstrates similar opening and partial closure but with much smaller excursions of the nostrils (Negus, 1958). This may also be seen during periods of rage and fear. In facial paralysis, patients not infrequently complain of unilateral nasal obstruction of the paralyzed side due to a loss of the dilator effect of the nasalis muscle.

Defects of the nares that interfere with the airflow may or may not be attributed to a single factor (Figure 6–4). Usually, they result from a combination of abnormalities about the boundaries of the nostrils. A careful evaluation of all possible causative factors is therefore essential to obtain a good functional result with surgical correction (Foman, Silver, Gilbert, and Syracuse, 1948).

THE INTERNAL VALVE

The nasal valve was first described by Mink in 1903 and is the passage between the lower margin of the upper lateral cartilage and the septum and the most important regulator of nasal airway resistance. In the normal nose, this is the narrowest portion of the upper airway. The nasal valve, also known as the ostium internum (Table 6–1), becomes depressed during quiet inspiration and widens on quiet expiration. This action controls the inspiratory airflow, changing it from a column to a

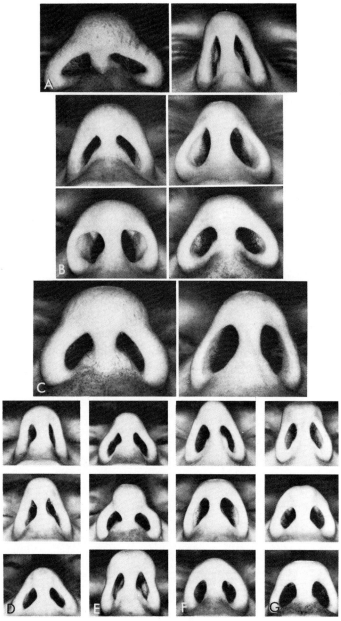

Figure 6–3. *A,* Different nasal widths in two European men. *B,* Different nostril shapes in European noses. *C,* Different nostril and alar cartilage thicknesses in two European men. Different alar base marginal shapes with *(D)* almost straight, *(E)* curved, *(F)* symmetrically arched, and *(G)* almost angular margins.

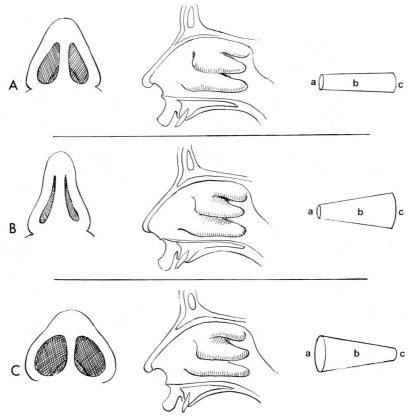

Figure 6–4. Control of pressure differentials by the nares. *A,* Normal nares: (a) nares; (b) sinuses; (c) choanae. *B,* Constricted nares, accentuating negative and positive pressures. *C,* Abnormally large nares, diminishing negative and positive pressures. (After Fomon and associates, 1948.)

TABLE 6–1   SYNONYMS FOR THE INTERNAL NASAL VALVE

Os internum	Nasal valve
Ostium internum	Valve region
Limen nasi	Valve area
Limen vestibuli	Flow limiting segment
Liminal chink	Area 2
Liminal valve	

After Kern, 1973

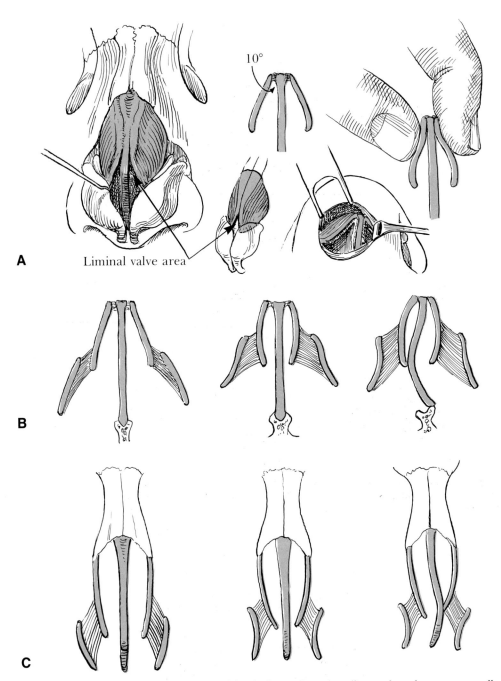

A   Liminal valve area

B

C

Figure 6–5.   *A,* Internal nasal valve region between caudal end of upper lateral cartilage and nasal septum normally subtends an angle of 10 degrees. Narrowing, closing, or depressing this angle closes the internal valve and increases nasal airway resistance.

B, Cross sections, and *C,* sagittal sections demonstrating anatomic-physiologic relationships in the valve area. The upper edge of the alar cartilage slightly overlaps the lower edge of upper laterals, with a fibrous attachment between them. Column 1, quiet inspiration demonstrating gentle closing. Column 2, forced inspiration with accentuated closing of the valve. Column 3, forced inspiration with a deviated septum. No external deviation need be visible and with narrowing of the nose during rhinoplasty the problem can be exacerbated. (After Gorney, 1977.)

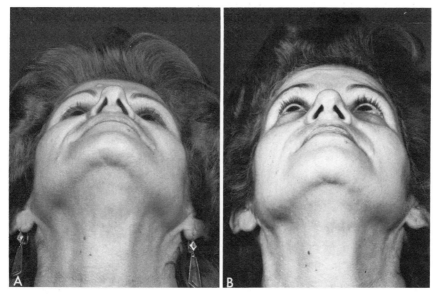

Figure 6–6. *A,* Patient with alar collapse resulting from total removal of alar cartilages during rhinoplasty. *B,* Following bilateral conchal cartilage grafts to the alae, nasal obstruction is lessened on inspiration.

sheet of air, thereby giving shape, velocity, direction, and resistance to the air currents (Hinderer, 1977).

The junction between the upper lateral cartilages and the septum are intimately related near the nasal bones and fused dorsally to the septum. However, the caudal end of the upper lateral cartilage is attached by an aponeurosis to the septum and flares away from it at an angle of 10 to 15 degrees (Figure 6–5). Free movement is allowed by this aponeurotic attachment, the septum being the fixed portion of the valve. Since this terminal portion of the upper lateral cartilage is not firmly attached to the septum, shortening of the cartilage excessively during rhinoplasty may narrow the angle or disrupt the function of the valve; indiscreet removal may result in pinching. On the other hand, unremoved projecting ends of upper lateral cartilages caused by an error or omission in a rhinoplasty may block the airway (Goldman, 1966).

Because of the importance of the nasal valve area and of preserving sufficient mucosa, some rhinoplasty surgeons advocate the subperichondral approach to separating the septum from the upper lateral cartilages. This technique is felt to minimize the possibility of scar and synechiae formation, which can occur more easily in dividing and resecting the mucosa and cartilage. However, in experienced hands, dividing the upper lateral cartilage from the septum with judicious removal of excess mucosa and cartilage has not resulted in a higher incidence of obstructive complications.

There is a form of inspiratory nasal obstruction in which the nasal valve and cartilaginous vault collapse at small, negative intranasal pres-

sures. Clinically, this entity has been described as "alar collapse" (Figure 6–6). If the upper and lower lateral cartilages are involved, the entire cartilaginous wall collapses and the nostrils appear as slits. If the collapse is limited to the upper lateral cartilages, the central portion of the nose may assume a pinched appearance (Bridger, 1970). This phenomenon can be demonstrated by gently compressing the lower lateral cartilages above the nasal tip. The resulting airway resistance can be felt immediately.

Probably the most common cause of alar collapse is excessive removal of the lower lateral cartilage during rhinoplasty. Correction of nasal obstruction secondary to alar collapse is difficult, and the various methods have been reviewed by Walter (1969, 1973). Treatment has varied from the use of breathing exercises to the insertion into the nostrils of special self-holding dilators fashioned from hairpins or wires. Injections of paraffin to stiffen the alae and implantation of various metal and plastic materials have also been attempted. The use of cartilage or composite grafts (Walter, 1973, 1969) has been the most successful.

Nasal airway obstruction at the internal valve can be caused by a variety of anatomic deformities (Figure 6–7). A deviated septum in the area of the nasal valve may be the cause of a malformation of the upper lateral cartilage. Any postoperative, posttraumatic, or postinfectious scarring may lead to web formation or narrowing in the region of the valve. These deformities may be aggravated by drooping or retraction of the columella or spurs and deviations of the maxillary crest and anterior nasal spine. The important relationship of the ce-

NASAL VALVE PATHOLOGY

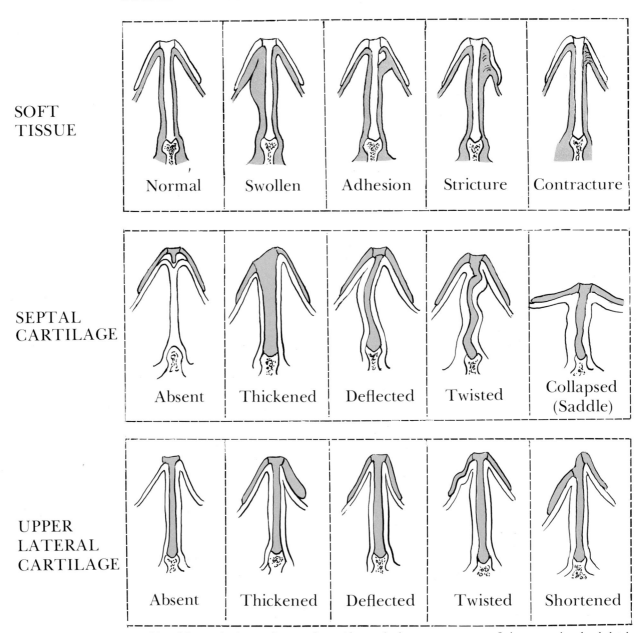

Figure 6–7.   Abnormalities of the nasal valve may be secondary to changes in the mucocutaneous soft tissue covering the skeletal structures of the nasal valve (top row), nasal septum abnormalities or deficiencies (middle row), and upper lateral cartilage deformities and injuries (bottom row). (After Kern, 1975.)

phalic border of the alar cartilage and the caudal edge of the upper lateral cartilage has been emphasized by Gorney (1977) (see Figure 6–5). A septal deviation at this point narrows the valve area and aggravates obstruction on inspiration.

THE SEPTUM

Of the surgical procedures for correction of nasal obstruction, none has been more abused than the submucous resection of the nasal septum. Since its development and popularization in the early part of the 20th century, the operation has not only been advised for every deviated septum regardless of symptoms (Spector, 1959) but has been recommended to treat every condition from headache to emphysema (Horton, 1973).

It is not necessary to correct an asymptomatic septal deviation merely to achieve a "cosmetic" septum, and the existence of a prominent spur does not always warrant removal. Angulation and curvature of the nasal septum is the rule rather than the exception, and man seems to be unique among animal species in possessing this deformity (Negus, 1958; Fry, 1976). Anatomic studies of 2152 skulls by Mackenzie in the Museum of the Royal College of Surgeons showed deformity of the bony septum in 1657, or about 75 per cent (Thompson and Negus, 1948). Further studies by Zuckerkandl demonstrated crests or spurs of bone projecting from the septum into one or the other nasal cavities in about 20 percent of skulls (Romanes, 1964). Schaeffer (1920) stated, "Indeed, deflection of the human nasal septum is so common that one almost thinks of it as normal anatomy."

Anyone who has broad experience in rhinoplastic surgery can attest to the fact that some patients with a grossly deviated septum are free of symptoms of nasal obstruction most of the time. Occasionally, a patient may complain of obstruction on the side opposite the septal deviation. In addition, the persistence of nasal obstruction following submucous resection of the septum is not uncommon. From the surgeon's viewpoint, the operation has been successful since he has removed the septal obstruction; but the patient all too often may be disappointed with the effectiveness of the operation as he still has difficulty breathing through his nose.

The concern of surgeons with deviations of the nasal septum has less relevance today than it did in the past. From a functional viewpoint, a deviated septum must be evaluated in its relationship to the structures that are lateral to it — the upper lateral cartilages, nasal bones, and turbinates (Williams, 1954). The importance of the cartilaginous septum and its relationship to the upper lateral cartilage in forming the internal valve has been stressed. Conceivably, a septal deviation could be necessary for the creation of a valve in a given nose with a particular upper lateral cartilage. By straightening the septum, the distance between it and the upper lateral cartilage could be altered sufficiently to interfere with proper nasal airway resistance (Williams, 1954).

Similarly, a deviation of the septum that has developed gradually is frequently accompanied by compensatory hypertrophy of the inferior turbinate and septal tubercle on the concave side. This compensation tends to maintain fairly equal nasal airway resistance in both nasal cavities. In performing a septoplasty or submucous resection, the patency of the airway on the concave side of the nasal cavity must be estimated, and if necessary, the appropriate surgical procedure must be performed simultaneously on the inferior turbinate (Konno, 1973). After correction of the septal deformity, however, the turbinate hypertrophy usually resolves spontaneously.

A minor high deviation of the septum that was asymptomatic prior to rhinoplasty may become symptomatic after lowering the nasal dorsum and tip. On the other hand, merely correcting a septal deviation in a narrow nose may not result in an adequate airway, since only a complete rhinoplasty with lowering the vault in combination with septoplasty will accomplish the desired functional result (Walter, 1973). An excessively high septum may stretch the upper lateral cartilages, thereby narrowing the angle between the septum and cartilages and predisposing to collapse of the valve on inspiration. This condition is sometimes referred to as "tension nose."

Some of the clinical abnormalities and indications for surgical correction of the septum include dislocations (Figure 6–8), deviations, spurs, and ridges. The rhinoplasty surgeon should not have a fixed method for correction, but he should be familiar with the combinations and variations of septal surgery. Today, nasal septal reconstruction with preservation of as much cartilage as possible is preferred to the classical submucous resection. Ersner (1948) analyzed several hundred submucous resections and reported that whenever the cartilaginous portion of the septum was involved, the end results of the orthodox Killian procedure were generally unsatisfactory. In this operation, the semirigid cartilaginous medial wall is exchanged for a relatively flaccid membrane with less stability. During inspiration, a slight pressure difference between nostrils may be sufficient to produce collapse of the membrane into one nostril.

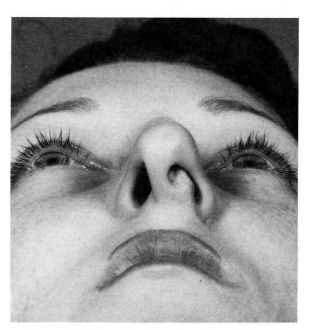

Figure 6–8. Complete obstruction of nasal airway from dislocated caudal end of cartilaginous septum.

Today, it is preferable to maintain the resiliency and stability of the cartilaginous septum whenever possible (Bridger, 1970), and also to maintain it as a potential donor site for cartilage. In reconstruction of any given septum, proper evaluation of nasal structures prior to and during surgery is essential in order to accomplish and maintain the proper relationships so that the nose will function as an integrated unit. This requires knowledge of the relationship of the septum to the upper lateral cartilages, the nasal bones, the turbinates, and the tip (Williams, 1954).

Little has been written about the various functions of the nasal septum. To state merely that the septum is the nasal partition creating two cavities, each a distinct and complete entity, is an oversimplification. The septum helps create and support the nasal dorsum and provides a hard wall in the nasal cavity important for maintaining resistance to air currents. It also forms part of the nasal valve and serves as a resisting terminal for the cyclical excursions of the turbinates (Williams, 1953). In conjunction with the upper lateral cartilages and turbinates, the septum regulates the airflow and creates eddies of air currents; with the nasal bones, it helps protect the cranial vault.

THE TURBINATES

The turbinates are thin semicircular bones covered by a dense, adherent periosteum and a thick, highly vascular mucous membrane. These scroll-like laminae project and overhang from the lateral nasal wall and incompletely subdivide each nasal cavity into a number of groove-like passages, the nasal meatuses. The main functions of the turbinates are filtration, humidification, and warming of inspired air. They also protect the respiratory passages against noxious agents by reflex swelling and obstruction of the nasal passages when stimulated. According to Little (1963), the inferior turbinates are most susceptible to enlargement and the most common cause of nasal obstruction.

The inferior turbinate is composed of a fibroelastic stroma rich in cavernous sinusoids, whose expansile and contractile functions are to regulate a controlled volume of warmed air into the lungs. Abundant elastic tissue with circular and spirally arranged bundles of smooth muscle supports the walls of the sinusoids (Figure 6–9). A rich capillary network opens into these sinusoids, which in turn drain into deeper venous plexuses. A type of erectile tissue is thus formed by this vascular arrangement (Lichtenstein and Norman, 1971).

Indeed, the similarity between the sinusoidal tissue of the inferior turbinate and the erectile tissue of the penis is well documented (Mackenzie, 1884). The middle and superior turbinates possess numerous mucous glands but very few cavernous spaces. Their function seems to be moistening of the air by the efficient production of mucus.

The turbinates are exceedingly sensitive, and the vasomotor supply is from both divisions of the autonomic nervous system. Sympathetic stimulation causes intense vasoconstriction, reduction in erectile tissue, and widening of the airway. Vasodilatation, vascular engorgement, and narrowing of the airway result from parasympathetic stimulation (Lichtenstein and Norman, 1971). The vasomotor control of the nasal mucous membranes is most active in the second decade of life, and it is apparently closely associated with the physiologic changes of puberty (Dutrow, 1935).

The pathology of an enlarging turbinate is the progression of hypertrophy to hyperplasia to polypoid degeneration (Little, 1963). In hypertrophy, there is a physiologic response with engorged sinusoids and hyperactive glandular structures. Although the connective tissue cells of the tunica propria are edematous, there is no increase in their number. Chronic hypertrophy leads to hyperplasia with thickening of the epithelial layer and infiltration of the tunica propria with connective tissue cells of all ages as well as lymphocytes. The reparative process brings new blood vessel formation and fibroblastic proliferation (Little, 1963; Sanders, 1971). The advanced stage leads to the formation of polyps, which are edematous areas of mucosa so engorged with interstitial fluid that their weight and the pull of gravity expand these areas away from the nasal walls (Sanders, 1971).

Although obstruction of the airway may be secondary to enlarged middle and superior turbinates, more commonly the anterior third of the inferior turbinate partially or totally occludes the airway. Little (1963) stated that the common denominator in the production of hypertrophied turbinates is stimulation from chemical, thermal, mechanical, or nervous stimuli. In their study of reactions within the nose during varying life experiences, Holmes and associates (1950) listed eight common stimuli that could provoke vascular engorgement and nasal obstruction:

1. Contact with infectious agents
2. Inhalation of irritant dusts or chemical fumes
3. Inhalation of pollen or other substances to which the patient is sensitive
4. Life experiences provocative of conflict, resentment, or frustration

Middle turbinate

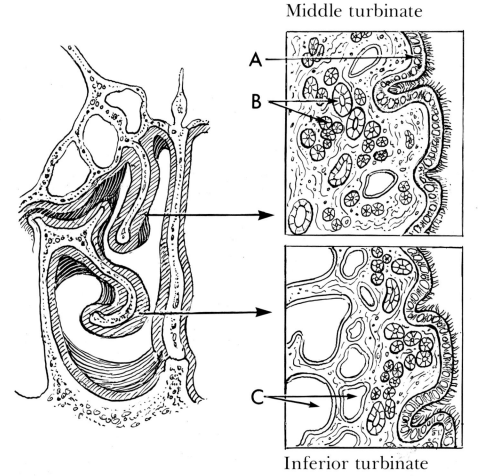

Inferior turbinate

Figure 6–9. Histology of the middle and inferior turbinates. *A,* Ciliated respiratory epithelium. *B,* Mucous and serous glands. *C,* Cavernous sinuses. The middle turbinate contains numerous mucous glands but very few cavernous sinuses compared with the inferior turbinate.

5. Chilling of the body surface
6. Menstruation and pregnancy
7. Sexual excitement
8. Strong odors and bright lights.

Changes in posture may also affect turbinate size, primarily because of the gravity effect of venous flow (Rundcrantz, 1969). Patients with unilateral nasal obstruction usually avoid sleeping on the patent side, as the downside turbinates engorge due to the decrease in venous outflow and the upside turbinates shrink.

The degree and chronicity of turbinate obstruction range from the normal transient swelling of the turbinates — which occurs when passing from a cold to a hot environment — to the chronically enlarged turbinate — which develops on the contralateral side of a markedly deviated septum. Although in most instances only the soft tissues of the turbinate hypertrophy, hyperplasia of the bony portion may also occur.

ANTHROPOLOGIC CONSIDERATIONS

Noses in each race and ethnic group are basically different, unless that group has become diluted enough to lose much of its original identity (Rogers, 1974). It is of interest and may perhaps be important to correlate a patient's ethnic origin with his contour anatomy and his nasal function.

Rogers (1974) reviewed various nasal configurations and basic ethnic differences (Figure 6–10). Vertical, oblique, and horizontally directed nostrils are characteristic features of three basic nasal types: leptorrhine (narrow nose), mesorrhine (medium nose), and platyrrhine (broad nose). Narrow or leptorrhine nostrils are more commonly found in the Northern European and Mediterranean (white) races; obliquely directed or mesorrhine nostrils are chiefly characteristic of the yellow races; and flat, platyrrhine nostrils are most frequently seen in the black and brown races.

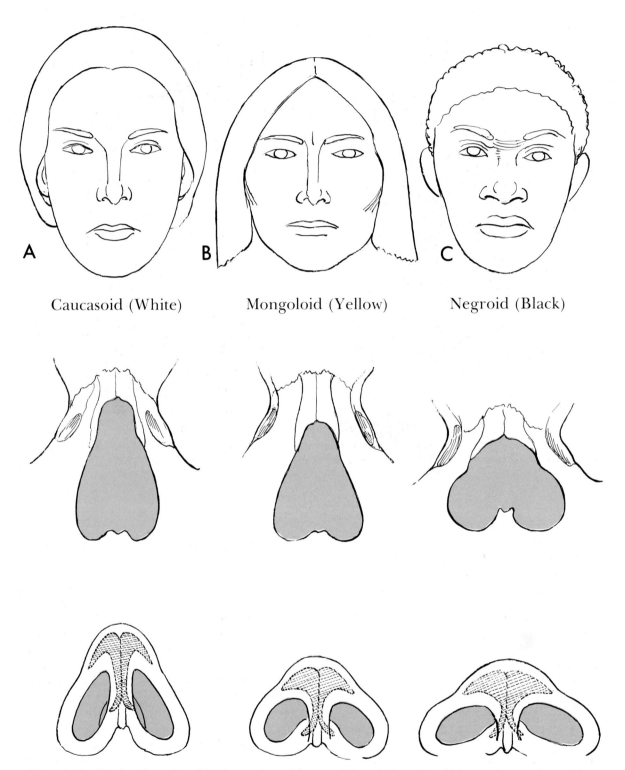

Caucasoid (White)   Mongoloid (Yellow)   Negroid (Black)

Figure 6–10.   Nasal configuration of the three major racial groups. *Column A,* Caucasian with long and narrow leptorrhine-type nostrils and narrow, bony nasal aperture. *Column B,* Mongoloid with narrow, obliquely directed or mesorrhine nostrils. *Column C,* Negroid with broad, somewhat flattened or platyrrhine nostrils and widest bony nasal aperture.

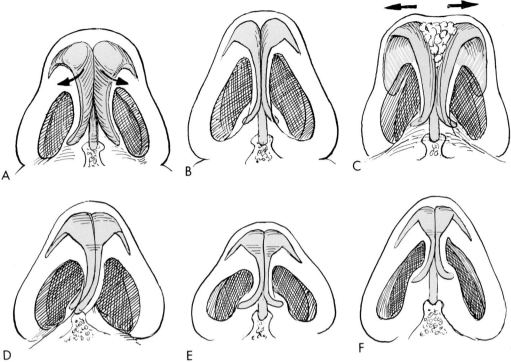

Figure 6–11. Differences in shape of nasal septum: wide columella and septum *(A)*, narrow columella and septum *(B)*, wide midseptal or columellar groove *(C)*, septal bases — deficient *(D)*, low *(E)*, and high *(F)*. (Reproduced from Ziegelmayer, G.: Äussere Nase. *In* Becker, P. F. (ed.): Humangenetik, Stuttgart, Georg Thieme Verlag, 1964. Used with permission.)

There is also a notable difference in the nasal cartilages of different races. According to Barelli (1977), the upper lateral cartilage of the black nose is small and triangular, and the lower lateral borders show no projection (Figure 6–11). The cartilage normally extends all the way to the end of the septum. In contrast, the upper lateral cartilage of the Caucasian nose is large, trapezoidal, and the caudal borders have different projections; the cartilage attachment does not extend to the end of the septum. The normal relationship in Caucasians of the upper lateral cartilage to the septum at the distal one third is approximately 10 degrees, forming the internal valve that accounts for approximately 50 percent of airflow resistance in the Caucasian. Bridger (1970) suggested that in the black or wide, platyrrhine nose, the inferior turbinate is the most important airflow regulator. Variations in shape of the alar cartilages have been well documented by the studies of Natvig and associates (1971) and Schmalix (1968).

It has been stated that a deviated septum is a common and frequent occurrence. This is true for the majority of European and Caucasian noses (Schwarz and Becker, 1964). However, septal deviation is seldom observed in non-Caucasian populations, as noted in studies of Japanese, Negro, and American Indian noses (Rogers, 1974). Joseph (1967) measured septal thickness at the valve area

in 300 patients and made the following observations: total septal width in the leptorrhine nose was 5 to 8 mm, and in the platyrrhine nose, 10 to 13 mm.

Anthropologists have used the nasal index for the purpose of distinguishing various races. Essentially, this represents the relation between the total length of the nose and its maximum breadth as measured at the pyriform aperture:

$$\text{Index} = \frac{\text{greatest breadth}}{\text{greatest length}} \times 100$$

Williams (1956) found that on the average, the width between the pyriform aperture was 4 mm greater in the Negro than in the Caucasian skull (Figure 6–12). There was also a significant difference in the average distance of the pyriform crest above the floor of the nose in the two races. In the Caucasian, the inferior turbinate inserts on the lateral nasal wall approximately 23 mm from the nasal floor, whereas in the black, the distance is only approximately 17 mm. The shape and size of the nostrils seem to have a direct relationship to the width of the pyriform aperture. Some authors have postulated that the configuration of the nose is related to climatic conditions (Negus, 1958). Thus, the wide, platyrrhine nose is associated with a hot climate and the narrow leptorrhine nose with

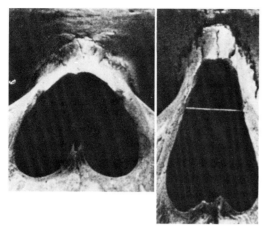

Figure 6–12. Very wide and very narrow openings of the nasal bones.

a cold, dry climate. Bridger (1970) suggested that the expanded nostrils in blacks might physiologically provide a greater physical endurance.

Cottle (1960) felt that the nose of the Caucasian is especially efficient as an air warming apparatus, whereas the black nose is more effective as an air cooling apparatus. Williams (1954) concluded that Negroid type nostrils in Caucasians may not be conducive to good breathing; likewise, Caucasian type nostrils and pyramids may not allow good breathing in black races. Cottle (1955), Fomon, and associates (1949) and Williams (1954) have suggested that from a reconstructive surgical standpoint, the surgeon must evaluate and alter the shape and size of the nasal cavity and vestibule so that these structures will function physiologically more in keeping with the patient's ethnic characteristics.

It should therefore be evident that not only must the rhinoplasty surgeon evaluate the nose in terms of surgical techniques, but he must also have a basic understanding of the individual and combined relationships of the various structures that make up the entire nose. As Rogers stated, "The modern anthropological approach to an understanding of nasal anatomy and physiology can give us a refreshing new insight into a facial feature which we as plastic surgeons have all too often considered only from a purely surgical standpoint."

CHANGE IN NASAL AIRWAY RESISTANCE AFTER RHINOPLASTY

Following infracture or lowering of the nasal dorsum in the normal nose, the main air current is only slightly lowered and nasal airway resistance is not significantly affected (Konno, 1973). The rea-

son for this is that the area mainly affected by the procedure is restricted to the narrow supralateral portion of the nasal cavity; the widely patent middle and lower portions are left undisturbed. A careful study of the human skull and coronal sections through the nose (Ritter, 1973) demonstrates this.

Webster and associates (1977) recommended a "curved" lateral osteotomy to avoid excessive medial displacement of the lateral walls of the nose after hump removal. This technique leaves a triangular piece of bone at the pyriform aperture intact just superior to the level of the inferior turbinate, theoretically avoiding medial displacement of the lateral wall and impingement on the airway. Our own experience with a standard lateral osteotomy in thousands of rhinoplasties has not demonstrated this to be a cause of postoperative nasal obstruction.

Numerous causes of nasal obstruction may occur following rhinoplasty either as a sequela of the surgery or exacerbation of some underlying factor (Figure 6–13). The most common include hypertrophied turbinates, persistent septal deviation, intranasal adhesions and webs, alar collapse, and inadequate tip support. The causes and treatment of many of these conditions have been reviewed by Goldman (1966) and more recently by Beekhuis (1976).

EVALUATING A PATIENT FOR NASAL OBSTRUCTION

The etiology of nasal obstruction can usually be determined from a careful history followed by a thorough physical examination including anterior and posterior rhinoscopy. The history provides an important clue, and it must be determined if environmental factors are responsible for nasal symptoms. Common irritants are tobacco smoke, automobile exhaust fumes, and lack of humidity in heated rooms during the winter months. Changes in the temperature humidity index may also act as a stimulant. Table 6–2 lists some of the problems found in the five nasal areas (Figure 6–14).

According to Goode (1977), in the absence of prior nasal surgery or trauma, nasal obstructive symptoms occurring at ages 20 to 60 years are rarely due to abnormalities of the septum or external nose. Since the nose completes growth by about age 18, symptoms secondary to congenital septal deflections or external narrowing or collapse should have appeared by that time. With the aging process, there is drooping of the nasal tip along with some loss of the upper lateral cartilage

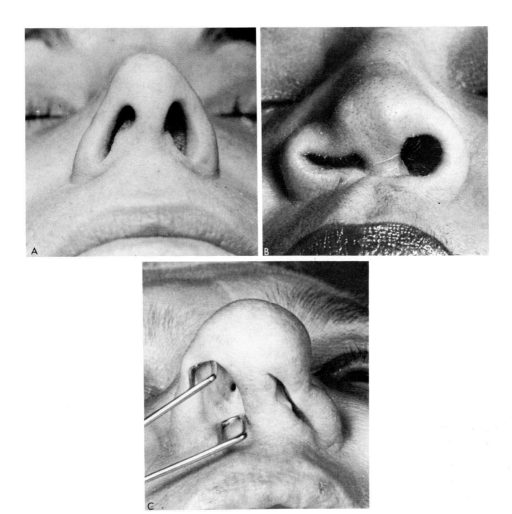

Figure 6–13. Some post-rhinoplasty causes of nasal obstruction.

A, Excessive removal of lower lateral cartilage, resulting in unilateral alar collapse.

B, Total removal of lower lateral cartilage with collapse and deformity of nostril.

C, Extensive scarring and contraction at the internal nasal valve.

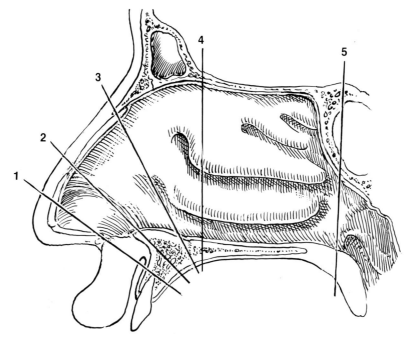

Figure 6–14.   The nose is sometimes divided into five areas by rhinologists. Area 1 (vestibular area) is that portion of the nasal vestibule that may be obstructed by the columella, membranous septum, or caudal end of the cartilaginous septum. Area 2 (nasal valve area) is bounded by the caudal end of the upper lateral cartilage, soft tissue overlying the pyriform aperture and floor of the nose, and the nasal septum. Area 3 (attic area) is immediately above and behind the internal valve under the bony vault of the nasal bones. Area 4 (anterior turbinate area) is the turbinate area also bounded by the bony and cartilaginous septum opposite the turbinates. Area 5 (posterior turbinate area) is that portion of the septum located adjacent and caudal to the choanae.

TABLE 6–2   SOME SPECIFIC PROBLEMS AT THE FIVE NASAL AREAS

Area 1 (Nasal Vestibule)
Birth defects
Trauma at birth
Slight trauma (frequent small bumps)
    on nose (especially in childhood)
Adult injuries
Surgical injuries
Soft-tissue infections and
    vestibular crusting

Area 2 (Valve)
Frequently combined with area 1 problems
Associated with problems of areas 3 and 4
Tension nose
Flattened nose
Synechiae at the valve from previous
    surgery, burns, and packing
Associated with twisted-nose problems

Area 3 (Behind and Above Valve)
Trauma with little evidence of
    external deformity
Trauma with obvious evidence of
    external deformity
Overgrowth of bone

Perpendicular plate that bends
    the cartilage
Hypertrophy of mucosa in swell body areas
Neoplastic growths

Area 4 (Turbinate)
Spurs and ridges (bony or cartilaginous)
Combined with vomer and perpendicular
    plate deformities
Paraseptal cartilage
Synechiae
Turbinal engorgement, hypertrophy, or other
    anatomic enlargement
Polyps (single or multiple)
Neoplasms

*Area 5 (Adjacent and Caudal
to Choanae)*
Spurs (bony or cartilaginous)
Choanal atresia
Hypertrophied posterior turbinate tips
Solitary or multiple polyps
Neoplasms (primary in nose or encroachment
    by tumors arising in the pituitary gland
    or sphenoid sinus)

After Kern, 1975

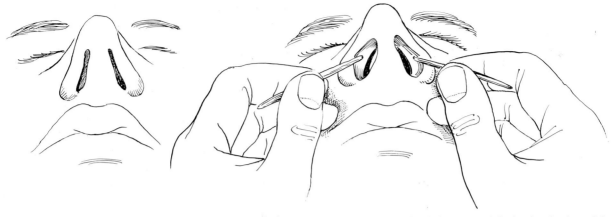

Figure 6–15. Test to evaluate "alar collapse" for surgical correction. Applicators hold alae outward during inspiration. If the volume of air increases significantly on inspiration, cartilage grafts to alae may provide some relief. (After Cinelli, 1971.)

strength, which can lead to some inspiratory collapse of the alae. Surgery or trauma to the nose usually produces symptoms immediately or up to one year afterward. It is essential to remember that in the 20- to 60-year age group, in the absence of surgery or trauma, the septum is not changing but the turbinates probably are (Goode, 1977).

Most authors agree (Goode, 1977; Little, 1963; Baker and Strauss, 1977) that the most common cause of nasal obstruction is a gradual, chronic enlargement of the turbinates usually secondary to vasomotor, allergic, or irritative rhinitis. A history of hay fever or allergic disorders should forewarn the surgeon of a potential postoperative exacerbation of nasal obstruction. Patients with vasomotor rhinitis should be told that a rhinoplasty may accentuate nasal symptoms.

After a careful history is taken, the next step in the examination should be inspection and palpa-

tion. Observe closely the base of the nose and the flare of the nostrils during quiet and forced respiration, in order to assess alar collapse and widened medial crurae (Figure 6–15). Study the size, shape, and direction of the alae and nares for symmetry, general configuration, and narrowing (Figure 6–16). Is the nasolabial angle acute or open? Is the tip drooping or retroussé? Palpation of the bony and cartilaginous nose should be done meticulously and delicately. Determine whether the cartilages are thick, thin, or absent. The lobule of the nose should be pushed from one side to the other to study the shape and direction of the caudal septum.

After insertion of the speculum, the mucous membranes, the size and consistency of the inferior turbinates, and the position and mobility of the cartilaginous septum should be assessed and recorded. The nasal valve must be studied for its

Figure 6–16. In a patient with a long nose and nasal obstruction, gently raising the tip may assess whether shortening the nose will improve respiration. (After Cinelli, 1971.)

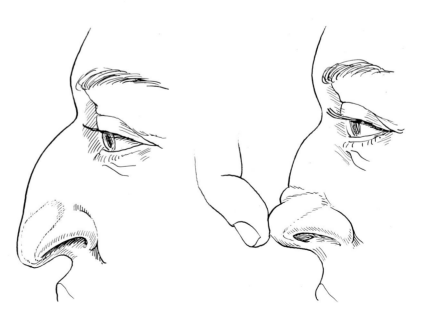

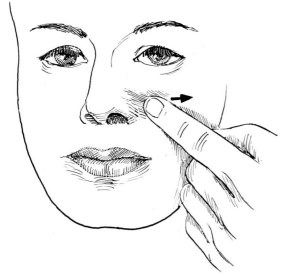

Figure 6–17. Simple clinical test to confirm the presence of an abnormality of the nasal valve (Cottle sign). During quiet inspiration, the cheek is drawn laterally, carrying the upper lateral cartilage away from the septum, thereby opening the angle of the nasal valve. If the airflow is improved through the tested side, the Cottle sign is positive, indicating an abnormality of the nasal valve. A "false-negative" sign may occur if the valve is occluded by scarring of the upper lateral cartilage to the septum. A "false-positive" sign may occur in alar collapse secondary to excessive removal of the lower lateral cartilages.

angle and mobility, and the floor of the nose must be evaluated for strictures (Figure 6–17). A thorough examination of the anterior and posterior nose should be made to evaluate nonturbinate causes of nasal obstruction such as septal perforations, polyps, tumors, synechiae, strictures, and atresias. Structural abnormalities of the nasal septum, nasal pyramid, internal valve, or alae may cause obstructive symptoms that mimic those seen in chronic turbinate disease (Goode, 1977). Often, a combination of factors may be present, contributing to nasal symptoms.

Since the septum of the normal nose is rarely straight, the significance of septal deflections in patients with hypertrophied turbinates may be difficult to assess. Intranasal findings may be varied, and thus they require careful evaluation. An allergy may be the cause of nasal obstruction when a deviated septum or medial displacement of the inferior turbinate is thought to be responsible. Structural deformities often have an associated allergic component adding to the obstruction. If a structural abnormality such as a deviated septum warrants correction and the patient also has findings of allergic or vasomotor rhinitis, he should be told that the operation will improve but not cure his nasal obstruction. Removal of the anatomic deformity may also facilitate medical treatment. A narrow nasal cavity with a moderately deviated

septum may limit turbinate enlargement and predispose a patient to obstructive symptoms as the turbinate hypertrophies. A septoplasty in these patients might improve the airway by allowing more room for the turbinate to enlarge (Goode, 1977).

There are several methods to help estimate the effectiveness of surgical therapy in relieving nasal obstruction. These are best accomplished if the patient has obstructive symptoms at the time of examination. Following a careful evaluation, a vasoconstrictive agent such as 0.25 percent Neo-Synephrine-soaked cotton pledget should be placed along the inferior turbinates for several minutes. The pledgets are removed and the patient's nasal breathing is reevaluated both at rest and during rapid, deep respiration. Complete relief of obstructive symptoms following inferior turbinate shrinkage confirms a turbinate etiology; partial relief may indicate chronic hypertrophic rhinitis with poor response to vasoconstrictor, a significant septal deviation, or other intranasal abnormalities as causes. Similarly, a vasoconstrictor may be applied to the middle turbinate and the nasal airway may again be reassessed. Occasionally, a high septal deflection or middle turbinate enlargement may be the cause of obstruction singly or in combination with inferior turbinate enlargement (Goode, 1977). Mabry (1978) reported on the value of using intranasal steroids in patients with allergic or vasomotor rhinitis and septal deviation. Many patients obtain a subjectively normal airway with this technique and do not require septal surgery.

Finally, some patients are aware of the financial gain from a deviated septum, as health insurance usually compensates for corrective surgery of a deformity causing nasal obstruction. However, a patient who alters complaints preoperatively for financial gain may have little hesitation to do so postoperatively.

MEASUREMENT OF OBSTRUCTION

Numerous methods have been described for the measurement of nasal obstruction and airflow. Qualitative tests involve such simple means as listening in order to differentiate in the tone of air going through each nostril, having the patient breathe against the examiner's hand, and observing the condensation from each nostril on a highly polished mirror (Glatzel's mirror test). Although these tests may offer some help when combined with a careful history and rhinoscopic examination, they are gross and qualitative at best.

Many quantitative methods have been devised

for the purpose of research. The most popular of these is rhinomanometry, which measures the amount of air pressure and the rate of airflow in the nasal airway during respiration. Most authors prefer posterior active rhinomanometry for research investigation. In this method, a nasal mask on which a pair of pneumotachometers measures the velocity of nasal airflow through both nasal cavities and the transnasal pressures is used. This technique closely approximates the physiologic state by maintaining the spontaneous respiration of ambient air while not interfering with the resistance at the valve, alae, or turbinates (Kern, 1973).

Although much information about nasal physiology has been learned from rhinomanometry, it has limited clinical value at present. It can aid the observer in differentiating between structural and mucosal disturbances of the airway, but it cannot select a candidate for surgical intervention (Kern, 1973). Rhinomanometry can be used to evaluate a patient preoperatively and postoperatively following structural changes. However, in an organ such as the nose — which is a dynamic respiratory system in constant change — absolute figures are impossible to obtain.

TURBINATE DISORDERS

Surgical techniques of septoplasty and submucous resection will be reviewed (see Chapter 11). However, since turbinate disorders are undoubtedly the most common cause of nasal obstruction,

a more complete description of the pathology and treatment follows.

Infectious Rhinitis. The common cold is the most frequent cause of infectious rhinitis and nasal obstruction (Figure 6–18). Turbinate edema occurs secondary to vasodilatation and increased capillary permeability. There is also stromal infiltration with inflammatory cells and shedding of ciliated epithelium. This condition usually responds well to fluids, rest, antihistamines, and time.

Allergic Rhinitis. According to Norman (1973), allergic rhinitis is the most common immunologic disorder and affects an estimated 13 million Americans. Hinderer (1963) stated that 80 percent of patients with nasal complaints have some form of allergic rhinitis, and that the same percentage of patients with anatomic deformities also have a potential or active allergic rhinitis.

True allergic rhinitis is an antigen-antibody induced hypersensitivity reaction with the turbinates and nasal mucosa acting as the shock organ. Turbinate engorgement follows with nasal obstruction and rhinorrhea. The classical rhinoscopic findings are a pale, edematous turbinate and watery secretions. Allergic rhinitis usually occurs in a seasonal form associated with pollens or fungal spores. Skin testing is frequently positive, and the patient's response to desensitization is generally good.

Perennial or nonseasonal allergic rhinitis implies multiple hypersensitivities to airborne inhalants (Stahl, 1974). Frequently, the offending aller-

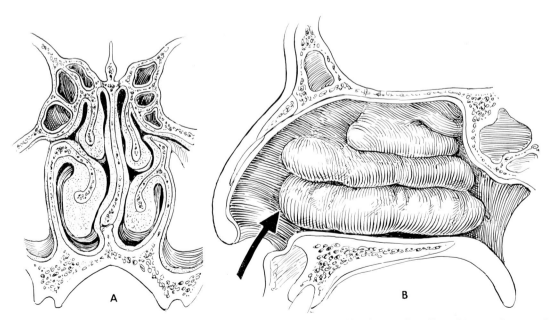

Figure 6–18. *A,* Severe crowding of the airways occurs in vasomotor states with edema and swelling of the membranes. This is by far the commonest cause of airway obstruction. *B,* The air current is blocked at the anterior nose.

gens are difficult or impossible to identify. House dust, animal danders, or occupational dusts such as flour or chalk are some of the more common causes. The patient's response to desensitization is often poor. Air pollution and the temperature-humidity index seem to influence the symptomatology, and this may represent an overlap of vasomotor rhinitis.

Vasomotor Rhinitis. Vasomotor rhinitis implies an inability of the autonomic nervous system to evoke an appropriate vasomotor response from the nasal mucosa to various stimuli (Reed, 1963). It can be induced by a variety of emotional or endocrine factors or mechanical or chemical irritants (Holmes and associates, 1950; Wolf, 1951). These stimuli do not provoke an antibody reaction. The typical vasomotor response of the nasal mucosa is a profuse, watery discharge with partial or total nasal obstruction, which may be episodic or chronic and bilateral, unilateral, or alternating from side to side. Symptoms are usually perennial but may come and go several times a day. The nasal mucosa may appear normal or boggy, and sometimes the clinical picture may be indistinguishable from that of allergic rhinitis. A good allergic history is usually not obtained, however, and the allergic workup is negative.

Hyperplastic or Hypertrophic Rhinitis. This is the end result of chronic mucosal swelling of the inferior or middle turbinates, and it may be caused by chronic infections or allergic and vasomotor rhinitis. An etiology is often not discovered (Jaffe, 1974). The mucosa of the turbinates may touch the septum as well as the floor of the nostril, causing complete obstruction. Characteristically, the mucosa undergoes minimal shrinkage even when treated with strong topical vasoconstrictors. This condition is usually best treated with a surgical approach.

Rhinitis Medicamentosa. This is a commonly overlooked cause of nasal obstruction. The prolonged use of sympathomimetic nose drops or sprays leads to tachyphylaxis, resulting in a rebound phenomenon of vasodilatation, engorgement of the mucosa, and nasal obstruction. The stronger the solution of nose drops or spray, the greater the rebound. After several months of chronic usage, red, swollen turbinates that respond poorly to the spray or drops develop. Treatment involves discontinuing use, but it often takes several weeks or months to recover (Dolowitz, 1971). The local use of intranasal corticosteroids has been a useful adjunct in managing patients with rhinitis medicamentosa.

Numerous other parenteral drugs have been implicated as a cause of turbinate hypertrophy and nasal obstruction, and these have been reviewed by Blue (1968), May and West (1973), and Stahl

TABLE 6–3   COMMON DRUGS THAT MAY PRODUCE NASAL OBSTRUCTION

Therapeutic	
Aspirin	May activate peripheral chemoreceptors that control the vascular bed, causing turbinate engorgement
Rauwolfa (Reserpine)	Produces nasal congestion and rhinitis by its cholinergic action
Lycopodium	An absorbent powder used as a coating for pills; may cause nasal stuffiness
Estrogens, Progestins (Birth Control Pills)	Produce engorgement of nasal mucous membranes
Antithyroid Drugs	May cause engorgement of nasal mucous membranes
Xanthenes (Caffeine, Aminophylline)	Direct effect of vasodilatation on vascular musculature
Social	
Alcohol	Causes engorgement of nasal mucous membranes
Cocaine	Initially causes vasoconstriction followed by rebound congestion; chronic use may lead to septal perforation
Marijuana, Hashish	Respiratory tract irritants that often cause nasal stuffiness
Tobacco	Mucous membrane irritant that also impairs nasal ciliary action

After May and West, 1973

(1974). Table 6–3 summarizes some of the common parenteral and "social" drugs causing nasal obstruction. We live in a society oriented to medicines and drugs, and any patient with nasal obstruction should be carefully questioned about their use thereof.

Postrhinoplasty Rhinitis. After rhinoplasty, postoperative nasal obstructive symptoms are common. Almost all patients experience partial nasal obstruction from transient edema of the mucosa, coagulated blood, or crusting along the incision lines. This type of obstruction usually resolves spontaneously in several weeks without treatment.

Patients with allergic disorders or vasomotor rhinitis may experience exacerbation of nasal obstruction postoperatively. In a review of 1000 consecutive rhinoplasties, Beekhuis (1976) found that approximately 10 percent of patients developed a persistent enlargement of the inferior turbinates postoperatively, causing an obstructive vasomotor rhinitis. The obstruction usually began at the time of surgery and persisted for several months if left untreated. Intranasal steroids were the treatment of choice, and the majority of symptoms resolved with their use.

Atrophic Rhinitis. Atrophic rhinitis is a rare condition of unknown etiology, but it may be due to chronic infection. There is gradual and progressive atrophy of the nasal mucosa, and lack of moistening secretions leads to crusting that accumulates and causes nasal obstruction. The crusts harbor bacteria at their bases, and with the associated poor aeration and drainage, a foul odor (ozena) results. It has often been stated (Barelli, 1977, 1978; Cottle, 1978; Goode, 1977) but apparently never documented (Courtiss et al., 1978) that a similar syndrome may occur following excessive surgical removal of the turbinates. Treatment is usually daily intranasal saline irrigation and appropriate antibiotics. Surgical correction is sometimes successful by the use of nasal implants to widen the septum, thereby narrowing the airway, or by moving the lateral wall medially by osteotomies and bone grafts.

Other Forms of Rhinitis. Patients under chronic emotional stress in life situations of anxiety, hostility, and frustration may also develop obstructive swelling and hyperemia of the turbinates, and this syndrome may be one of the most difficult to diagnose. On the other hand, the nasal neurotic is usually easily identified by his excessive preoccupation with sniffing or nose blowing (Goode, 1977).

A "nasal neurosis" may be initiated by any experience that draws the patient's attention to his nose. He will inhale with great force and insist that the resulting noise is due to nasal blockage, despite all objective evidence that the nasal passages are clear (Brown, 1951). Persistence of forced inhalation causes a reflex congestion of the membranes, which must react to filter, warm, and moisten this fast-moving air. The patient becomes increasingly conscious of his nose; mucus is forced toward the nasopharynx, causing a postnasal drip. Often, this type of patient will resort to nose drops or sprays or submit to surgery, usually turbinectomy.

Greater air space may satisfy this type of patient, or his neurosis may demand more of an airway. According to Brown (1951), the original Benzedrine inhaler developed an entire generation of nasal neurotics, many of whom were physicians given inhalers free of charge. The clear, cool sensation of an open nose gave a sense of euphoria that was habit forming. The only desirable treatment for this combination of symptoms is patient reeducation.

MEDICAL TREATMENT OF TURBINATE DISORDERS

Antihistamines and Sympathomimetics. Antihistamines are commonly employed for temporary relief of allergy and nasal obstruction. In addition to histamine antagonism, they have an atropine-like action that is helpful in drying excessive nasal secretions. Hundreds of antihistamines are on the market, and there is no single universally effective compound. Usually, several preparations must be tried by each patient before an acceptable one is found. Antihistamines are of little benefit in cases of chronic nasal obstruction, and their effect is generally incomplete and of short duration. With prolonged use, they seem to lose effectiveness, and changing to another antihistamine occasionally restores effectiveness. In patients with seasonal allergic rhinitis, approximately 80 percent obtain relief with antihistamines. For maximal benefit, the drug should be taken in the morning and continued throughout the day (Goode, 1977).

A disadvantage of antihistamines is the high incidence of side effects, estimated to occur in 20 percent of patients (Dolowitz, 1971). The central nervous system effects are the most prominent. Sedation occurs with the highest incidence and is a common side effect of all antihistamines (Goodman and Gilman, 1975).

Sympathomimetic drugs such as ephedrine, pseudoephedrine, and phenylpropanolamine may counteract the drowsiness associated with antihistamines, and in some cases, combined preparations are effective. Their primary mode of action is to stimulate alpha receptors to produce vasoconstriction of the turbinate vessels. Their use, however, is short term, and they may produce undesirable effects such as nervousness, insomnia, and palpitation, which may be more troublesome than the nasal obstruction (Blue, 1968).

Immunotherapy. In patients with seasonal allergic rhinitis, desensitization is a well established and accepted method of treatment. However, patients with allergic, vasomotor, and hypertrophic rhinitis tend to respond poorly to desensitization. Furthermore, the extended time required for effective results from this treatment tends to make it unpopular and undesirable with patients about to undergo rhinoplastic surgery.

Nosedrops and Nasal Sprays. Along with the oral antihistamines and decongestants, nose drops and nasal sprays are the most commonly employed drugs for treating nasal obstruction. They are of transient benefit in patients with acute infectious rhinitis, and prolonged use is to be condemned as it leads to rebound congestion and rhinitis medicamentosa.

Corticosteroids. Corticosteroids have been used for over 25 years for the treatment of allergic and vasomotor rhinitis and nasal polyps. They may be administered orally, intramuscularly, or intranasally (spray or injection). Used orally or intramuscularly for short periods, corticosteroids may be very effective in the treatment of seasonal allergic rhinitis. The side effects, however, are well known, and close monitoring of dosage and tapering off is required. Steroid sprays such as dexamethasone aerosol (Turbinaire Decadron*) have also been reported to control the symptoms of perennial allergic rhinitis effectively (Chervinsky, 1966; Gibson and associates, 1974). Improvement is temporary, however, and suppression of adrenal function with the doses recommended has been reported (Norman and associates, 1967). Furthermore, some patients may respond adversely to the propellant vehicle. Recent success has been reported with the use of aerosol and beclomethasone dipropionate for the long-term management of allergic rhinitis (Cockcroft and associates, 1976; Mygind, 1977). One risk is the patient's developing a dependence on the spray, and prolonged use could possibly lead to atrophy and septal perforation. The use of intranasal injections of corticosteroids is discussed under surgical therapy.

Other Factors. Temperature and humidity changes are important in the therapy of some cases of allergic and nonallergic chronic rhinitis. Al-

though the normal nose can tolerate a wide range of temperatures and humidity, the abnormal nose cannot (Proetz, 1941). Excessively warm, dry air can cause drying of the mucous membranes and pharyngeal mucosa. Adequate hydration and use of a humidifier can often alleviate this problem. Tobacco smoke or house dust might also be factors that are easily eliminated. Sleeping on several pillows or elevating the head of the bed will minimize the turbinate venous congestion as well as help gravity flow of mucus from the nasopharynx.

SURGICAL TREATMENT OF ENLARGED TURBINATES

Of the surgical approaches currently used for the treatment of enlarged turbinates, virtually all are controversial, few are permanently curative, and most have a risk of serious complications. Many rhinologists (Cottle, 1978; Barelli, 1978) feel that subtotal or total removal or destruction of the turbinates interferes with the essential nasal functions of humidifying, warming, and filtering of inspired air. The consensus among nasal physiologists (Proetz, 1941; Cottle, 1978) is that the turbinates be retained as far as practical in their normal positions and with their surfaces intact. Therefore, medical therapy should be tried initially and a conservative approach should be taken prior to surgery.

The main criticism of destruction or resection of the inferior turbinates is the alleged sequela of rhinitis sicca. It is felt that excessive removal of the inferior turbinate allows for a jet of inspired air to impinge on the nasal mucosa, leading to drying, destruction of the cilia, and infection. Some authors have mentioned a syndrome similar to atrophic rhinitis (Proetz, 1941), and senior rhinologists such as Cottle (1978) and Barelli (1978) state that they have treated such patients. Apparently, the difficulty may not present until many years following turbinectomy. Nevertheless, in a thorough review of the literature, Courtiss and associates (1978) were unable to find a documented case.

Recently, some surgeons (Fry, 1973, 1976; Courtiss and associates, 1978) have recommended turbinectomy routinely for enlarged or crowded turbinates causing nasal obstruction. They have not experienced the complication of rhinitis sicca, and Courtiss et al. postulate that this untoward sequela may or may not have been seen years ago, and that it most likely followed surgical resection that was performed after caustics had failed or in the presence of extensive chronic sinusitis in the preantibiotic era. Regardless of the recent favor-

---

*Merck, Sharp & Dohme.

able reports, historical experience and physiologic principles advocate a conservative attitude toward amputating or destroying the turbinates until longer followup is obtained. Another distinct disadvantage of turbinectomy is the high incidence of postoperative hemorrhage reported to occur in about 10 percent of patients (Goode, 1977).

Anesthesia

Surgery of the turbinates may be performed as an office procedure or in combination with a rhinoplasty or septoplasty. Adequate local anesthesia is important, along with a vasoconstrictor to minimize bleeding. Topical anesthesia is first obtained with 5 percent cocaine solution. The entire turbinate is then infiltrated with several ccs of 1 or 2 per cent lidocaine with epinephrine 1:100,000.

INTRANASAL STEROID INJECTIONS

Since the first descriptions (Wall and Shure, 1952; Sidi and Tardiff, 1955) more than 25 years ago, the intranasal injection of steroids has proved to be an effective method for rapidly relieving nasal obstruction secondary to severe allergic or vasomotor rhinitis, rhinitis medicamentosa, and acutely enlarged nasal polyps. The mechanism of action appears to be a purely local antiinflammatory response. There is inhibition of edema, fibrin deposition, and sinusoid engorgement, as well as fibroblast and capillary proliferation. The inflammatory response is inhibited whether the inciting agent is mechanical, chemical, or immunologic (Goodman and Gilman, 1975).

Several days following the first injection, the mucosa begins to return to a normal pink color. Edema subsides, and there is also a decrease of secretions. Following several injections, the turbinates often appear fibrous (Simmons, 1960). Pretreatment and posttreatment biopsies of the inferior turbinates by Simmon (1960) demonstrated a reduction in the sinusoids, disappearance of edema, and a reduction in the thickness of the connective tissue layer.

Indications. The relief of nasal obstruction caused by engorgement of inferior turbinates in chronic allergic and vasomotor rhinitis is the prime indication for the use of intranasal steroids (Baker, 1972). For seasonal allergic rhinitis, this type of therapy should be considered as an adjunct rather than a replacement for an allergic workup and desensitization. Intranasal steroids have also proved to be of great benefit in the treatment of obstructive rhinitis of the vasomotor type seen in the postrhinoplasty patient (Beekhuis, 1976). Some surgeons (Mabry, 1978) have employed intranasal steroid injections routinely at the conclusion of all rhinoplasties and intranasal surgery and have been impressed with the diminution of postoperative edema as well as the absence of symptoms of allergic and vasomotor rhinitis for several weeks following the surgery. Some of the other uses are outlined in Table 6–4.

TABLE 6–4   INDICATIONS FOR INTRANASAL STEROID INJECTIONS

---

1. Chronic Hypertrophic and Vasomotor Rhinitis:
   Improvement or relief in almost 80 percent of patients

2. Severe Nasal Allergy:
   For acute seasonal flare-up or severe symptoms despite hyposensitization

3. Post Rhinoplasty or Intranasal Surgery:
   Reduces postoperative edema and symptoms of allergic and vasomotor rhinitis

4. Acutely Enlarged Nasal Polyps:
   For temporary relief of airway obstruction; not recommended as a substitute for polypectomy or sinus surgery

5. Rhinitis Medicamentosa:
   Allows discontinuance of nose drops; antihistamine or decongestant should also be given for prn use

6. Differential Diagnosis:
   Of nasal obstruction — in nasal allergy plus deviated septum, reduces turbinate engorgement to allow evaluation of the role of the septum in subjective obstruction
   Of headache — may relieve headache secondary to pressure by septal spur or sinus "congestion"

After Mabry, 1978

The advantages of intranasal steroid treatment over other forms of therapy are:

1. It is nondestructive, as opposed to turbinectomy or cauterization
2. It is physiologic and does not interfere with the normal ciliary action and mucus secretion
3. There is no rebound phenomenon
4. There are rare contraindications, since there is no significant rebound phenomenon
5. The total amount of steroid required is small compared with the oral or parenteral dose required to obtain similar benefit.

Technique. Intranasal steroid injection is simple, rapidly accomplished, and, when performed properly, virtually painless. Two cotton

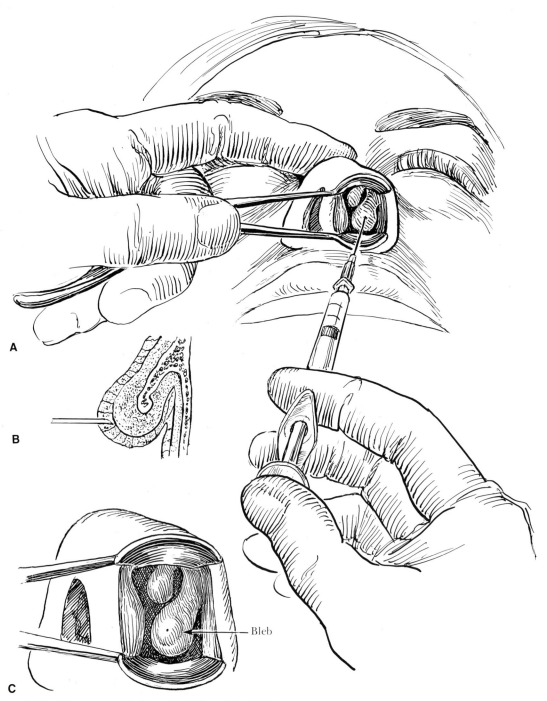

Figure 6–19. The proper technique of injection of the inferior turbinate. *A,* A 1.5-inch 25-gauge needle is inserted intramucosally in the anterior tip of the inferior turbinate. *B,* Cross section demonstrating that only the bevel of the needle need be inserted. *C,* Approximately 0.3 cc of steroid suspension is injected slowly and without force to form a bleb (similar to a PPD test).

pledgets moistened with a 5 percent cocaine solution or 2 percent lidocaine with epinephrine 1:100,000 are placed along the anterior-medial aspect of each inferior turbinate, and they remain in place for about five minutes. Using a tuberculin syringe and a 1.5 inch, 25 gauge needle (the solution will not flow readily through a smaller gauge) with 0.3 to 0.5 ml of prednisolone tertiary-butyl acetate (Hydeltra-TBA*) 20 mg per ml or triamcinolone acetonide (Kenalog†) 40 mg per ml is injected intramucosally in the anterior tip of the inferior turbinate (Figure 6–19). Only the bevel of the needle is inserted to be certain that the injection is given intramucosally. If necessary, the needle tip may be moved submucosally during injection to deposit the steroid without force more easily (Mabry, 1978).

The injection is made slowly, and the mucosa can be seen to swell and turn pale as it fills with steroid solution. *Rapid injection or excessive pressure must be avoided.* Several articles and textbooks have described an intraturbinate injection, and there are reports of the needle being buried to its hilt in the turbinate during injection. This is unnecessary and dangerous because of the marked vascularity of the concha and the risk of intravascular injection. When the needle is withdrawn, a dry cotton pledget is inserted into the nostril to apply slight pressure on the turbinate and to minimize bleeding from the puncture site, which usually stops within a few minutes.

Results. The onset of relief of nasal obstruction is often noted within 24 to 48 hours following injection and may last for intervals of several months to a year. If symptoms are not relieved after the first injection, treatment may be repeated in several weeks. Patients with severe hypertrophic or allergic rhinitis may require another injection one month later, with repeat injections at three-month, six-month, and twelve-month intervals. For the past 20 years, the preferred steroid has been prednisolone tertiary-butylacetate (Hydeltra-TBA), which is extemely insoluble and has a long duration of action, taking several months to be absorbed or dissipated. Other long-acting corticosteroids such as triamcinolone acetonide (Kenalog) have also been effective (Mabry, 1978). Because of the larger particle size of hydrocortisone, it should not be employed for intranasal injections.

The overall experience with intranasal steroids for the relief of nasal obstruction secondary to vasomotor, hypertrophic, and allergic rhinitis has been gratifying; Simmons (1960) reported

*Merck, Sharp & Dohme.
†E.R. Squibb Co.

78 percent improvement in 419 patients, Baker and Strauss (1962) reported 75 percent benefit in 487 patients, and Mabry (1978) reported 83 percent effectiveness in 276 patients. None of these authors reported any serious complications or side effects of the treatment.

Complications. Complications associated with intranasal steroid injections have been reported, the most serious being temporary amaurosis or permanent blindness. Mabry (1978) reviewed the reports and mechanisms of visual complications following these injections and found two documented cases of permanent visual loss. On the basis of reported clinical experience, he concluded that the likelihood of visual complications following intranasal steroid injections is 0.0067 percent. Mabry pointed out that, undoubtedly, many hundreds of thousands of intranasal steroid injections have been carried out without complications in the past and have not been reported in the literature. Other reports include those of Kabaker (1975), with an estimated 36,000 injections, and Peisel and associates (1975), with over 1000 injections, all with no untoward reactions. McCleave and Goldstein (1977) reported on two instances of transient visual blurring out of a total 60,000 injections.

The mechanism of visual complications has been postulated as a vasoconstrictive or embolic phenomenon via the rich anastomoses between the ophthalmic artery and branches of the sphenopalatine artery (Rowe and associates, 1967) (Table 6–5). This complication is not limited to intranasal injections, and during 1963 and 1964, there were reports from Sweden by Von Bahr (1963) and from France by Baran (1965) of acute uniocular loss of vision following injections of steroids into the scalp for alopecia areata. This was explained on the basis of anastomoses between the superficial temporal artery and branches of the ophthalmic artery (Selmanowitz and Orentreich, 1974). Also, very large quantities of steroid solution (up to 8 cc) were used. Besides amaurosis following steroid injections, transitory or permanent loss of vision has been reported following local anesthetic and nerve block injections in dental, oral, nasal, and orbital procedures (Blaxter and Britten, 1967; Cooper, 1962; Markham, 1973; Walsh and Hoyt, 1969). During the early 1900's, visual loss was reported to occur following paraffin augmentations of the nasal and orbital regions (Hurd and Holden, 1903).

McGrew and associates (1978) have reported two other cases of sudden blindness, each following injection of a mixture of lidocaine and steroid into the tonsillar and pterygopalatine fossae. They

TABLE 6–5 OPHTHALMIC ARTERY BRANCHES IN USUAL SEQUENCE*

Group/Distribution	Branches in Sequence	Comment
Group 1/Ocular-orbital	Central Retinal a and Ciliary aa	Retinal a originates independently or in common trunk with medial and/or lateral posterior ciliary aa (and occasionally with muscular a); anastomotic twigs on pial covering of optic nerve
	Lacrimal a ⟶ Sub-branches ⟨ Muscular aa / Lateral palpebral aa / Recurrent meningeal a	
	Muscular aa	
Group 2/Extraorbital-terminal	Supraorbital a	To frontoparietal scalp
	Ethmoidal aa	To sinuses and nose
	Medial palpebral a	
	Supratrochlear (frontal) a	To medial frontal scalp
	Dorsal nasal a	

*The a indicates artery; aa indicates (multiple) arteries.

After Selmanowitz and Orentreich, 1974. Simplified outline of the sequence in which arterial branches of the ophthalmic artery arise. Ocular accidents following scalp and intranasal injections have been explained by forceful retrograde flow into the regionally appropriate arterial branches in group 2, followed by dissemination of the injected material via group 1 branches. It remains uncertain in particular cases whether the accidental injections were intraarterial or intravenous.

investigated the mechanism with animal studies by injecting various substances into the carotid circulation of dogs. Injection of steroid alone resulted in no retinal changes; however, combining the steroid with epinephrine (either with or without lidocaine) caused severe retinopathy. A combined injection of steroid and epinephrine should therefore be avoided.

Selmanowitz and Orentreich (1974) and Mabry (1978) have assessed the role of steroid particle size in producing retinal embolization. The larger the particle in suspension, the larger and more consequential the vessel it may block. Hydrocortisone suspension contains particles from 50 to 200 micra and should therefore not be used for injections in the head and neck. Particle dimension of methylprednisolone acetate (Depo-medrol 40 mg per ml), triamcinolone acetonide (Kenalog 40 mg per ml), and prednisolone tertiary-butylacetate (Hydeltra-TBA 20 mg per ml) has been much reduced for the currently available suspensions. According to Selmanowitz and Orentreich, analysis of sample batches indicate that most particles were less than 8.5 micra in these suspensions. However, they emphasize that sedimentation and agglomeration of particles may occur when the suspension is allowed to stand, and therefore thorough agitation prior to injection is important.

The risks of visual complications with intrana-

sal steroid injections are minimal and are far outweighed by the therapeutic benefits. When the steroid is injected correctly intramucosally into the anterior tip of the inferior turbinate, the results have been gratifying and complications have been negligible. These technical guidelines should be followed:

1. Use topical vasoconstrictor to diminish the size of the turbinate vasculature
2. Use a small diameter needle (25 gauge)
3. First aspirate to insure that the needle is not intravascular
4. Inject only the anterior tip of the inferior turbinate slowly and with minimal pressure
5. Attempt to balloon or blanch the mucosa, indicating an intramucosal injection
6. Never inject a single bolus deeply into the turbinate.

SCLEROSING SOLUTIONS

Submucosal and intramucosal injections of sclerosing solutions such as sodium morrhuate have been employed to treat enlarged turbinates, although these are destructive in that they cause fibrosis and scarring. A 5 percent solution of sodium morrhuate is used, and no more than 0.6 cc is infiltrated into the turbinate. Following injection, significant edema and rhinorrhea occur and persist for three to four weeks. Crusting may also occur. Usually one inferior turbinate is injected at a time, the other being injected several months later (Goode, 1977). The technique may be repeated when necessary.

CHEMICAL CAUTERY

Over the years, agents such as phenol, fuming nitric acid, silver nitrate, and trichloroacetic acids have been used to streak the turbinates in an attempt to shrink them. Relief is usually temporary, and repeated use can result in chronic tissue destruction, fibrosis, and altered nasal physiology, which may produce symptoms of atrophic rhinitis (House, 1951).

ELECTROCAUTERY

Electrocautery can be used topically or submucosally. With surface cautery, the turbinates are streaked with a hot wire electrode. This is followed by edema and crusting for up to three weeks. With submucosal cautery, a needle electrode is inserted submucosally along the entire length of the medial aspect of the inferior turbinate and is slowly withdrawn, using continuous current. The procedure is usually repeated in a second plane to produce a linear submucosal coagulation. Extreme care must be taken to avoid contact with the turbinate bone, which could injure the periosteum and result in discomfort and sequestration (Richardson, 1948; House, 1951). Excessive coagulation may lead to massive slough, secondary hemorrhage and prolonged healing. Fibrosis and scarring of the turbinates result from this treatment and the effect usually lasts from two to twelve months or more.

CRYOSURGERY

Cryosurgery of the inferior turbinates results in freezing the hypertrophic mucosa, which then gradually slough over a period of four to eight weeks, leaving a smaller turbinate with normal appearing mucosa. Complications reported by Ozenberger (1970, 1973) include perforation of the nasal septum, secondary hemorrhage, and delayed healing. In Goode's experience with 60 cases (1977), there was no significant bleeding or osteonecrosis. Improvement is reported to last up to a year, and the procedure may be repeated.

OUTFRACTURE

Outfracture of the inferior turbinates has been advocated as a method of improving the nasal airway. The turbinate is first fractured upward and inward toward the septum with an instrument such as the Goldman bar. It is then fractured toward the lateral nasal wall, where it may be held in place for a few days with nasal packing. Simple crushing of the turbinate bones has also been recommended. Overall experience with these methods has shown temporary, minor improvement at best, as the turbinate usually returns to its previous position, and the basic pathology — hypertrophy and hyperplasia of the soft tissue — is not corrected.

VIDIAN NEURECTOMY

Vidian neurectomy has been recommended by Golding-Wood (1961, 1973) as a treatment for chronic vasomotor rhinitis with rhinorrhea. A transantral approach to the vidian nerve is used, which requires general anesthesia and is difficult technically. The neurectomy destroys the secretomotor supply to the nasal mucosa, but the lacrimal gland is also enervated. This results in the unfortunate side effect of a dry eye, which requires the use of artificial tears. Golding-Wood (1973) reported 94 percent complete relief in 242 patients who were followed for 5 to 15 years. He emphasized that patient selection must be meticulous in order to rule out allergic rhinitis, which does not respond well to this treatment. The magnitude of this operation, however, must be weighed against the significance of symptoms and potential risks.

SURGICAL EXCISION

Amputation of the inferior turbinate is one of the oldest methods practiced to correct nasal blockage by swollen turbinates, and criticism of this procedure by rhinologists has been severe. Nevertheless, there has been renewed interest in this technique, and some authors (Fry, 1973, 1976; Courtiss and associates, 1978) have found it successful, causing only minimal complications or sequelae. This "surgical attack" is not recommended until adequate allergy management and conservative therapy — including antihistamines and intranasal steroid injections — have been given an adequate trial.

Two surgical approaches are possible. The first is a simple excision of hypertrophied mucosa and bone. The turbinate is fractured toward the septum and a traction suture is placed in the anterior end. An angled scissor is then used to resect mucosa and bone (Figure 6–20). The portion of turbinate removed should be based on the amount of hyperplasia present; usually, 30 to 80 percent is removed (Goode, 1977). In general, a conservative resection is recommended, and radical resection flush with the lateral nasal wall should be con-

demned. Resection of the middle turbinate is not recommended. The raw edge of the turbinate should be covered with Gelfoam* to prevent hemorrhage, and Courtiss and associates (1978) recommend Avitene.† Goode (1977) reported postoperative bleeding in about 10 percent of cases

---

*Upjohn Co.
†Avicon, Inc., Fort Worth, Texas.

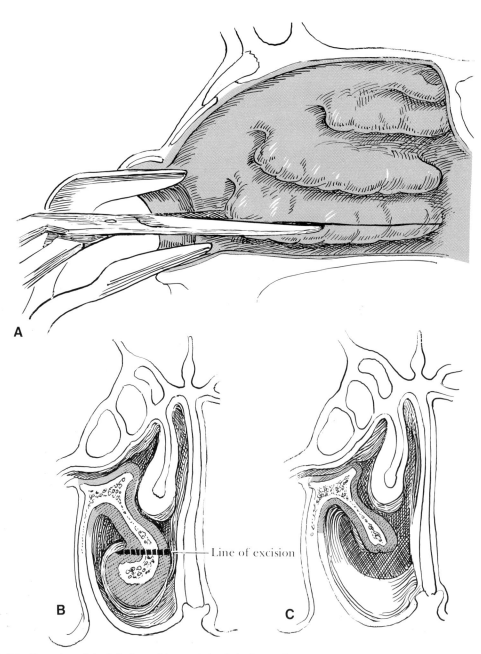

Figure 6–20.   Resection of the inferior turbinate. *A,* Angled scissors placed with a vertical orientation to resect a portion of the hypertrophied mucosa and bone. *B,* Gelfoam or Avitene should be used to cover the raw edge of the turbinate in order to help prevent hemorrhage. *C,* Final result after healing. Remaining turbinate soft tissue may hypertrophy again, causing obstruction.

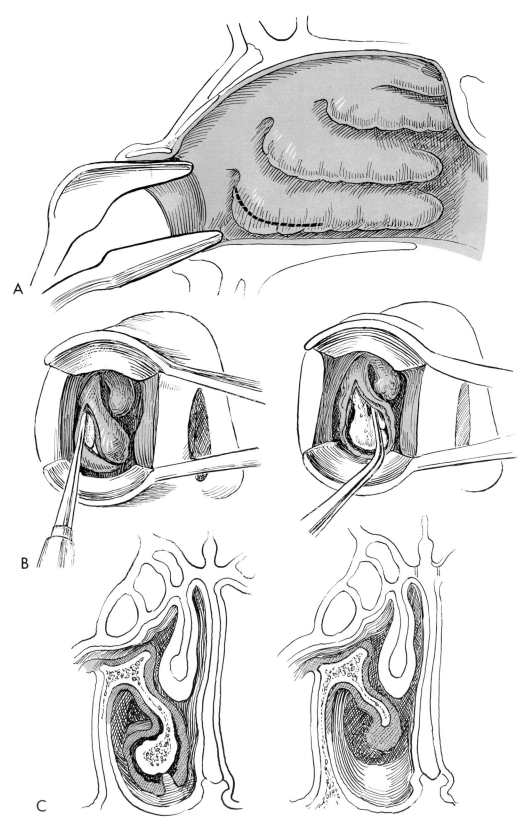

Figure 6–21. Submucous resection of turbinate bone. *A,* Curved incision down to bone over anterior inferior edge of the turbinate. *B,* Mucoperiosteum and submucosa elevated off medial and lateral surfaces of the conchal bone up to its attachment with lateral wall. *C,* Hypertrophied bone excised with angled scissors.

around the eighth postoperative day, and Courtiss and associates (1978) reported excessive bleeding in 3 of 88 cases, one requiring transfusion.

Most authors report subjective improvement in patients' symptoms, and on physical examination, a larger airspace is seen. It is not unusual, however, for regrowth of turbinate soft tissue to occur, and the operation may be repeated. When performing turbinate resection in conjunction with septal surgery, extreme care should be taken to avoid the occurrence of postoperative turbinal-septal adhesions.

The second surgical approach is a submucous resection of the inferior turbinate bone as recommended by House (1951), which avoids interference or destruction of nasal mucosa. A curved incision down to bone is made over the anterior inferior edge of the inferior turbinate (Figure 6–21). Using a Freer elevator, the mucoperiosteum and submucosa are elevated off the medial and lateral surfaces of the conchal bone up to their attachment with the lateral wall and as far posterior as possible (usually about 2 cm). Approximately one half to two thirds of the bony turbinate is excised with a large angled scissor (see Figure 6–21), and the nose is packed for several days. Healing is usually excellent, postoperative bleeding is rare, and patients with hypertrophied turbinate bone generally experience significant improvement.

SUMMARY

From the foregoing review, it might seem that rhinoplasty is a procedure fraught with danger of untoward physiologic alterations and complications. Nasal physiology, however, although of paramount importance, must not be confused with the overall aims of rhinoplasty. Aesthetic results are of as much concern to the surgeon as they are to the patient, and to overemphasize nasal function relative to nasal form is incorrect. Clinical experience has demonstrated that if care is taken, neither subjective nor objective symptoms or sequelae follow rhinoplasty.

The rhinoplasty surgeon must deal concomitantly with nasal function and nasal form and be aware of the consequences of overlooking either. He must have a basic understanding of the individual and combined relationship of the various structures that make up the nose. Relief of nasal obstruction is not achieved merely by increasing the luminal cross section of the nasal cavity. It depends more on maintaining or restoring the smooth, rounded contours of the vestibule and turbinates and avoiding interference with the nasal valve. This requires careful placement of incisions, preservation of mucous membranes, judicious handling of cartilages, and avoidance of unnecessary sacrifice of the septum or any other nasal structure.

(For references, see pages 453 to 455.)

Chapter 7

Preoperative Considerations

THOMAS D. REES, M.D., F.A.C.S.

THE NATURE OF RHINOPLASTY

Rhinoplasty is the most difficult of all operations for the young plastic surgeon to master; it is likewise the most difficult to teach. There are many reasons for this. Rhinoplasty is hard for the beginner to understand, since it is performed almost blindly and its success depends to a great extent on the tactile sense of the surgeon. It also requires a three dimensional concept. It is easy to provide an orderly, step-by-step operative technique; however, it is not so easy to teach the flexibility so frequently required to vary the technique for a given individual. The complexity is further compounded because it is often difficult or even impossible to predict the final outcome. Many factors combine to produce the result, including the skill of the surgeon, anatomic variations in the skin and subcutaneous tissues as well as in the cartilages and bones of the nose, healing idiosyncrasies, and the presence or degree of complications. It is the author's opinion that a certain artistic appreciation or ability to conceptualize operations in an artistic manner is an important attribute in order to become proficient in rhinoplasty. Most surgeons can be taught the technique, yet few become masters of the art. Nevertheless, most should be capable of producing an acceptable result, given the average patient.

One of the most difficult aspects of teaching rhinoplasty is to impart the limitations of each technique and the variable results that may occur due to the patient's physiognomy. Some of these limitations are predictable but others are not so clearly foreseen. One of the most common causes of failure in rhinoplasty (the indifferent or disastrous result) is the pressing desire of the surgeon to accomplish a "perfect" job. Frequently, such a result is completely outside the realm of possibility,

and in such a case the failure is produced by the inability of both the surgeon and the patient to accept the fact that there will be some limitation in the final result. The experienced surgeon readily accepts these limitations and stops when a maximal practical correction has been achieved, whereas the inexperienced surgeon will resist these limits and court defeat and an unsatisfactory result. The overoperated nose is a tragedy because reoperation is rarely able to achieve a satisfactory result; indeed, even minor improvement is frequently unattainable.

The routine (cookbook) patterned operation advocated by many surgeons is to be condemned; it is simply not possible to do a standard operative procedure on every patient and obtain satisfactory results. To attempt to correct each tip by the same technique shows a complete lack of understanding of the variations in size, shape, and direction of the alar cartilages, as well as a failure to appreciate the influence of the subcutaneous tissue and overlying skin on the tip structure of each patient. The surgeon must appreciate these limitations and problems and command at least three or four basic surgical approaches in order to treat the individual nasal plastic problem adequately.

The young surgeon is advised to study his patient carefully before surgery and to follow him postoperatively for several years, since only in this way can he learn surgical cause and effect. The final result of rhinoplasty is only evident after months or sometimes years, during which time the nose changes continuously. This long-term and gradual metamorphosis is extremely important for the surgeon to grasp, since overoperating occurs because of the surgeon's dogged determination to achieve a result that fits his preconceived vision of what the results should be, without a real appreciation of the healing process. This dimension of knowledge, unfortunately, comes only with experience.

PATIENT SELECTION

Most patients seek rhinoplasty simply because they want to improve the size and shape of their noses. Probably the most common request is for a reduction in size of part or all of the nose. This may mean simply the removal of a strong dorsal hump typical in noses of patients of Mediterranean descent (but also common in other Europeans), or the reduction of the size of the tip and augmentation of the profile height with an implant or autogenous graft common in Orientals and other non-Caucasians. In recent years, patients have shown more interest in achieving overall improvement in their facial structures rather than striving for a particular standard of nasal beauty such as the thin aquiline nose with a delicate or chiseled tip frequently referred to in past publications on the subject. In this context, it should be pointed out that in some ethnic groups, the presence of the nasal hump is a sign of beauty; however, the profile most desired throughout the world today involves a relatively straight dorsum or slight degree of retroussé. A much larger number of patients seen in consultation are more concerned with correcting deformities of the dorsum rather than those of the tip-columella-lip area. The patient's attention is easily focused on a hump nose deformity, which often eclipses the anatomic defect and visual impact of the lower nose. Excessive flare in the nostril is also usually considered a flaw. The "ideal" nostrils are thin and delicate with a slight flaring. Accentuation of the convex line of the columella resulting from excessive curvature of the caudal border of the septum or the inferior margins of the medial crura is also a cause of complaint.

It is exceedingly important for the surgeon to let the patient define his or her complaint. A hand mirror is useful for this purpose. The surgeon should refrain from injecting his own ideas or otherwise editorializing for as long as possible. In this way, he can gain a more accurate picture as to what is troubling the patient. The patient's analysis of his problem may be diametrically opposed to that of the surgeon. It is important for the surgeon to know what the patient hopes to achieve by the operation. By listening carefully to the patient's complaint, it is often possible for the surgeon to discern a deep, unresolved, and perhaps serious neurotic or psychotic attitude that would not only defeat the surgery but could plunge the patient into severe difficulties.

It is clear to all surgeons in this field that anatomic evaluation of the patient is very important but not nearly as important as the psychiatric evaluation. Since it is not always possible to ascertain an accurate psychiatric status of a patient in one consultation, the surgeon should not hesitate to suggest a second consultation if he feels the slightest doubt. The surgeon should also suggest that the patient seek psychiatric help, should such be strongly indicated. The latter is often easier said than done because of the demands on the psychiatrist's time. (This provocative, important, and difficult subject is covered in the section on psychologic considerations in plastic surgery.) Plastic surgeons everywhere are admonished to develop their skill of perception in this area to the highest degree possible.

It is obvious that the first key to a successful result is proper patient selection. Unfortunately, like the operation itself, wisdom in patient selection requires an accumulation of experience before the surgeon becomes adept. Refusing a patient for rhinoplasty can be an unpleasant and difficult experience. Nevertheless, if the surgeon honestly feels that the surgery is ill-advised for whatever reason, he should politely decline the operation. It is infinitely wiser to have a patient temporarily disappointed for being refused an operation than permanently upset after surgery because of disappointing results. The surgeon must learn to follow his intuition and conscience as well as his good judgment. The final decision is based on equal regard for the anatomic and the psychologic evaluation of each patient.

PATIENT EDUCATION

Patients and their relatives are more demanding today and generally better informed than ever before because of the continuous barrage of information on plastic surgery in magazines and news media. Much of this information can be misleading, and thus the patient may be under false impressions. It is incumbent on the surgeon to attempt by any reasonable means to inform and educate the rhinoplasty patient about the operation, what to expect, what complications may occur, and what he may look for in the postoperative course. In the case of minors, parents or other responsible adults should be educated along with the patient in order to avoid misunderstandings within the family. Various informative techniques are available such as letters, pamphlets, audiovisual aids, and so forth. A sample letter supplied to the author's patients is shown in Figure 7–1.

TO: MY PATIENTS
FROM: THOMAS D. REES, M.D.
RE: SOME FACTS FOR PATIENTS ABOUT COSMETIC SURGERY

You will do yourself a service if you read and re-read what
follows carefully, for here you will find answers to many of
the questions that are most often asked about plastic surgery
of the nose. Most of these questions are universally asked by
patients interested in this type of surgical correction.

The purpose of cosmetic surgery is to make you look as good as
it is possible for you to look. It cannot do more than that. If
you are expecting a transforming miracle from surgery, you will be
unquestionably disappointed. Plastic surgery is a combination of
art and science. Surgery is altogether not an exact science and
because some of the factors involved in producing the final result
(such as the healing process) are not entirely within the control of
either the surgeon or patient, it is impossible to warranty or
guarantee results. Surgical results from surgery on the nose, however,
are more predictable in some patients than others. This is
determined by a number of factors such as thickness and shape of
the bones and cartilage, the shape of the face, heredity, age, and
the thickness and condition of the skin. The skin is a highly
important factor influencing the result of nasal surgery for
thick skin precludes a delicate nasal tip. Every nose has a certain
combination of these anatomical features which influence the outcome
of the surgery and the predictability of the results. These will
be discussed with you during our consultation. No two noses are
the same; therefore the results of nasal surgery are never
exactly the same.

The nose is one of the main balancing features of the face and
sometimes an alteration of the size and shape of the nose should
also be accompanied by appropriate changes in other facial
structures to obtain the best results. The chin is often augmented
or altered along with the nose particularly if it is recessed or
small in size. During examination, your facial structure will
be evaluated and other appropriate recommendations made.

Now for specific questions:

(1) Who actually performs the operation?

continued...

Figure 7–1.

(2)

The operation on your nose will be done entirely by me. I perform
all surgery on my patients.

(2) Can complications occur from nose surgery?
Yes, however this type of surgery rarely produces serious complications.
The most common complication is nose bleed after surgery. Such
bleeding can be troublesome, but is fortunately uncommon, rarely
serious, and usually amenable to conservative treatment.
Infection is very rare. If infection occurs it is treated with
antibiotics. Occasionally a second operation may be done to
correct minor defects arising from the first, or to further improve
the breathing mechanism. Other complications and problems are very
rare, but will be discussed with you in detail if you desire.

(3) Why are preoperative photographs important?
Just as the chest surgeons cannot operate in an intelligent way
without x-rays of the chest, the plastic surgeon cannot operate
on the nose without medical photographs. These photographs are
not meant to flatter you. You probably will find it a harsh
photograph unsuitable for framing. The photos will show your
face in every detail. This aids greatly in the total evaluation of
your facial structure and the surgical performance of technical
variations in the surgery.
We do not show you the before and after photographs of other
patients. Such photographs can be misleading and are a confidential
part of the record. Besides, no two noses are the same.

(4) Are there external scars?
Nasal plastic surgery is accomplished through incisions inside
the nose which are not visible. Occasionally small external
incisions are made in the nostrils to reduce the size of them.
If these are necessary in your case, they will be explained to you.

(5) What type of anesthesia is used during the operation?
Local anesthesia is used for most nose operations. This does
not mean that the patient is fully awake. Various drugs are given
before you go to the operating room to make you sleepy and calm.
Very nervous or "squeemish" patients may be put to sleep temporarily
only while the local anesthetic is administered; however an expert
anesthesiologist is then required who charges separately for his
services. His fee is explained in the pre-operative instructions.
Despite the type of anesthesia selected, there will be no pain
during the operation.

(6) How long is the operation?
The actual operating time may vary, depending on the amount of
surgery necessary. A nasal plastic operation usually requires
about 30 to 60 minutes. A chin implant adds 15 to 20 minutes to
that time.

continued...

Illustration continued on the following page.

Figure 7–1. *Continued.*

(3)

(7) How long is the hospital stay?
The usual hospital stay is three days. Admission is always one
day prior to the operation at about 11:00 a.m. and discharge time
is about 10:00 a.m. the second or third day after surgery. Admission
to the hospital may seem unnecessarily early, but is necessary in
order to perform the required laboratory work and examinations by
the resident surgeon and anesthesiologist.
Although the room accommodations are booked well in advance of
admission, it may not always be possible to have the accommodation
you desire on admission to the hospital. Every attempt on my part
will be made to handle this problem to your advantage.

(8) Are bandages applied?
A cast or splint is applied over your nose and remains for
approximately one week. Light packs may or may not be inserted in
your nostrils. Packs are removed two days after the operation.
This maneuver is absolutely painless. Ice compresses are usually
applied to the eyes for several hours. These are thought to
help minimize swelling and bruising.
The splint covering your nose will be worn home after discharge
from the hospital. It is meant to protect your new nose and to
hold down the swelling. In this regard it is also important that
telephone calls and visitors be kept to a minimum for the first
48 hours after the operation. But post operative pain is rare and
whatever discomfort there may be is usually mild, short-lived and
easily handled with routine medication. All bandages are removed
in the office about one week after the operation.

(9) When are the stitches removed?
Any stitches in the nostrils are removed on the third or fourth
day after the operation. Stitches inside the nose are removed
about the ninth day. Stitches are always removed by my nurses.

(10) Who takes care of me after surgery?
Except on Fridays and over the weekends, you will be visited every
day in the hospital by me. If for unforeseen reasons, I am unable
to visit you, you will be seen by one of my staff. There is an
expert team of associates and assistants always in attendance, who
are continuously in touch with me. It is also not possible for me
to visit you the night of admission to the hospital. Therefore,
it is important that any unresolved questions be discussed prior
to admission, if necessary by a further visit to the office.

(11) Are private nurses available?
Although not a necessity, some patients feel happier knowing
that someone will be with them following surgery. Some hospitals
require the patient to book private nurses at the time of admission.
At other hospitals we are able to arrange for nurses in advance.

continued...

(4)

In spite of booking well in advance of surgery, there is no
guarantee that nurses will be available because of the critical
shortage of such help.

(12) What happens in the postoperative period?
You must remember that before you see the improvement you are
expecting you will go through a standard postoperative period in
which you will look quite battered and bruised followed by another
temporary period of time when you may look strange to yourself.
This varies considerably with each individual but most patients
are quite presentable ten days after the operation when they can
go back to school or work. In some patients a slightly longer
period is required. I think you should also bear in mind that in
some patients undergoing nose surgery there is a temporary period
of slight emotional depression immediately following the surgery,
during the period of time when you look your worst. This is quite
normal and should not alarm you. It is not easy to look bruised and
swollen, particularly when natural expectations are towards improving
your appearance. Fortunately this period usually passes rather
quickly. Do not scrutinize your nose under the splint too closely.
Remember that it is swollen and taped in a high position so that it
may appear too short; however, after the bandages are removed,
the nose will "drop" slightly. During the first 10 day period,
your eyelids, cheeks, and upper lip may be swollen. The chin
too, particularly if an implant was inserted.
Many months are required for the final subtle changes in the
nose to appear; so be patient. This period may extend from 6 to
18 months or rarely even longer. Softening of the tip of the
nose occurs last.
The skin may be upset as the result of both the operation and
the bandages. Patients with acne may experience a flare-up.
Instructions for skin care will be given by me or my staff during
your postoperative office visits.
Athletic activities must be limited within reason for several
months. The nose is "healed" in about four or six weeks. At
that time swimming, tennis, golf, horseback riding and other
sports are permitted that do not involve direct body contact.
Body contact or team sports such as volleyball, football, wrestling,
etc. are prohibited for 3 months. Remember that if your new nose
is accidentally broken, it is easier to set the bones than it was
before the operation.
Your nose may seem stuffy or congested from time to time, for
several weeks after surgery. This reaction is normal. Do not
continuously use nose drops, however, as it is easy to become
habituated to them.
Do not take aspirin for two weeks before or after surgery, as it
may increase bleeding tendency. Tylenol may be taken.
Exposure to the sun is permitted in moderation immediately after
the operation. Avoid sunburn.
Mainly, common sense is required in regulating your activities
after surgery.

continued...

(5)

If you have any other questions be sure to get them answered
in advance by me or my office staff. Many members of my staff
have been with me for years and are thoroughly informed, trained
and able to answer questions that may occur to you. Well meaning
friends are not a good source of information. Find out everything
you want to know. A well informed patient is a happy one.

Thomas D. Rees, M.D., F.A.C.S.

It is important to realize that even the most exhausting efforts to educate the patient and to inform him may fall on uncomprehending ears. The amount of information retained or understood is often unpredictable. Dr. Michael Gurdin of California once remarked that many patients have "selective cerebration"—they hear only what they want to hear and discard the rest. This is probably a human failure common to all of us.

It is often particularly difficult to get the patient and family to grasp the simple fact that surgical reconstruction of the nose is not perfect and cannot be precisely diagrammed or blueprinted. They are often under the illusion that the opposite is true; that the surgery is similar to sculpting in wood or clay. Great pains should be taken to inform them that such is not the case and that perfection cannot be expected. If perfection results from the operation, it is more in the nature of an unanticipated gift than a realistic expectation.

THE FIRST CONSULTATION

One of the most difficult and sensitive parts of the operation begins at the first consultation with the patient. At this time, the surgeon must determine whether the patient is emotionally suited to the operation and to what degree the nose can be improved in contour. A poor decision at this time can result in the ultimate failure of the operation, even though a technically successful contour has been achieved. Of equal importance to the physical characteristics is the patient's concept of the outcome of the operation; this concept has to do with the self-image, so important in all of cosmetic surgery.

One of the key elements to consider at the first consultation, without benefit of exact psychiatric knowledge of the patient, is the demeanor and general physical appearance presented by the patient. A disheveled, overweight, sloppily dressed individual may experience a dramatic "turn-around" in self-esteem after surgery and improve the general appearance. On the other hand, a patient with such an initial presentation may be manifesting a more severe underlying neurosis that can be aggravated by the surgery.

If the patient is a minor, his interaction with his family (or responsible adults) is important to notice. It is not uncommon for a minor to be brought to the surgeon for rhinoplasty evaluation actually against his own wishes. Operating on such patients often ends in disappointment for all concerned and is not considered within the realm of good medical practice. The motivation for surgery should come from within each patient, not from pressure from other individuals. These signs are not difficult to pick up, particularly if any question addressed to a minor patient is immediately answered by the mother or father, giving the patient little opportunity to speak. It is my habit, in such instances to discuss the operation candidly with the patient, alone, in a separate room, away from the parents. It is then frequently possible to obtain a true reading of the patient's feelings.

At the first consultation, the patient is given a set of instructions, including the letter of information shown in Figure 7–1. At the conclusion of the consultation, the patient or legally designated adult must sign an informed consent, which indicates that such a letter has been read and is understood. The entire subject of informed consent has been discussed in many publications. It goes without saying that it is virtually impossible to inform each patient of every complication that could possibly follow a nasal plastic operation. The more common problems such as epistaxis, however, can and should be discussed. Also, as indicated in the letter of information, the patient is given the option to ask any further questions he or she has regarding possible complications.

PATIENT HISTORY

Several general medical facts can be especially pertinent for a rhinoplasty patient. A family history of bleeding tendency or a personal history of bruising or bleeding, particularly epistaxis, may indicate obscure blood dyscrasias. Although females do not have true hemophilia, they may carry the potential for excessive or even dangerous postoperative hemorrhage by virtue of disorders of their blood coagulation mechanism. The usual bleeding and clotting time tests are generally of little or no value in these circumstances, and a complete hematologic evaluation of the patient's coagulation abilities is indicated if suspicion of a bleeding tendency exists.

A history of allergic disorders, particularly hay fever or vasomotor rhinitis, warns the surgeon that such patients may have an exacerbation of such difficulties in the postoperative period, often prolonged for several weeks or months. Vasomotor rhinitis can be distinguished by the intermittent nature of the nasal obstruction, often shifting from side to side, especially while the patient is in bed. Submucous resection is by no means always the answer to difficult breathing; more observations on this problem are made in Chapter 6. The patient with a history or objective evidence of vasomotor rhinitis should be forewarned that the operation may accentuate his symptoms for a very long time. Surgery should be postponed if an active respiratory infection is present.

PHYSICAL EVALUATION

Although it is not possible to be absolutely accurate in predicting the result of rhinoplasty because of the many variables encountered, it is important for the surgeon to recognize certain anatomic problems that may pose difficulties during the surgery and will definitely limit the results to be obtained. He must learn to recognize just how these specific features will modify the outcome; many of these variations in anatomy have been discussed by numerous authors, but because of their importance they bear repeated emphasis.

Factors that may influence the result of rhinoplasty are the thickness of the nasal bones, the presence or absence of the nasion, and the thickness and position of the septum. If the nasal bones are thick, if the septum is shifted laterally at the level of the nasal bones, or if the septum is excessively thick in this area, the possible degree of narrowing of the nose along its dorsum will be severely limited. A high deviation of the septum, unless corrected, will be reflected by an external deviation of the nasal framework after completion of the operation.

Deviations of the cartilaginous septum of the nose pose the most challenging and difficult problem. Despite all possible surgical maneuvers, attainment of a completely straight dorsum may not be possible, and some curvature or external deviation of the nose may still be present after the operative procedure. It may also become apparent only after some weeks or months following the surgery. Lowering of the nasal profile during rhinoplasty may expose a deviation of the cartilaginous septum in the lower portion of the septum but not along its dorsal border. Trimming of redundant alar cartilages may also expose a crooked septum previously camouflaged by the lateral alar crura. The correction of a deviated septum will be discussed further, but it is important to recognize the septal conformation preoperatively in order to plan the corrective procedure carefully.

The mucous membrane should be shrunk with a topical vasoconstrictor during the preoperative examination so that all confines of the nasal cavity can be exposed. Patients with external nasal deformities, the result of septal deflections, should be advised that it may not be possible to obtain a completely straight nose and that they must be willing to accept a possibility of a persistent small deviation. If a straight nose is obtained, little criticism can be directed at the surgeon, whereas if a small deviation persists, the patient has been adequately warned.

The tip frequently presents the most technically challenging part of the procedure. It requires considerable experience to be able to evaluate the tip preoperatively and to predict with any degree of accuracy the postoperative result. Some tips pose more difficult problems than others, and indeed some of these prove insurmountable; these patients should not, in most cases, be accepted for surgery. The most difficult tips to correct are those in patients with thick oily skin, usually associated with an abundance of sebaceous glands and a marked excess of subcutaneous fatty tissue. This kind of tip has an amorphous appearance (the underlying cartilage may or may not be hypertrophic) and cannot impress its shape on the external aspect of the nose because of the thickness of the overlying tissues. The thick skin frequently obliterates the normal supra-alar groove; in patients presenting with this sign, great care must be taken in examination of the nasal tip.

Correction of such a nose should be approached with caution, since the results are apt to be indifferent. If excessive surgery is done in an attempt to reduce the tip, the results will frequently be marred by added deformity and scarring. Whereas a certain amount of improvement can be accomplished in such tips, it must be remembered that the memory of the patient and the patient's friends of the preoperative appearance can be very short, and what has been accomplished may be forgotten. Whether to accept a patient for surgery depends entirely on the surgeon's evaluation of the attitude of both patient and family, and it is frequently on the basis of the evaluation of this attitude that the patient is to be finally accepted or rejected for surgery.

It is well for the young surgeon, particularly one just starting practice in a community, to realize that he will be able to accomplish very little with conventional techniques operating upon such a tip and that if he becomes too aggressive with his surgery, it will result in a disaster for all.

Occasionally, despite the many obstacles to obtaining acceptable surgical results in patients with some of these difficult anatomic problems, we find that the patients who seem to be helped the least are frequently most grateful and pleased. This certainly has to do with self-image. Conversely, we may find a patient who has obtained a superb technical result to be highly dissatisfied. Such patients usually have emotional problems that require, at the least, psychotherapy.

The use of preoperative photographs is frequently helpful in discussing the proposed change with the patient. Careful retouching of a matte photograph can often illustrate the patient's wish to the surgeon, and at this time, it will occasionally become very clear that the patient's self-concept and image of what can be accomplished is grossly distorted. The surgeon must explore the depth and cause of this distortion and determine whether it can be channeled in a positive direction. The nuances of this type of situation are many, and clear guidelines do not exist. As the surgeon gains in experience, he will make fewer and fewer mistakes in patient selection, but he will probably never reach the point at which he makes no clinical misjudgments.

In my opinion, the use of preoperative plaster casts and moulages on which the proposed nasal change is sculpted or carved is both misleading and inadvisable. Such three dimensional carvings are usually more fancy than fact, and they frequently fail to convey the dynamic changes of the healing of the nasal tissues. The patient is apt to gain the impression from the plaster cast that the beautifully carved nose is exactly what to expect, and this expectation may turn quite sour if the result is not exactly reproduced. It is well to remember that such casts provide excellent exhibits at legal proceedings for those patients who favor litigation.

THE AGE TO OPERATE

It was long taught that one should not operate on the nose before the age of 16 in the female or 17 in the male. Most clinics now perform the operation at an earlier age, since there is no convincing evidence that the nose continues to grow significantly after the age of 15, except in some exceptionally immature individuals. Such signs of immaturity are often obvious at consultation. In the female, breast development is lacking and the menses have not begun. In the male, there is an evident lack of maturity shown by the pitch of the voice and the general body habitus. Surgery should be postponed in such individuals. Surgery in the older age group carries its own considerations.

THE YOUNGER PATIENT

In the younger rhinoplasty patient, handling the family is frequently more difficult than handling the patient. Nevertheless, if the patient is a minor, the family must be kept in the picture. Frequently, the parents insist upon the operation while the minor patient does not wish the change to be made. Under such conditions, it is both unwise and unethical to operate, since it is the primary job of the surgeon to help the patient; aiding the family is secondary. My policy in such an impasse is to advise the patient that when, if ever, he or she desires to discuss nasal plastic surgery, a further consultation is available but that, in the meantime, no surgery will be performed.

Another difficult situation with the young patient is when the patient desires surgery but the mother or father or both are vehemently opposed to the procedure. This can be most troublesome because someone is certainly not going to be pleased with the results, and frequently a transfer of this dissatisfaction from the parent to the patient may occur. A similar situation may exist between husband and wife; emotional and psychologic interplay may complicate proposed surgery and its results. Again it must be emphasized that when such problems are encountered, it is the surgeon's job to do his best for the patient. Thus, if consultation and careful appraisal of all relevant factors indicate the strong possibility of success, he should proceed with the surgery.

Such situations are difficult to resolve and can often present a long and trying road for the surgeon. Yet, when successful, they are part of the pleasure of cosmetic surgery. Every surgeon must be prepared to assume certain risks that must be weighed against the chances of success; indeed, every cosmetic operation is a risk of sorts. However, the rewards for both patient and surgeon are such that the risk is well worth taking, provided that the odds are not overwhelmingly weighted against success.

THE OLDER PATIENT

Rhinoplasty in the adult, particularly in the older adult, presents the surgeon with a different set of problems and challenges than nasal plastic surgery in the teenager (Rees, 1978). The mature nose is different in both form and function from that of the teenager. Furthermore, the emotional needs and expectations of the older patient seeking elective cosmetic surgery may be significantly different from those of the younger one. Rhinoplasty is an operation of deep consequence to the patient in middle age, more so than many other cosmetic operations such as blepharoplasty or rhytidectomy. The nose is a central and prominent landmark of the face, and as such it may have been the focal point of the patient's attention for so many years that the self-image may have become distorted to the extent that it completely masks the true appearance of the nose itself.

In any prospective rhinoplasty patient, the surgeon must determine emotional suitability as well as the degree to which the nose can be improved if successful postoperative results are to be achieved. However, among the older age group, social and psychologic factors are often considerably more important in patient selection than are anatomic factors. Therefore, preoperative evaluation of the older patient requires a more in-depth and time-consuming consultation than that required of the young. Often, two or more preoperative interviews are necessary, because important information, such as what the patient expects from the surgery, may not be as easy to obtain in the older person as it is in younger people, who have a tendency to be more open about their personal thoughts.

Good candidates for surgery want to do something positive for themselves. Many patients in the older age group are healthily motivated, emotionally sound, and among those most pleased postoperatively. A positive approach on the part of the patient often demonstrates itself during consultation by a statement such as, "I have wanted my nose done since I was very young, but only at this time have I arrived at a position where I am able to have it done, because improved finances and a lessening of my family duties and responsibilities now make it possible."

On the other hand, the patient who opens the interview with a negative approach such as, "I have always considered myself ugly. I can't stand the way I look and I want to do something about it," or the patient who has recently lost a spouse through death or divorce, is a poor candidate, and regardless of the aesthetic outcome of the surgery, he or she is likely to be dissatisfied with the postoperative results.

Any older patients who might be considered emotionally "borderline" in terms of suitability for surgery should be referred for psychiatric evaluation before a decision of whether to operate is reached. It goes without saying that patients who show clear signs of deep underlying emotional illness or psychosis should be gently but firmly refused operation. To operate on such patients is an open invitation to disaster for patient and surgeon alike.

In years past, many surgeons categorically refused to perform cosmetic rhinoplasty on older patients. Although few surgeons today would support this polarized attitude, it is still important to recognize the need for cautious and thorough evaluation of the motives of older patients, with particular attention to the patient's self-image, in seeking cosmetic surgery.

Anatomic Considerations

In addition to dealing with a different set of psychologic, social, and emotional factors in the older as opposed to younger rhinoplasty patient, the surgeon must anticipate some very real anatomic and physiologic differences.

As a natural consequence of the aging process, the skin of the nose loses a certain amount of elasticity and becomes dehydrated, thickened, and redundant. It is therefore less apt to redrape itself smoothly over a reformed bony and cartilaginous framework. Furthermore, minor blemishes such as telangiectases and keratoses are more apt to appear with age and must be treated accordingly. However, the skin of the older individual generally heals with thin, soft scars, so external incisions are more feasible and acceptable in these patients. In addition, the skin of the tip is less apt to be subject to intensive hormonal barrage as it is in the teenager; it will have fewer sebaceous glands, unless a rhinophymatous condition exists; and it may well be less prone to postoperative swelling in the supratip region.

The membranes lining the nose of the older patient are, in general, less likely to be involved in intense vasomotor activity such as is often seen in the younger patient. With age, the effect of allergens decreases, the erectile tissue becomes atrophic, and unless a significant bony or cartilaginous obstruction is present, fewer breathing problems (except those attendant on living in our polluted urban societies) are likely to be present.

Perhaps of most significance to surgeons in the operative procedure, however, are the biophysical changes in the bone and cartilage resulting from the aging process. Cartilage, although much less affected by aging than bone, can become calcified or ossified, making remodeling more difficult. Changes in the bone density and tensile strength, however, are more likely to affect the outcome of rhinoplasty in the older individual than possibly any other anatomic factor. The bones of the older individual are brittle and very apt to splinter and fragment, despite all attempts to achieve clean osteotomy lines. The current emphasis on a greenstick infracture of the nasal bone after lateral osteotomy, a highly acceptable technique in most young patients, becomes fraught with potential difficulties in the older individual. Every effort should therefore be made to obtain clean and thorough osteotomies, and the use of a very sharp osteotome where fracture lines are required is recommended. For example, when superior osteotomy is indicated, the author makes a percutaneous puncture at the root of the nose with a fine and very sharp 2-mm osteotome.

Even with such careful and precise sculpting, fragmentation and comminution of the nasal bone are not uncommon in the older patient. Therefore, as a further safeguard, the skin and periosteum over the external surfaces of the nasal bones should not be undermined until the infracture has been accomplished. In this way, the danger of extensive comminution with loss of fragments into the pyriform aperture is minimized. Should the bones comminute, they still remain attached to the skin and periosteum, and they can be molded as in traumatic fractures to achieve an acceptable result.

Radical operations on the septum, including the time-honored Killian submucous resection, should be performed very selectively in the older patient, and then only when severe obstructive conditions exist. Such procedures in the older patient carry a high morbidity risk and a greater possibility of troublesome or serious hemorrhage. For example, extensive surgery of the posterior septum can result in severe hemorrhaging from sclerotic ethmoid vessels, which may be exceedingly difficult to control. The surgeon must remember that the vascular changes that occur in the older patient — as well as hypertension, which is frequent in this age group — may lead to such bleeding problems.

Finally, it is important to emphasize that the entire concept of rhinoplastic surgery in the older patient must stress conservatism. Not only are minimal elevation of the tip and gentle changes with conservation of all tissues more desirable in the older age group, but radical changes in appearance are more difficult to accept by the patient — and more difficult to correct by secondary surgery. (Incidentally, in a certain number of older patients who are having face lift and eyelid surgery, a slight elevation of the nasal tip, without disturbing the nasal skeleton, provides a salutary effect in the overall appearance. All facial tissues fight the effects of gravity as aging occurs, and the nose is no exception.)

PREPARATION AND SURGERY

The routine use of prophylactic antibiotics before and after surgery is a frequently debated point, but in nasal surgery, where infections — although rare — are critical, it would seem wise to take advantage of every precaution; a thrombosed cavernous sinus with infection is a grave problem never to be forgotten. The author provides a high blood level of antibiotics intraoperatively, after which they are discontinued. Keflex is the current favorite.

Recent knowledge that aspirin and aspirin-containing drugs may inhibit the agglutination of platelets may have contributed to a reduction in hemorrhage by withdrawing such compounds for several days before surgery.

Recently developed tests of blood coagulation help us to identify occult bleeding problems. Curtailment of a routine submucous resection in every operation significantly reduced postoperative morbidity, particularly in the older patient.

INPATIENT OR OUTPATIENT?

Rhinoplasty can be done either on a hospital inpatient or outpatient (ambulatory) basis. There is a growing trend toward performing rhinoplasty on an outpatient basis in many localities because of the reluctance of insurance companies to compensate for aesthetic nasal surgery and the need to economize on costs of surgical care. Rhinoplasty can be safely performed on an outpatient basis provided a properly equipped operating suite and good postoperative care is available. Hemorrhage and drug reaction are the main concerns following rhinoplasty. Hemorrhage can occur up to two weeks after surgery, at a time when most inpatients have been discharged from the hospital. Epistaxis is rarely significant and can be handled readily on an outpatient basis in most cases. Drug reactions usually occur within the first few hours following the operation. Early detection of a drug reaction during the immediate postoperative period in a suitable recovery facility is important in order to institute appropriate therapy.

Patients who require particularly complicated nasal operations or who have associated general health problems might best be treated in the hospital. Some patients (as well as their surgeons) feel more secure in a hospital setting. In the last analysis, the choice depends on economic factors, individual preferences, and availability of a proper and safe facility. There is little doubt that the trend toward outpatient surgery will continue as long as the costs of hospital care continue to soar.

The only topical skin preparation that is required is a thorough soap and water wash of the face 12 hours before surgery and once again just before surgery. The author prefers a hexachlorophene soap for this procedure. Patients troubled with chronic pustular acne may be sustained on prophylactic antibiotics, since many are on low-maintenance doses for long periods.

PREMEDICATION

In rhinoplasty, the premedication combination is most important, particularly if local anesthesia is to be used. A relaxed, sleepy, and cooperative patient is apt to remember the experience, if indeed memory persists at all, without fear or discomfort, whereas the undermedicated or improperly medicated patient has only a disturbing and frightening memory to impart to friends.

The medication should be given sufficiently far in advance of the procedure so that the patient is well relaxed before transportation to the operating room. Too frequently, patients placed on the schedule "to follow" are sent for with only a few minutes of time remaining for the floor nurses to administer the premedication. Such patients usually arrive in the operating room tense, worried, and anxious because the medication has not had enough time to take effect. Often, it is not until the surgery is nearly completed that the medication finally works, so that during the most feared part of the procedure, in the period when sedation is most needed, the effects of the premedication are absent.

The use of intravenous valium in the operating room for the undermedicated or anxious patient has proved to be quite effective in recent years; 5 to 10 mg administered slowly may be required. Valium is also highly effective as an antidote to and a preventative of cocaine intoxication.

Serious cocaine reactions are exceedingly rare but can be dangerous and sometimes fatal; therefore, they must be treated instantly and vigorously. Reaction to cocaine is often heralded by anxiety, excitation, and tachycardia followed in severe cases by grand mal seizures. Such reactions are similar to the systemic effects of epinephrine. If a cocaine reaction is suspected, appropriate therapy should not be delayed. Specific treatment includes the immediate intravenous administration of barbiturates or diazepam (Valium), the immediate establishment of an adequate airway, and oxygen inhalation therapy. Endotracheal intubation and cardiac resuscitation may be required in severe forms of intoxication. These measures are more fully described in the chapter on anesthesia.

POSITIONING THE PATIENT

Positioning the patient for rhinoplasty is important. Hands should be lightly restrained; the table end is elevated so that the head is above the level of the heart. This simple maneuver is very important in diminishing bleeding during the procedure. The patient should be placed on the table so that the table break falls in the lower back region. This will enable the trunk and head to be raised to produce more postural hypotension if this should prove necessary. A foot plate should always be used to prevent sliding of the patient during surgery, and this should be adequately padded both for comfort and to prevent inadvertent grounding of the patient in this region should an electric cautery be used during the operation (Figure 7–2).

The operator should learn to adjust the height of the table and the distance at which he operates so that he may work most comfortably. For most surgeons with normal or corrected vision, the table is best located at elbow height.

A good light source is mandatory. I prefer to have the whole face lighted directly from above, with a second light directed from below to illuminate the interior of the nose. When extensive septal work is done, I prefer to use electric head lights rather than head mirrors and reflected light. However, this is a matter of individual preference. Fiberoptic "cold" lighting has been adapted for use for the dorsal nasal retractor of the Aufricht type, this instrument providing excellent illumination of the nasal interior (Figure 7–3).

The skin is prepared with pHisoHex and benzalkonium chloride (Zephiran) solution. The area will also have been washed with pHisoHex the night before surgery during the patient's preoperative preparation. Draping is done with the traditional towels and a split sheet, but it is important that the drapes expose the entire face. Obscuring the forehead and chin will prevent the operator from appreciating the full nuances of facial contour. The nasal vestibule hair is trimmed and the external nares are cleaned with cotton-tipped applicators soaked in Zephiran solution (Figure 7–4).

ANESTHESIA

Local anesthesia is generally used, although general anesthesia can be employed in extremely apprehensive patients. Hypotensive anesthesia insures a dry field, but this technique requires the service of an expert anesthesiologist well versed in

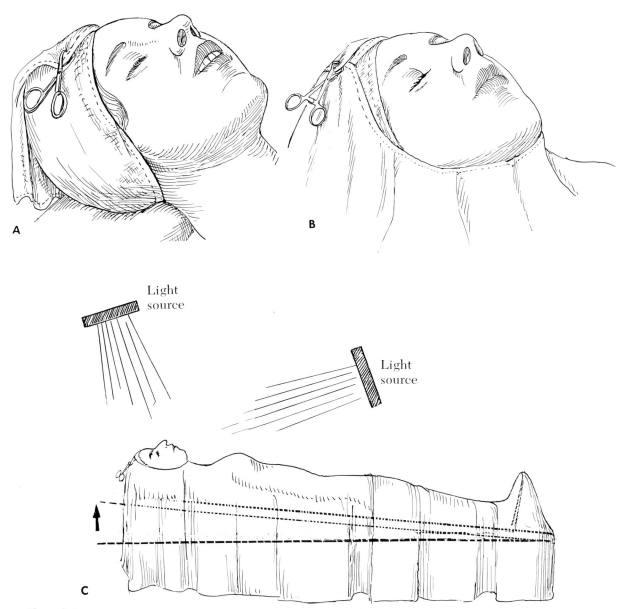

Light source

Light source

Figure 7–2. *A,* The optimum position of the patient on the operating table, with the head of the table elevated by about 10 degrees. The overhead lights are so arranged that one shines directly down onto the nasal dorsum and the other projects its beam into the external nares to illuminate the inferior of the nose.

B, The patient's hair is draped back and held by a towel; it is important that the forehead be exposed in order that a true appreciation of the patient's full face can be attained during surgery.

C, A split drape is drawn about the patient's head (again note the importance of exposing the full face), leaving the mandibular borders exposed.

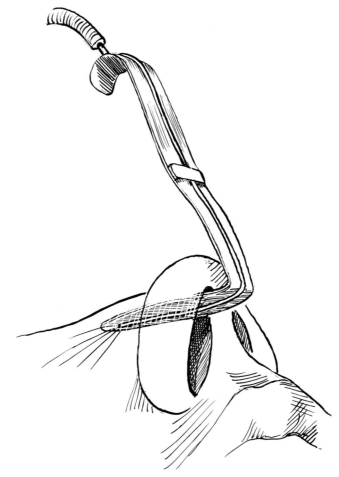

Figure 7–3. The fiberoptic Aufricht retractor provides excellent exposure and vision of the dorsal nasal framework. After revision of the profile, small defects of the bone or cartilage can be seen and corrected. Many secondary operations are prevented.

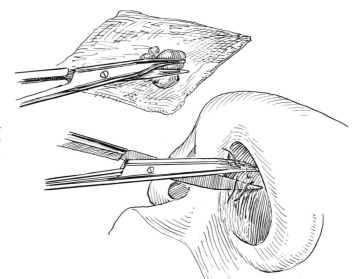

Figure 7-4. The nasal hairs are clipped after preparing the nares with Zephiran solution. The blades of a Stevens scissors are smeared with petrolatum so they will catch the severed hairs.

its use. Hypotensive anesthesia for use in elective plastic surgery was pioneered and perfected in England, primarily at the Queen Victoria Hospital and Plastic Center, East Grinstead. Ethrane has proved to be a safe and effective inhalant for general anesthesia and reduces bleeding to a minimum.

For local anesthesia, I favor topical cocaine and infiltration with lidocaine. Flattened pledgets of cotton moistened with 4 percent cocaine, or a mixture of 10 percent cocaine mixed equally with epinephrine 1:1000, are wrung out almost dry, since only small amounts of cocaine are required to produce excellent topical anesthesia (Figure 7–5). About three such pledgets are placed in the nose. It is important to get one well along the floor beneath the inferior turbinate. A middle pack extends along the floor adjacent to the middle turbinate. Most importantly, the superior pack must be placed high in the apex of the triangle formed by the septum and the lateral walls of the nose, for it is here that anesthesia is not always complete, caus-

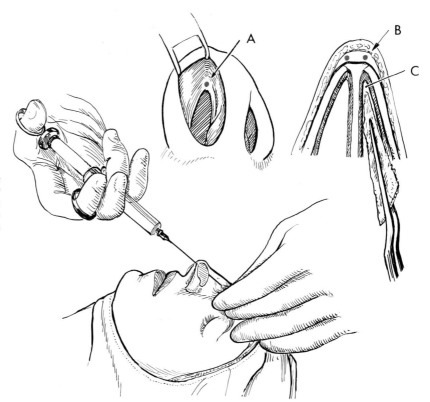

Figure 7–5. Placement of a cocaine pack high between the angle formed by the lateral wall of the nose and the septum (C) is most important to provide full topical anesthesia of the mucosa, since this area is often neglected.

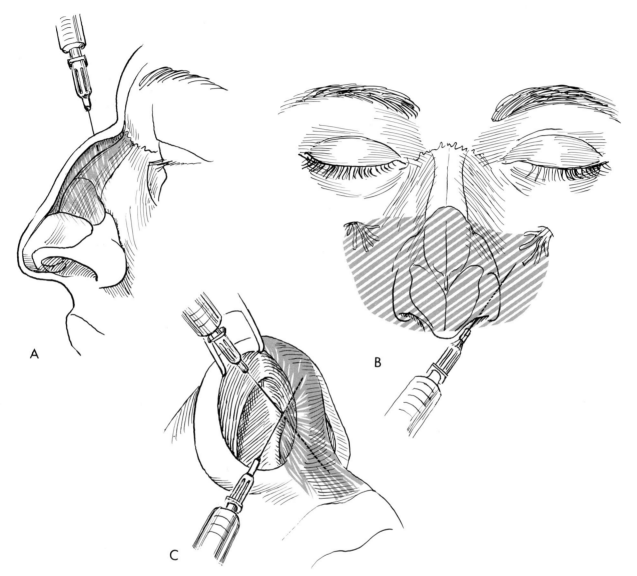

Figure 7–6. *A,* The dorsum of the nose is injected percutaneously with a 30-gauge needle. A minimum volume, only about 2 ml, is required to provide anesthesia and hemostasis for the entire dorsum! Larger volumes only distort the architecture by "blowing up" the soft tissues, making it difficult for the surgeon to evaluate the osteocartilaginous structures of the nose.

B, The sensory distribution of the infraorbital nerves are blocked by field fire injection in the general area of exit of the nerve. The needle should be introduced to the periosteal level. Actual blockage of the infraorbital nerve in the canal is convenient, but unnecessary.

C, The membranous septum is anesthetized by direct injection.

Only 6 to 10 ml maximum of local anesthetic solution need be injected to accomplish this initial anesthesia. Larger volumes are unnecessary, since they only distort the tissues and increase the possibility and severity of toxic manifestations.

ing pain during the operation. These packs should be left in place for a full five or ten minutes. They can then be replaced with one-quarter–inch gauze packing. It is unnecessary to leave cocaine in the nose throughout the operation. This only increases the potential amount of absorption and toxicity. Preoperative medication with Valium helps prevent or minimize cocaine intoxication.

Lidocaine and carbocaine are excellent local anesthetic agents for nasal surgery because of their quick action and prolonged anesthesia. For nasal surgery, I use 2 percent lidocaine with epinephrine added so that a solution of 1:60,000 is obtained. As with cocaine, it is important to keep the total dosage as low as possible. It is entirely possible to obtain excellent infiltration anesthesia with 6 ml of this solution, 10 ml at most.

The dorsum is infiltrated first, followed by field blocks just lateral to the pyriform aperture (Figure 7–6). If the infraorbital foramina can be located without undue delay, intraforaminal blocks are done. The base of the nose is blocked by infiltration with 1 or 2 ml near the nasal spine. It is helpful to wait at least five minutes for the anesthesia and the epinephrine to take effect before beginning surgery. Patience is rewarded by a much drier field. Apprehensive patients may be given a short-acting barbiturate, such as Brevital, during the time necessary to give the injections. Intravenous Valium can also be used for this purpose.

When anesthesia is complete, the nose is packed with one-inch gauze soaked in saline. This packing prevents blood and debris from draining into the posterior pharynx during the procedure.

(For references, see pages 450 to 453.)

Chapter 8

The Osteocartilaginous Vault

THOMAS D. REES, M.D., F.A.C.S.

THE OPERATION

The technical operative steps undertaken in any given patient must vary to accommodate the specific combinations of deformities present. An overall plan must be firmly in the surgeon's mind, but he should not slavishly follow a routine series of steps learned from a textbook or teacher. The modern rhinoplasty operation varies significantly in subtle ways from the technical steps generally taught in the past. What is different about the modern operative procedure? Variations are mostly minor in nature yet substantial in effect. Obvious as it may seem, one must remember that the nose is but one structure of the entire face, although it is the most prominent feature. Accordingly, it is important to evaluate the surgically draped face and the major external anatomic landmarks of the nose prior to beginning the operative procedure itself. Figure 8–1 illustrates some of the important points in this evaluation. For many years, Aufricht and others have emphasized the importance of viewing the nasal profile through a mirror that sometimes reflects defects and angles that are not otherwise easily discernible. It is also helpful to mark the forwardmost point of projection of the alar cartilages so that their relationship to the nasal profile is established, in reference to the postreduction profile. Diastasis between the alar cartilages should be noted before injection of local anesthesia. Identifying the forwardmost projection of these cartilages is facilitated by the thumb and long fingers.

The most prominent forward projection points of the domes are shown in Figure 8–1, *C* and *D*.

INCISING AND SKELETONIZING THE NOSE

Incisions are designed to preserve lining and soft tissue. The critical soft triangle of the tip as well as the membranous septum should be protected. Some surgeons advocate submucosal dissection of the entire chondrocutaneous skeleton including the upper lateral cartilages (see Figure 8–8). Such a technique has the obvious theoretical advantages of preserving the integrity of all lining structures, preventing cicatricial stenosis of the airway at the internal valve, and promoting an "exteronasal dissection" plane facilitating the use of dorsal grafts of bone or cartilage. In the author's opinion, however, it is more theoretical than practical.

Schematic steps in the nasal plastic operation (Figure 8–2) may be carried out in any sequence deemed necessary by the operator. Each surgeon develops his own operative approach to rhinoplasty. The order of the procedure, whether the surgeon first removes the hump, trims the tip cartilages, or does the submucous resection (if one is to be done) is not vital in the usual case. It is the author's belief, as has been stated and emphasized in other chapters of this book, that each procedure should be adapted to suit the individual needs at hand. At times, it makes more sense to operate on

114

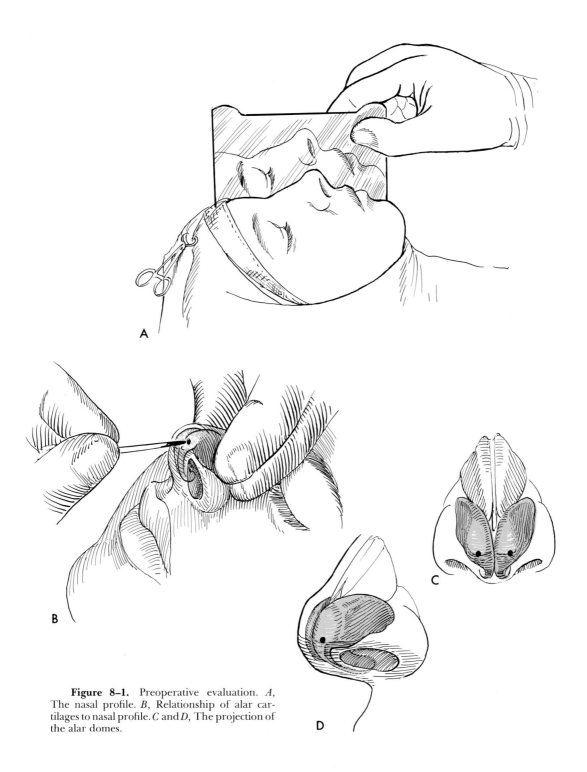

Figure 8–1. Preoperative evaluation. *A,* The nasal profile. *B,* Relationship of alar cartilages to nasal profile. *C* and *D,* The projection of the alar domes.

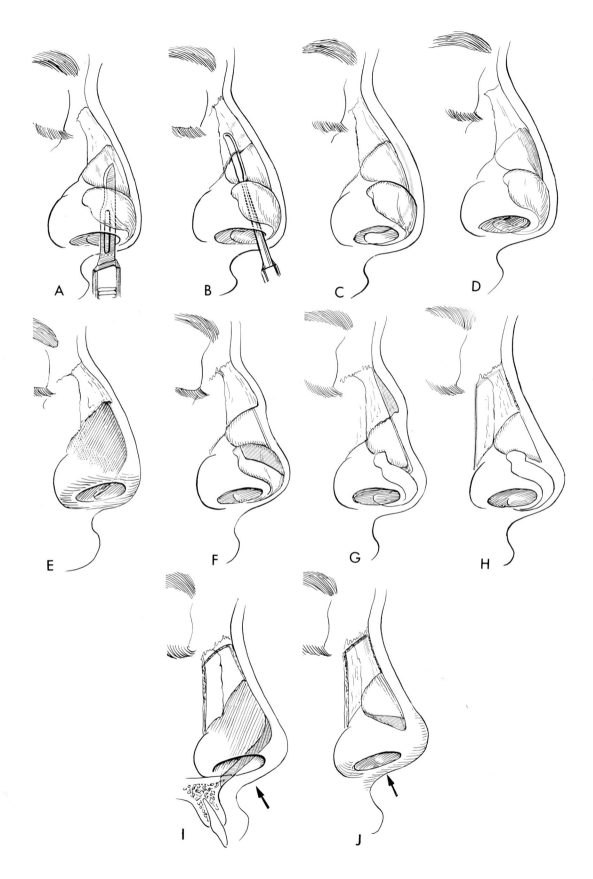

Figure 8-2. *See legend on the opposite page.*

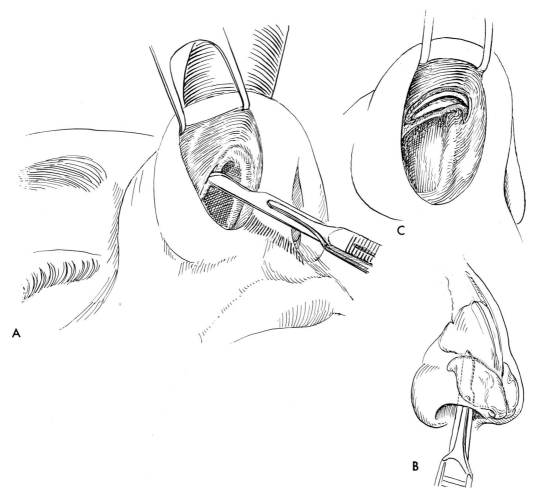

Figure 8–3. *A,* With the nostrils retracted by double-pronged retractor and under direct vision, a #15 blade is inserted into the intercartilaginous groove at its lateral extremities and carried forward toward the dorsum between the lower margin of the upper lateral cartilage and the upper border of the lateral crus of the alar cartilage. An optional incision preferred by some surgeons, such as Millard (1965) and Pitanguy (1965), is to proceed directly with an intracartilaginous incision into the lining of the lateral crus, which will mark approximately the cephalic level of resection of the redundant cartilage.

B, As the intercartilaginous incision is carried toward the septal angle, where it will be extended into the membranous septum, the knife blade is angulated more deeply and the dissection is continued in a plane just superficial to the lateral surface of the upper lateral cartilages.

C, The incision gapes slightly, showing the edges of the cartilages.

Figure 8–2. *A,* Intercartilaginous incision and raising of the soft tissues from the upper lateral cartilages.

B, Raising the periosteum from the nasal bones.

C, Transfixion incision, which may be complete or incomplete.

D, Modification of the dorsal borders of the upper lateral cartilages.

E, Modification of the dorsal border of the nasal septum in its cartilaginous portion.

F, Resection of part of the lateral crura of the alar cartilages in the nasal tip plasty.

G, Modification of the osseous dorsal border.

H, Lateral osteotomy and in- or outfracturing procedure.

I, Shortening of the caudal border of the cartilaginous septum, with or without modification of the nasal spine.

J, Shortening of the caudal borders of the upper lateral cartilages.

See illustration on the opposite page.

the hump before the tip. At other times, conditions warrant a reversal of these steps.

The traditional first incision in the rhinoplasty operation is separation of the covering tissues from the underlying osteocartilaginous framework. It is made in the clearly visible groove formed by the overlapping of the upper lateral cartilages with the alar cartilages (Figure 8–3). The tissues are then raised (Figure 8–4). Elevation of the periosteum is shown in detail in Figure 8–5.

Some surgeons attempt to incise the periosteum at the lateral extremity of the planned hump removal and to sweep both periosteum and soft tissues toward the midline in the belief that the periosteum will be removed along with the nasal hump. Whether this maneuver is truly effective is

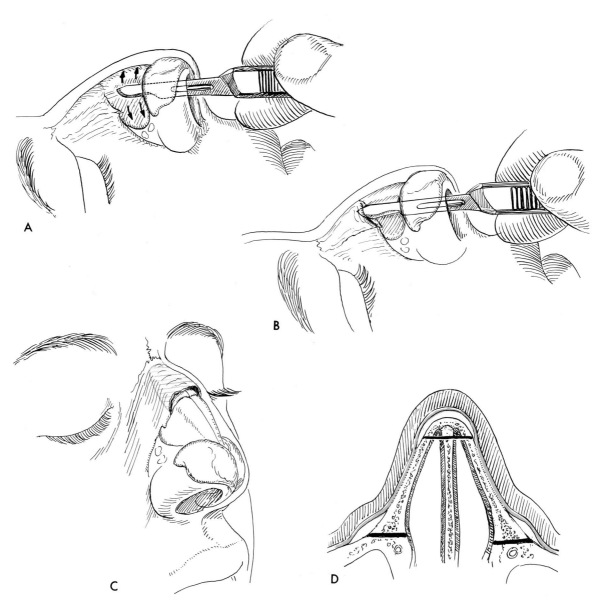

Figure 8–4. *A,* The intercartilaginous incisions on either side are joined by a sweeping motion of the #15 blade, with great care being taken not to injure the dermis, which can result in subdermal scarring with contour defects such as pits and depressions of the skin postoperatively. The soft tissues are elevated over the lateral cartilages. A Joseph's double-edged knife may also be used for this maneuver.

B, The subcutaneous sharp dissection is carried to the inferior borders of the nasal bones, where the periosteum is incised to allow penetration of the periosteal dissector.

C, The periosteum is elevated.

D, The horizontal dark lines indicate the proposed level of hump removal and lateral osteotomy. The lateral osteotomy is planned in the thicker portions of the frontal process of the maxilla.

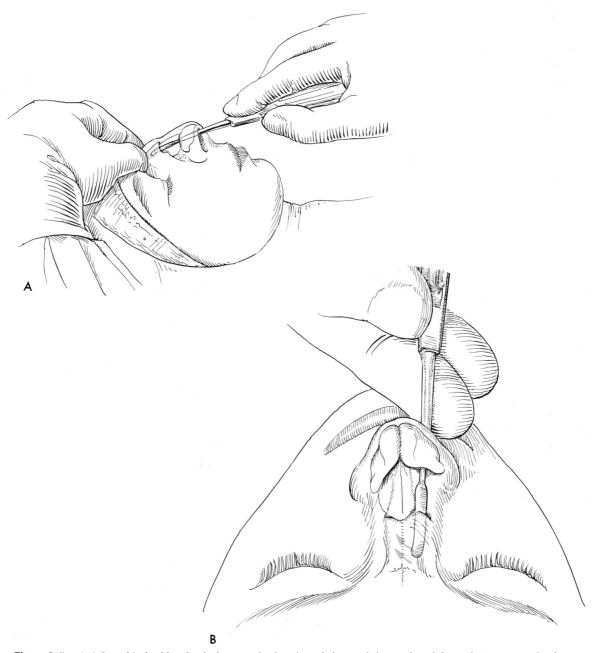

Figure 8–5. *A,* A Joseph's double-edged, sharpened subperiosteal elevator is inserted, and the periosteum over the dorsum of the nose as high as the nasofrontal bone is scored. This dissection is also accomplished by a sweeping motion from side to side since the elevator is sharpened on both its lateral edges.

B, Care must be taken not to perforate the dorsum of the skin while elevating the periosteum. The elevator should be kept parallel to the midline of the nose during this maneuver. It must be appreciated, as has been shown in anatomical studies by Broadbent and others, that a clean elevation of the periosteum over the dorsum is rarely accomplished; rather, the periosteum is more often than not shredded and disrupted since it is thin and extremely adherent to the underlying nasal bone.

difficult to know, particularly in the small hump excision where small amounts of tissue are removed. However, when the hump is large, it would seem well worth the effort. In any event, attempts at subperiosteal dissection insure maximal soft tissue preservation of the skin.

It is important to elevate the soft tissues over the hump only to the lateral limits of the planned hump excision (see Figure 8–46). The nasal bone plates are best left attached to the periosteum and skin in the event of inadvertent comminution during lateral osteotomy, in which case they could easily fall into the nasal vault and result in a disruption of the dorsum with saddling (see Figure 8–17). The method for undermining the soft tissues of the nose is illustrated in Figures 8–6 and 8–7.

With the nose thus skeletonized, there are a number of options available to the surgeon as to the sequence of operative steps. Some prefer to proceed by lowering the bony profile of the nose. Separation of the upper lateral cartilages from the septum is deferred by some surgeons but advocated by others. The technique of submucosal dissection is shown in Figure 8–8.

The author believes that separation of the upper lateral cartilage from the septum is an important step in the operative procedure and should follow skeletonizing the nose before any further direct surgical attack is made on the osteocartilaginous structures. Careful separation of the cartilages flush with the septum, and meticulous reconstruction of the internal valve (the triangle formed by the upper lateral cartilages and septum) rarely presents a problem unless excessive cartilage and mucosa were removed, in which case a web can form.

Once the upper lateral cartilage has been freed from the septum, the surgeon must determine the order of the rest of the operative procedure. Possible choices are hump removal, tip plasty, lateral osteotomies, or correction of septal deflection. Even in the hands of the expert operator, a change in the sequence may produce a significantly different result. Lipsett (1959) has emphasized that at times, a smaller amount of dorsal hump can be removed if the septum has first been shortened — an important consideration in any patient with a minimal hump deformity and a drooping nasal tip.

If the caudal margin of the septum is prominent so that the tip is encroached upon or the columella is displaced inferiorly or laterally, it is best trimmed at this time. The design of the excision of the caudal margin varies, depending on the deformity and on the extent of desired elevation of the nasal tip. To the novice, it cannot be overemphasized that this excision must always be conservative. Always underestimate the cartilage to be excised and later, in the terminal stages of the operation, adjust the cartilage to the new nasal contour. The short, chopped-off nose or the retracted columella that may result from excessive resection of the caudal border of the nasal septum is at best difficult to repair and quite frequently impossible to improve.

When both the caudal border of the septum — at its point of junction with the nasal spine — and the nasal spine itself project into the columella-lip angle, the lip appears foreshortened or tethered. This deformity may be further aggravated by the presence of a large dorsal hump. Resection of the caudal border of the septum together with the hump promotes relaxation and an apparent lengthening of the lip. If the nasal tip is to be elevated significantly, a triangular resection is done, with the base of the triangle at the septal angle. Where the lip is to be released with no or minimal elevation of the nasal tip, the triangle segment to be resected is reversed, the base lying at the nasal spine, which is resected at this time. By combining these resections, the operator may correct a variety of deformities in this region.

The decision whether to proceed with hump removal or tip remodeling from this point depends to a great extent on which of these two structures dominates the nasal deformity. On rare occasions, it is necessary to modify only the nasal tip, without osteotomy or hump resection. This is not a common situation, and some modification of the bony structure is usually necessary. The surgeon should look most critically at the result of a tip modification before deciding that no changes are necessary in the nasal framework (Figure 8–9).

Reduction of the nasal dorsum (hump) after skeletonization of the nose is the first logical sequential step in the operation. However, overresection with excessive removal of bone and cartilage results in exaggerated retroussé or even saddle nose deformity; therefore, correction of the tip deformity is often accomplished prior to hump removal. This provides a more accurate assessment of the amount of septal hump removal required. Whether the bony dorsum is reduced by rasp, osteotome, or saw is of little consequence in experienced hands; however, it cannot be overemphasized that, in the author's opinion, reduction of the hump with sharp cutting rasps or finely honed osteotomes is both easier to master and more accurate than the more inexact saw technique. Reduction of the nasal profile (the osteocartilaginous vault) is discussed in some detail in the following section.

Text continued on page 132.

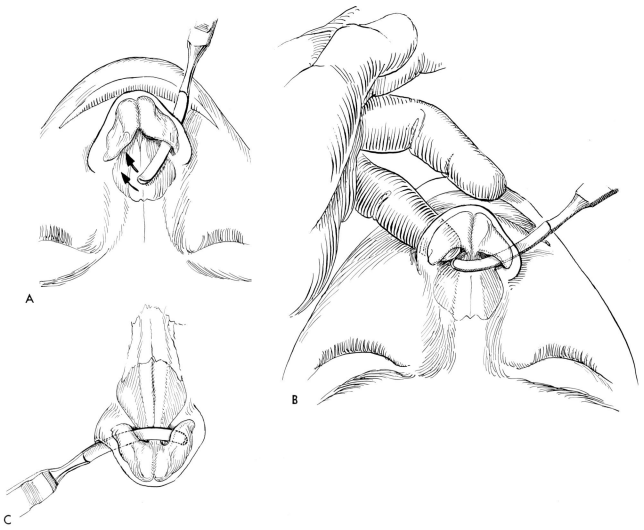

Figure 8–6. *A,* A semi-curved transfixion (button) knife is introduced through the intracartilaginous incision on either side and swept over the dorsum of the septum toward the septal angle, where it is angled downward, hugging the caudal margin of the septum and severing the few remaining soft tissue attachments of the nasal coverings to the nasal structure.

B, Guiding the transfixion knife over the septal angle is facilitated by gentle upward pressure on the ala by the operator's little finger. If undue force is exerted at this point, it is not difficult to incise completely through the columella. A Rethi incision is acceptable in some patients when especially planned, but is not acceptable if accidental.

C, As the transfixion knife reaches the septal angle and is angled toward the nasal spine, the dull (convex) border of the knife should hug the edge of the cartilage to preserve as much membranous septum as possible. Experience will aid the operator in attaining this tactile sense.

Illustration continued on the following page.

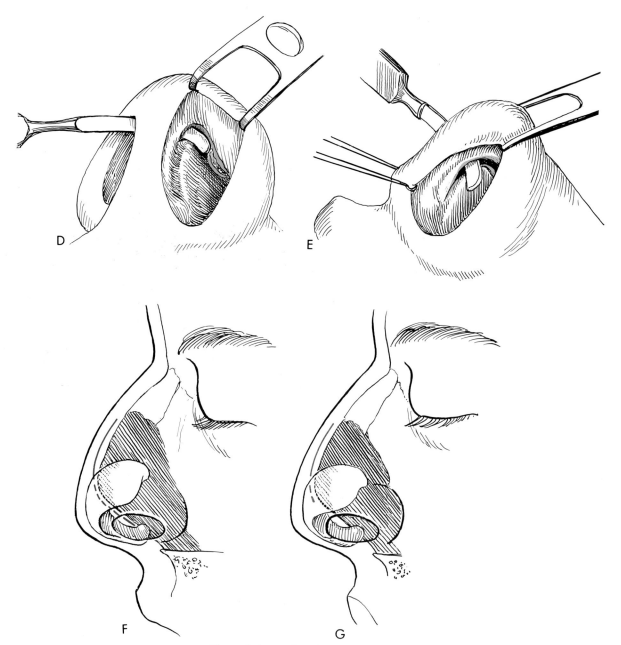

Figure 8–6. *See legend on the opposite page.*

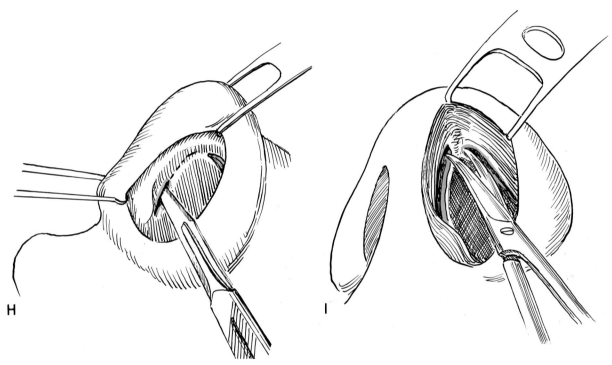

H

I

Figure 8–6 *Continued.* *D* and *E,* Preservation of the soft tissues of the columella and membranous septum is facilitated by retracting the nasal tip with a double-pronged retractor and inserting two hooks on either side of the base of the columella, exerting downward traction, putting the membranous septum on a stretch.

Completion of the transfixion incision provides mobility of the tip during the operative procedure.

F, The line in red indicates the soft tissue undermining.

G, H, and *I,* Soft tissue undermining can stop just short of the septal angle, facilitating use of an alternate transfixion incision made in the membranous septum with a #11 blade. The stab wound is extended in a cephalic direction, where the remaining soft tissue connections are severed with scissors.

Figure 8–7.   *A,* The membranous septum incised and the completed transfixion incision inspected.

B, A periosteal elevator is passed along the nasal dorsum to verify its freedom from attachment to underlying tissues and the completeness of the transfixion incision.

C, The nasal tip is dislocated from its normal position and the prominence of the dorsal border of the nasal septum and nasal bones is brought into view.

The question of whether to do a complete or an incomplete transfixion incision is frequently raised. In the majority of cases, a complete transfixion incision is preferred, as this frees the soft tissues from the nasal skeleton and permits much more complete exposure of the nasal dorsum. A complete transfixion incision is of further benefit in mobilization of the tip so that the alar cartilages may be more easily manipulated during the operative procedure and surgical access to the nasal spine and septum is gained.

It has been argued that a complete transfixion incision should not be made because healing of the wound will result in straight-line contracture, pulling the tip inferiorly. In practice, however, this theoretical problem does not overcome the excellent mobility achieved by completing the incision, and it has not proved to be an undesirable feature.

See illustration on the opposite page.

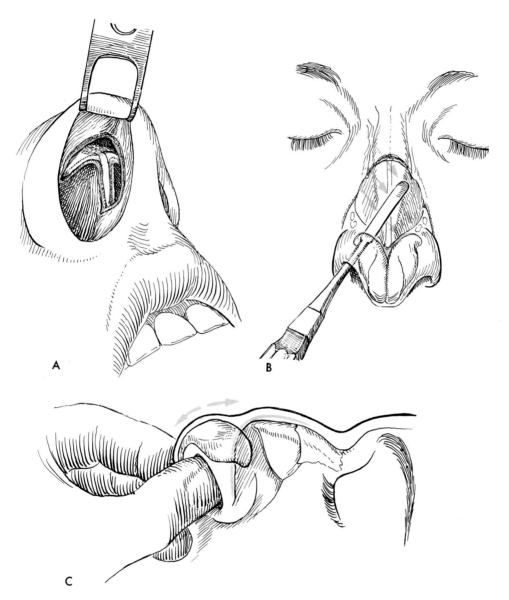

Figure 8–7. *See legend on the opposite page.*

Figure 8–8.   Jost, Anderson, Pollett and others advocate a submucosal dissection of the lower lateral cartilages and septum. They reason that by such a technique there is less likelihood of scarring of the mucosa, with synechia, distortion, and airway disturbances.

A, An incision is made just through the cephalic portion of the alar cartilage near its overlap with the upper lateral cartilage.

B, The incision is indicated.

C, After the transfixation incision is made, the mucoperichondrial flap is elevated from the septal border.

D, The dissection is continued toward the junction with the upper lateral cartilages and the septum.

E, The mucoperichondrial flap is dissected from beneath the inferior margin and surface of the upper lateral cartilages.

F, The conjoint flap is reflected into the nasal cavity on either side, leaving the bare cartilage support-free for adjustment as required.

G, The upper lateral cartilages are incised, and the septum can also be trimmed, all without disturbing the mucosa, which is intact.

The technique is appealing in that it preserves lining; however, the operative time is increased, and sometimes elevation of the flaps is not easy and may be associated with considerable bleeding.

See illustration on the opposite page.

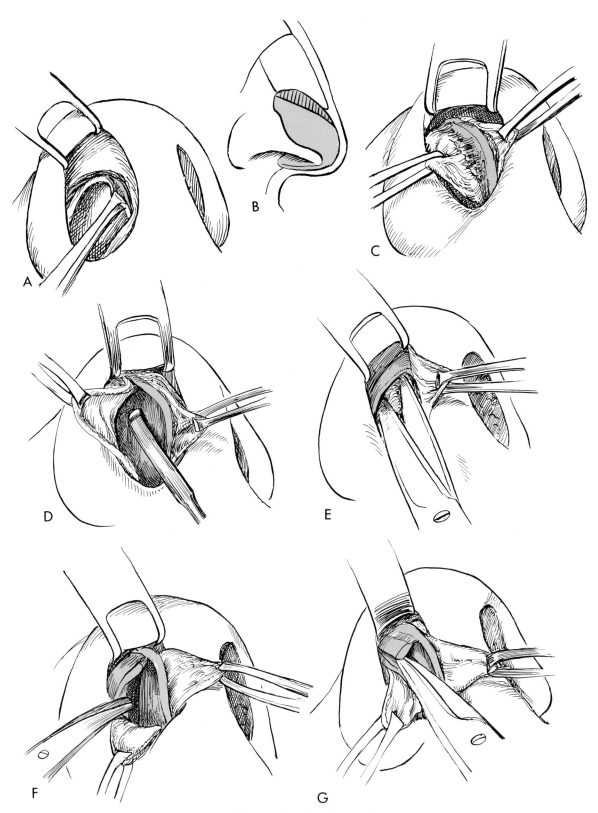

Figure 8–8. *See legend on the opposite page.*

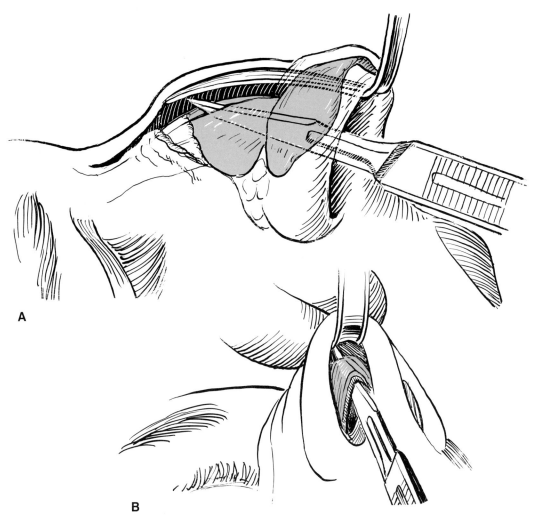

A

B

Figure 8–9.   Minimal or small humps are mostly cartilaginous. *A, B,* The upper lateral cartilages are cut free from the septum (flush) with a # 11 blade.

Illustration continued on the opposite page.

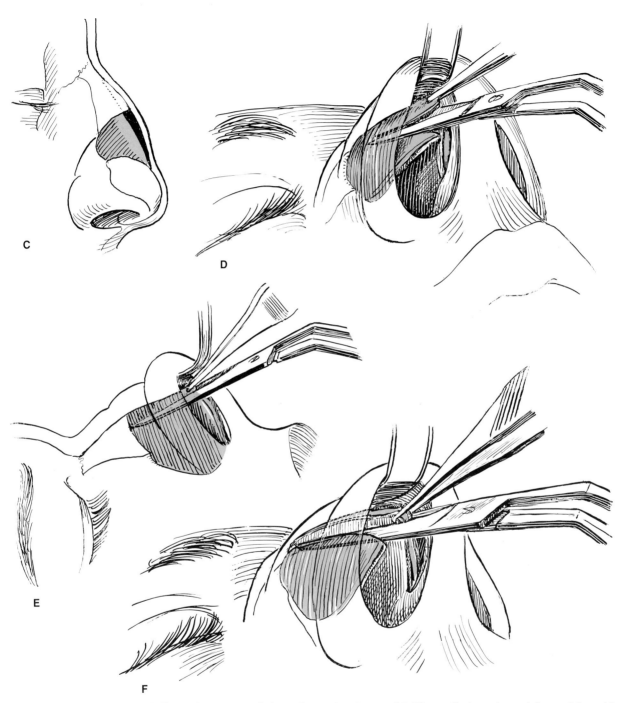

Figure 8–9 *Continued.   C* indicates the amount of planned resection. *D, E,* and *F,* The cartilaginous hump is lowered first with sharp angled scissors.

Illustration continued on the following page.

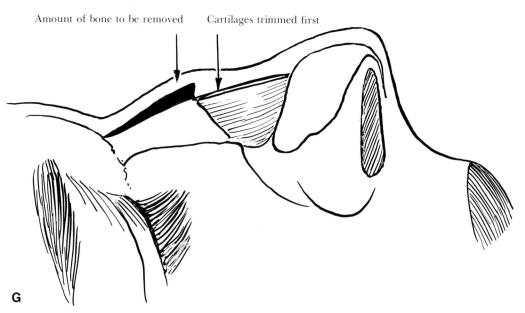

Amount of bone to be removed   Cartilages trimmed first

G

Figure 8–9 *Continued.*   *G*, The amount of bony hump to be removed is now clearly seen in bas relief. At this point, the tip and lower nose are usually remodeled before final reduction of the bony hump.

Illustration continued on the opposite page.

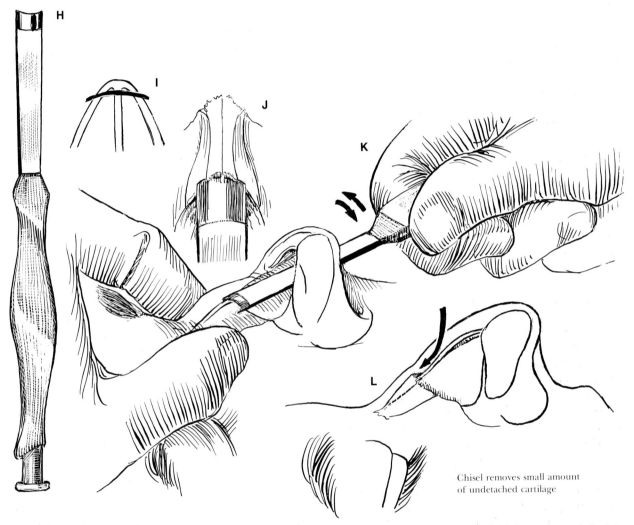

Chisel removes small amount
of undetached cartilage

Figure 8–9 *Continued.* *H–L,* The minimal bony hump is removed with the manually controlled chisel. Precise control of the depth of the cut is thereby maintained by varying the angulation.

REDUCTION OF THE PROFILE

The author prefers a sharp osteotome for resection of the nasal hump because it is usually possible to be more accurate with one. The osteotome can be angled quite exactly to fit the requirements of each operation; it is especially useful in deepening the nasofrontal angle. Use of the saw is particularly difficult in removing a small hump. The surgeon tends to turn the saw too far in order to gain purchase on the bone, and all too frequently, excessive bone removal is the result.

A further advantage to the osteotome is that a cleaner cut is produced with less dust and less soft tissue debris in the wound. This debris can serve as a focus of infection. Of course, it is equally important for such debris to be removed following rasping to smooth the cuts of the osteotome.

Deepening the nasofrontal angle may be desirable after hump removal, but it is an extremely difficult feat because of the thickness of bone and shortage of skin in the region of the nasal root. Aufricht (1943) emphasized the importance of considering the nasofrontal angle in relation to the profile before completing the hump removal. He recommended that if the radix nasi is tangential to the frontosubnasal line, the angle be left undisturbed. If it lies in front of that line, a deepening of the radix is desirable.

After removal of the nasal hump, it is usually necessary to adjust the dorsal borders of the septum and the upper lateral cartilages to the new nasal bone profile line (Figure 8–9). The cartilages are trimmed with sharp septal scissors; the Taylor dural scissors with serrated edges are excellent for this purpose. Irregularities of the bony dorsum are rasped, and a further minor reduction of the height of the dorsum may be gained by this rasping (Figure 8–10). It is usually not desirable to reduce the hump directly by rasping unless it is quite small. However, once the operator has gained experience with the use of osteotomes, small humps are better managed by careful shaving with a very sharp McIndoe type of chisel controlled by manual pressure (Figure 8–11). By this means, the bony dorsum can be decorticated, and only a minimum of tissue will be left to be removed by the rasp.

Removal of the dorsal hump does not, and indeed should not necessarily, result in an open bony defect extending to the root of the nose. As will be demonstrated later in this section, it is often preferable to maintain the roof over the root of the nose and the cephalic portion of the bony hump and purposefully to produce only a narrowing infracture of the Greenstick type whenever possible.

The architecture of the root of the nose is thereby maintained. In very large bony humps that require considerable reduction, an open roof is unavoidable. Sometimes, in such large humps, a web of bone remains at the apex of the dorsal aperture that blocks adequate infracture. In such cases, a sharp osteotome or biting forceps can be used to remove the bony web. Superior osteotomies are also advantageous in such wide nasal roots to promote a clean infracture.

Piecemeal rasping of the bony hump with sharp rasps followed by excision of the redundant dorsal septum and upper lateral cartilages is an alternative but excellent technique for profile reductions (Figure 8–12).

MINIMAL RHINOPLASTY

The subtle or minimal rhinoplasty is an operation done to correct such minor problems as a very small hump, slight widening, or minimal deformities of the alar cartilages, caudal septum, or columella. Such irregularities can be quite distressing to some patients whose complaints assume proportions that at first examination seem quite unrealistic.

Such patients should not be refused surgery before a thorough history, physical examination, and photographic study have been completed. Careful study of the photographs with these patients and inquiries about their aspirations will often make clear to the surgeon that the patient has a real problem and that there is a realistic approach to its solution.

Minimal surgery requires considerable experience and a gentle touch. Even when the surgeon possesses these qualities, the results still may not be entirely satisfactory. Because it is never possible to predict the final result of rhinoplasty, it is vital that patients be fully informed of this factor of uncertainty.

However, many minimal rhinoplasties produce gratifying results, although the physical change accomplished is small. A minor revision in the appearance of the nose can effect a great change in the patient's overall facial appearance — a point of particular importance to those who must work before the camera's critical eye.

Minimal rhinoplasties must be carefully planned to meet the requirements of each patient. Often, a small readjustment or excision of alar cartilage is all that is required, or a minor dorsal modification may accomplish the desired correction. However, in most patients, the entire rhinoplasty operation must be done, but with particu-

Text continued on page 139.

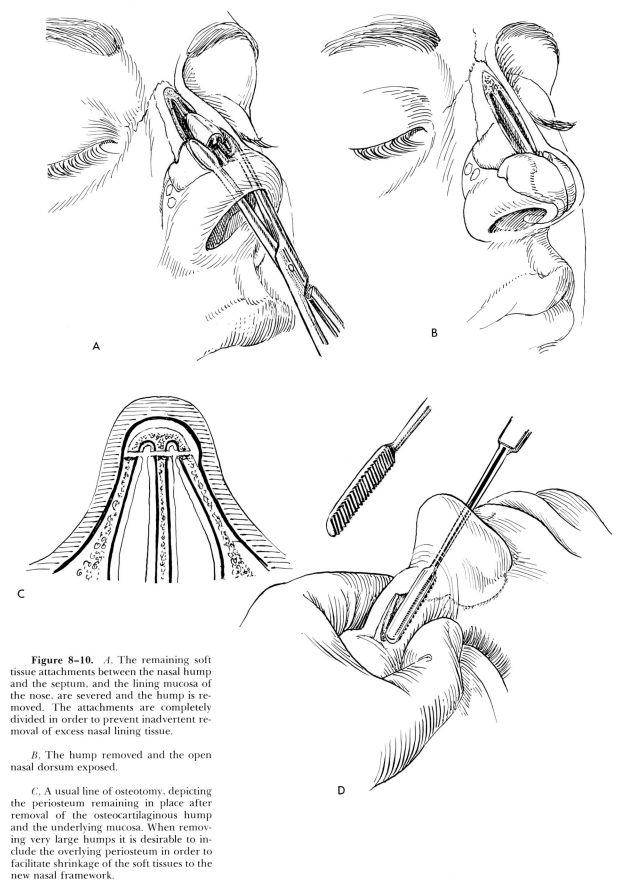

Figure 8–10. *A*, The remaining soft tissue attachments between the nasal hump and the septum, and the lining mucosa of the nose, are severed and the hump is removed. The attachments are completely divided in order to prevent inadvertent removal of excess nasal lining tissue.

B, The hump removed and the open nasal dorsum exposed.

C, A usual line of osteotomy, depicting the periosteum remaining in place after removal of the osteocartilaginous hump and the underlying mucosa. When removing very large humps it is desirable to include the overlying periosteum in order to facilitate shrinkage of the soft tissues to the new nasal framework.

D, Irregular bony surfaces are smoothed with a rasp; the sharp edges are rounded to simulate the normal convexity.

Figure 8–11.   Removal of the osseous hump after reduction of the cartilaginous profile.

A, The Cottle osteotome, which has gently curved edges that make it more difficult to penetrate the overlying skin.

B, The Cinelli osteotome; two guarded prongs protect the skin.

C, The McInode-Cinelli chisel, whose rounded corners protect the overlying skin. The advantage of the osteotome over the chisel is that the direction of the cut can be changed without withdrawing it and reinserting it in a different direction.

D, The portion of the nasal hump to be resected.

E, The Cottle osteotome placed in contact with and along the line of the resected dorsal border of the septum.

F, The osteotome is gently tapped in to resect the osseous hump.

See illustration on the opposite page.

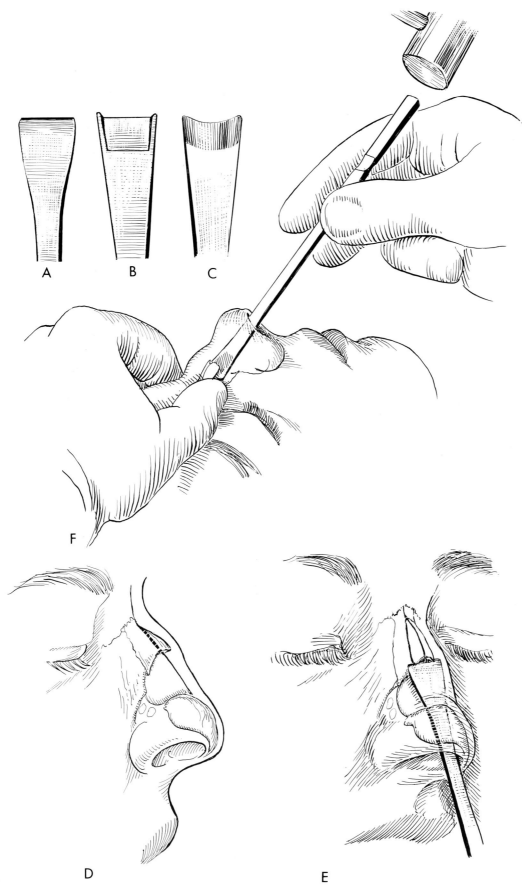

A   B   C

F

D   E

Figure 8–11. *See legend on the opposite page.*

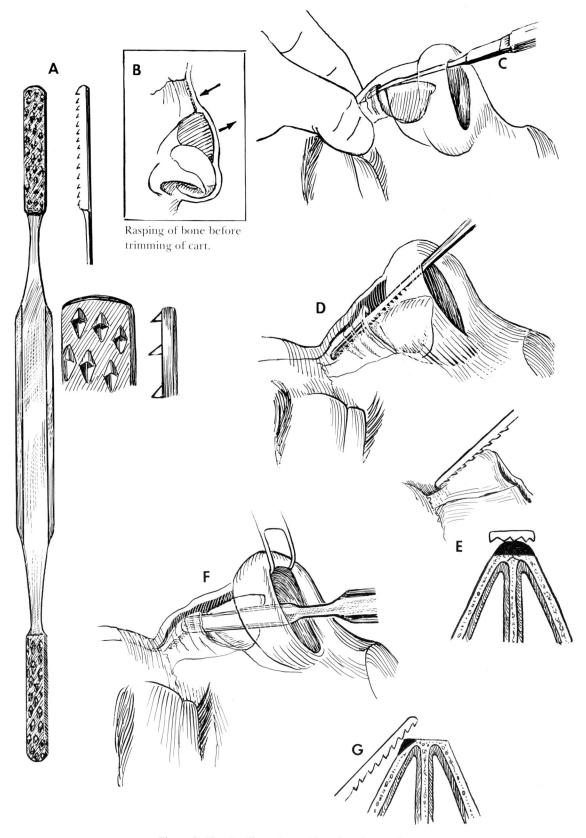

A

B

Rasping of bone before
trimming of cart.

C

D

E

F

G

Figure 8–12. *See illustration and legend on the opposite page.*

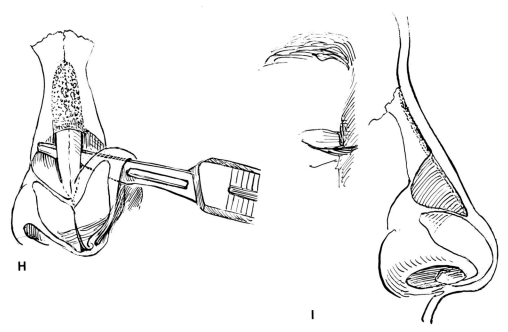

H

I

Figure 8–12.   Another excellent and accurate method of piecemeal hump resection championed by Sheen insures a conservative result by first rasping the bone and subsequently trimming the cartilaginous dorsum with a blunted scalpel blade. This technique attains the same ends as that shown in Figure 8–9, but the order of steps is simply reversed.

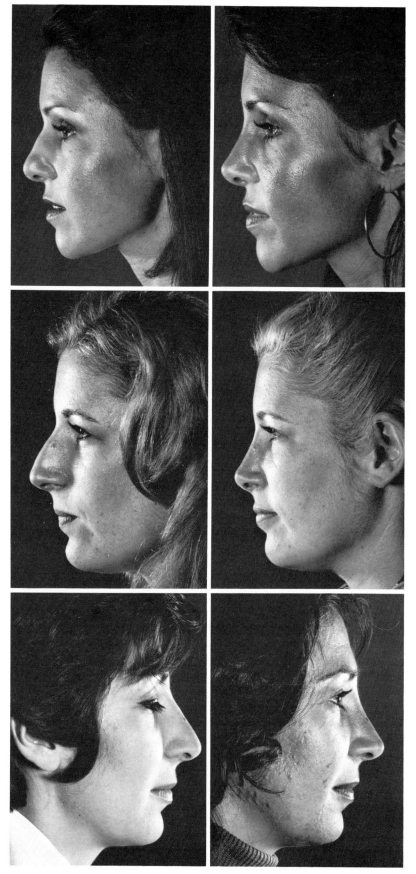

Figure 8–13.

lar emphasis on removal of minimal amounts of tissue. It is in such patients that only those most expert in the use of a saw should attempt to resect a dorsal hump by this method, and it is here that I prefer to use only the sharpest of osteotomes and chisels to remove fine slivers of bone and cartilage. The McIndoe hand-held chisel is excellent for this purpose.

When the surgeon prefers a rasp as his instrument of choice, the bony hump is first rasped away, followed by lowering the cartilaginous portion of the hump with either a small scalpel or right-angled scissors that are curved on the flat (see Figure 8–11).

When removing such small pieces of bone or cartilage, the angle at which the chisel or osteotome is directed is of utmost importance. Chisels may not be redirected once the cut is started; they must be completely withdrawn and a new cut

begun. The osteotome, however, may be shifted slightly by raising or lowering the handle, and until one becomes experienced, it is the safer of the two instruments. If a mallet is used, only light taps should be delivered in order to guard against a sudden, unplanned dip of the sharp instrument into the nasal dorsum.

On occasion, a lateral osteotomy with a 2- or 3-mm osteotome and infracture may result in sufficient narrowing of the nose without disrupting the dorsum. When there is doubt about the wisdom of this procedure, the surgeon should resort to medial osteotomy without dorsal resection, followed by lateral osteotomy.

The photographs of patients in Figure 8–13 demonstrate the principle of minimal or conservative rhinoplasty with careful lowering of the osteocartilaginous profile by osteotome or rasp and corresponding adjustments of the lobule.

Text continued on page 144.

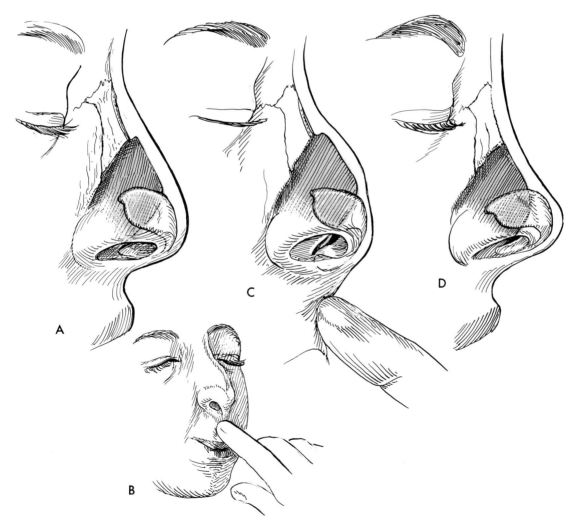

Figure 8–14. *A,* An estimate is made of the amount of excess cartilage by inferior traction of the upper lip by the surgeon's finger *(B).* The dorsal border of the septum is brought into prominence *(C),* and the nasal tip cartilages are dislocated from the septal angle. *D,* New profile line established.

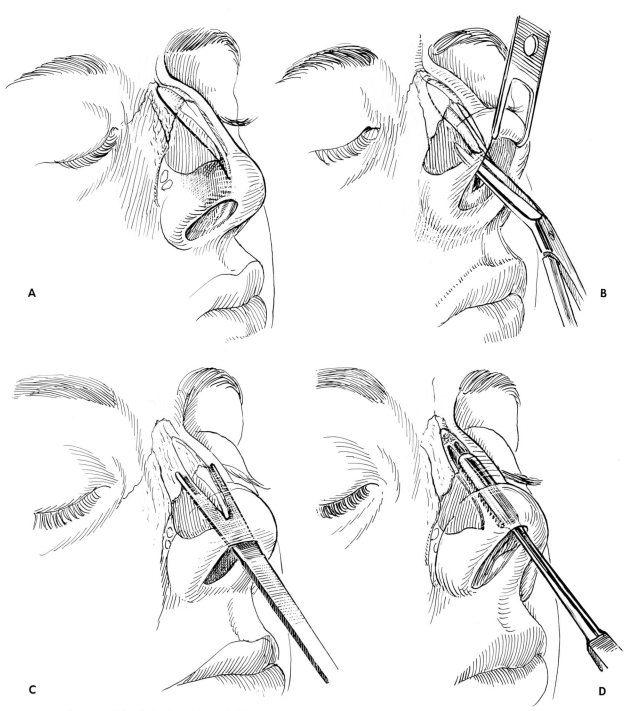

Figure 8–15. *A,* The desired excision is indicated by the solid line.

B, The excision is begun by preliminary cuts in the cartilaginous hump. This must be *conservatively* estimated. If the cartilage reduction is insufficient, more can be removed later in the procedure, but if too much is removed, the dorsum must be augmented by free graft replacement.

C, The osteotome is introduced and the excision accomplished.

D, Rough edges are rasped.

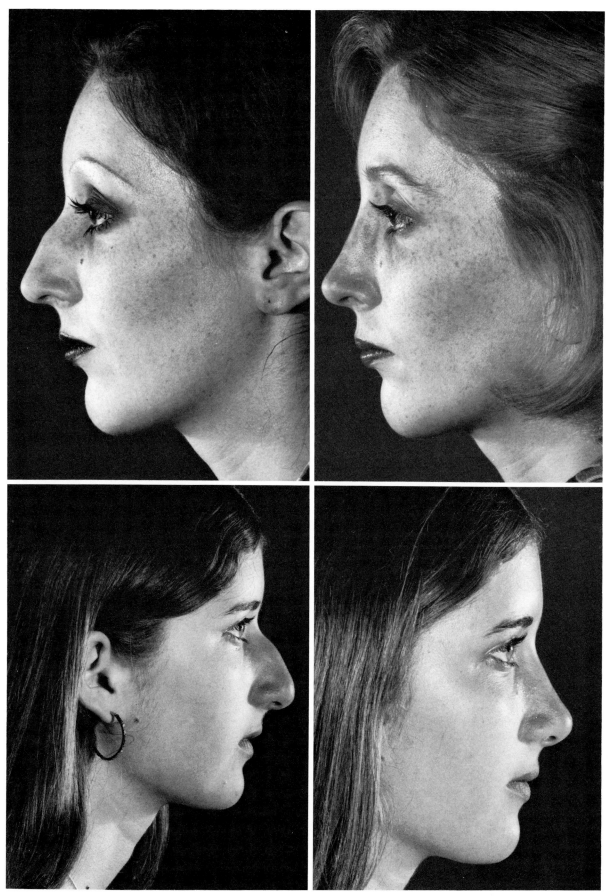

Figure 8–16.

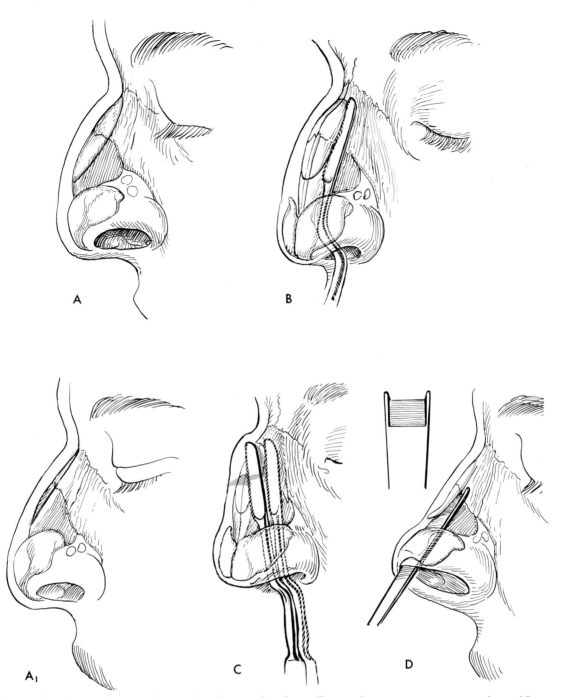

Figure 8–17. *The saw technique. A,* in a very large hump such as the one illustrated, a saw or an osteotome can be used for removal. The osteotome is particularly useful when the nasion is quite deep. The solid line represents the desired resection of the nasal dorsum.

A₁, In a small dorsal hump, the line of excision desired is indicated by the solid line.

B, The nasal saw should be introduced so that the blade lies flat and at almost a right angle to the underlying nasal bone. Care must be taken to maintain the saw at this exact angle while performing the osteotomy. It is best to gain purchase at the uppermost portion of the hump near the base of the nasion.

C, If the operator does not maintain the saw at exactly the right angle and with control, it is difficult to gain accurate purchase to begin the osteotome, and the saw tends to slip over the dorsum of the hump.

D, When the amount of reduction desired is minimal, it is easy to see that an osteotome is to be preferred because of the exact control it affords. In this instance, an inexperienced operator using a saw could easily create a saddle deformity by failing to accurately control the angle of the saw cut. Some surgeons prefer to begin the initial cut in the bone with a saw, then finish with a sharp osteotome.

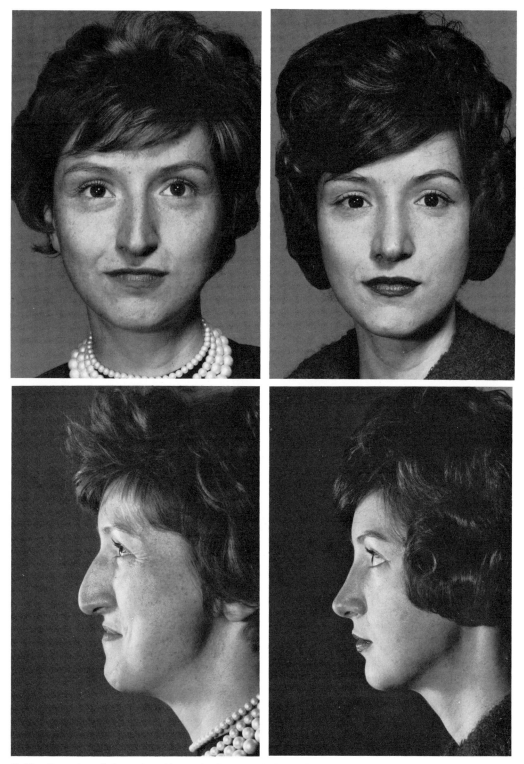

Figure 8–18.   Resection of a large dorsal hump by the saw technique. Tip elevation and lengthening of the upper lip were carried out after correction of the hump. A saw can be used for such large humps with little danger of excessive resection of bone and cartilage. The entire redundant osteocartilaginous dorsum can be removed in one piece.

When the bony hump is removed first by either rasp or chisel, the cartilaginous component of the hump projects forward and is brought into sharp focus. It is now understood by most surgeons that the cartilaginous hump is usually the largest component of the raised profile and in fact overshadows the bone. The recent trend toward conservatism in bony removal represents this clearer understanding of nasal anatomy.

The "trick" illustrated in Figure 8–14 is most helpful to the surgeon in estimating the amount of dorsal cartilage to resect after removal of the bony hump. It is also exceedingly helpful as a final step in the operation to determine if the dorsal septum has been lowered sufficiently. It is generally better to overcorrect the lower septum slightly in order to help avoid postoperative supratip swelling.

In addition to looking for obvious dorsal irregularities, the surgeon can often detect invisible ones by gently passing his finger along the dorsum from the nasofrontal angle to the septal angle. Inspection is aided by using an Aufricht retractor, which enables one to determine whether the excess of dorsum is due to the septum alone or involves the medial borders of the upper lateral cartilages. The addition of fiberoptic lighting to the Aufricht retractor has facilitated this procedure.

REDUCTION OF THE LARGE HUMP

Unquestionably, reduction of the large hump nose deformity poses less of a problem for the surgeon than does correction of the minimal hump. Nevertheless, one of the cardinal sins of rhinoplasty is excessive hump removal and the production of a beak-like deformity with excessive retroussé and saddling of the nasal dorsum. The key to accurate reduction is careful preoperative planning. The novice surgeon may find it helpful to draw external lines on the nose with marking solution to indicate the level of proposed hump removal prior to beginning the operation.

Reduction of the large hump lends itself to either piecemeal resection of the dorsal septum, upper lateral cartilages, and bone or removal of the entire osteocartilaginous hump en bloc.

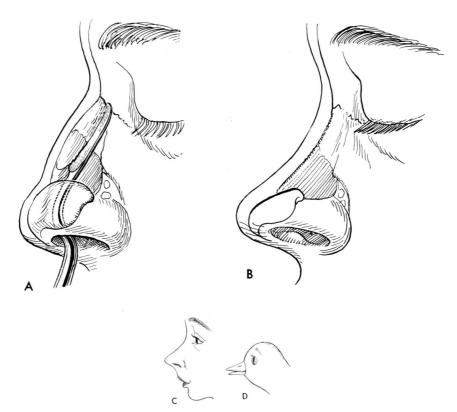

Figure 8–19. *A,* Resection of the osteocartilaginous hump in continuity by the nasal saw. With this technique the upper lateral cartilages are not detached from the nasal septum but are removed in continuity with the osseous hump.

B, Great care must be exercised in the use of the nasal saw, since it is easy for inexpert hands to remove too much of the nasal dorsum, as in this drawing.

C and *D,* Removal of excess nasal dorsum produces a so-called "birdlike" deformity.

Hump Removal En Bloc

En bloc resection of the osteocartilaginous dorsum in continuity with a sharp osteotome is shown in Figure 8–15. Great care must be taken not to angulate the osteotome too deeply toward the root of the nose in order to avoid excessive removal of bone or angulation thereof from side to side. Following all methods of hump removal, it is best to rasp away any small remaining spicules of bone or cartilage that may result ultimately in small, palpable, or unsightly irregularities in the nasal profile.

Strong dorsal humps, such as those shown in Figure 8–16, lends themselves well to en bloc removal with an osteotome.

The Saw Technique

The classical method of removal of a large dorsal hump with the Joseph saw is still preferred by many surgeons (Figure 8–17). When performed expertly, this technique produces acceptable results (Figures 8–18, 8–19, 8–20).

Humps that are mostly cartilaginous and thus involve the lower third of the nose primarily are best removed after tip plasty and in a most conservative fashion. Conversely, humps that are mainly osseous and involve the upper portion of the nose can be removed before tip plasty, when it is much easier to judge how much dorsum to remove.

Hump Replacement (Skoog)

Skoog (1974) advocated replacement of large osteocartilaginous humps in most patients with significant hump deformities (Figure 8–21). He believed that a more natural, rounded dorsum was provided by such a technique and that many of the objectionable features of hump removal such as irregular edges, asymmetry, postoperative lateral drifting of the nasal bones, and the "open roof syndrome" were avoided.

Repeated experience with such free grafts of dorsum indicate that they are almost uniformly successful. The graft is ideal and the bed is ideal — like to like. Such a technique should be used without hesitation during primary surgery if the surgeon removed too much hump or in cases such as the one in Figure 8–22 if he wishes to "slide" the hump to a new position. In this patient (Figure

Text continued on page 153.

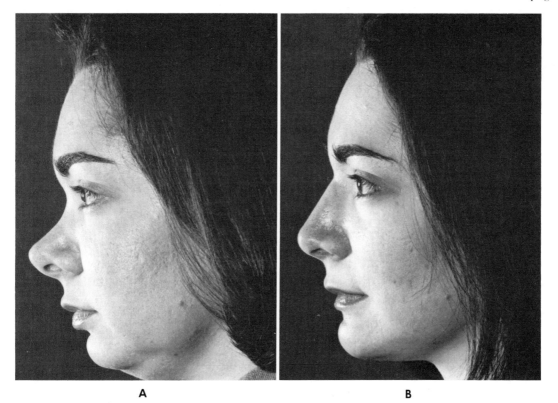

A   **B**

Figure 8–20. *A,* In this patient, too much of the dorsum was removed by the saw technique. The surgeon either did not recognize his mistake or did not know how to correct it. A severe saddle nose deformity was the result. When too much hump is inadvertently removed by saw or osteotome, it should be trimmed and reinserted to provide a dorsal substance. Skoog advocates such hump replacement in most cases.

B, The saddle nose deformity was repaired with an autogenous iliac bone graft (Dr. C. Guy).

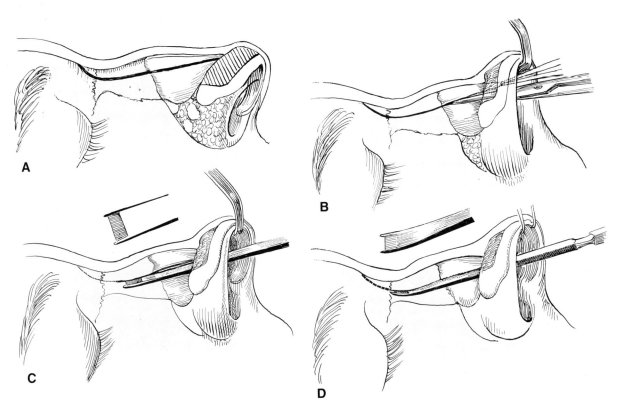

Figure 8–21.   *The Skoog Technique.*   *A,* The line of resection of the osteocartilaginous hump is indicated by the solid line. Note that it extends well up into the thick bone of the nasal root.

B, The initial cut into the upper lateral cartilages and the septal dorsum is made with an angled scissor and is similar to the standard osteotome technique.

C, The osteotome or chisel is inserted and driven toward the nasal root.

D, At the root of the nose, Skoog introduced a curved osteotome to gouge out the thick bone of this region.

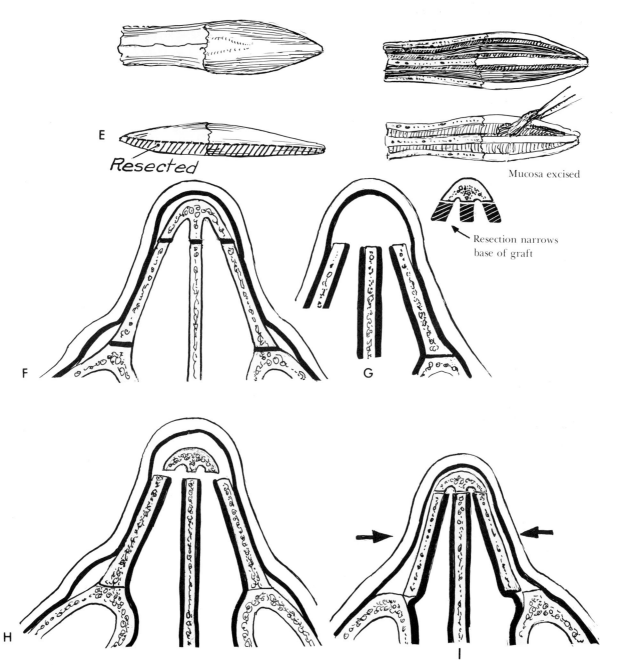

Mucosa excised

Resection narrows
base of graft

Figure 8–21 *Continued. E,* The grafts trimmed of all mucosa and cut down in size to reduce the dorsum appropriately.

F and *G,* The soft tissues are initially elevated only sufficiently to conform to the amount of dorsum to be resected, which is shown here in coronal section.

H, The reduced graft is inserted into the dorsal pocket.

I, The soft tissue flap is undermined sufficiently to fit snugly around the reinserted graft.

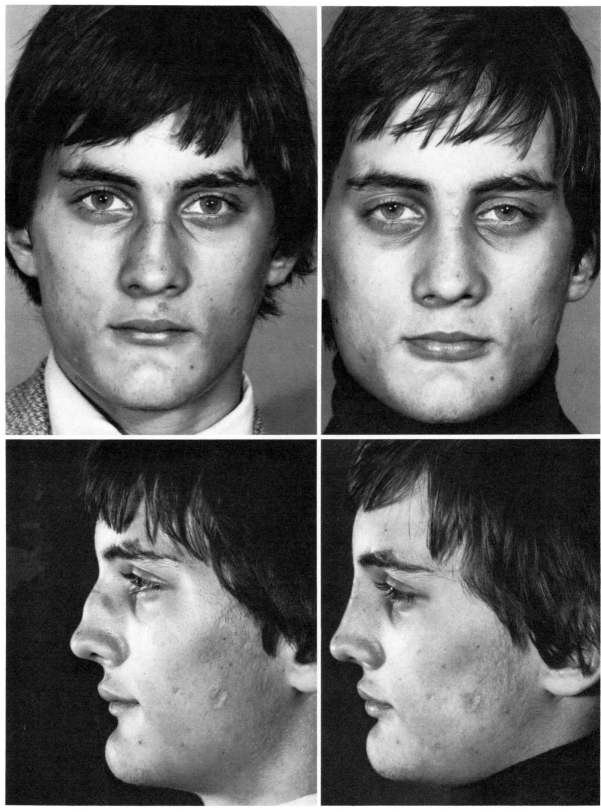

Figure 8–22. The Skoog technique was used to replace this strong dorsal hump in a new position.

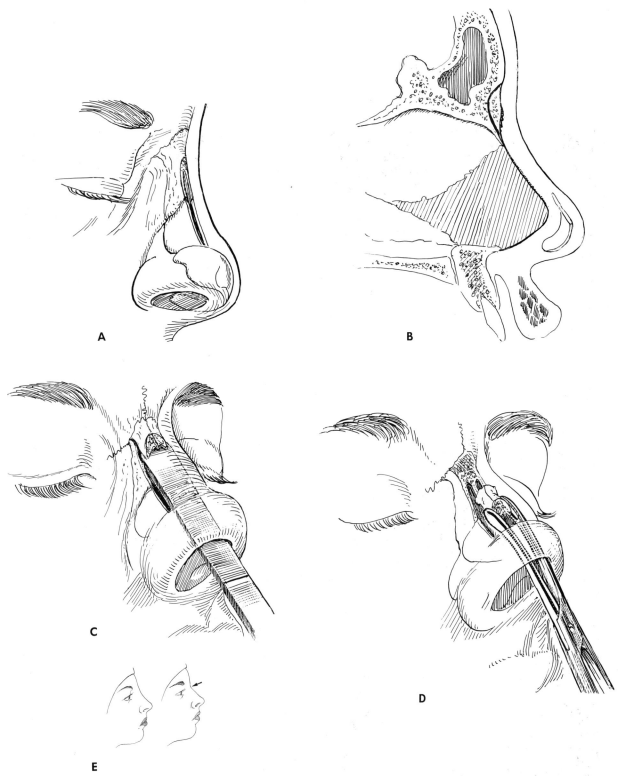

Figure 8–23. *A,* Excessive bone at the nasofrontal angle after an otherwise adequate removal of nasal dorsum.

B, The area of nasofrontal bone considered excessive, preventing the creation of a desirable new nasal profile.

C, A 10- or 12-mm. osteotome or chisel is passed along the new nasal dorsum and tapped into position. When adequate penetration of bone has been achieved, the instrument is levered slightly upward to produce a fracture at the upper end of the osteotomy.

D, The nasal bone is removed with the Converse forceps.

E, A common form of profile resulting from failure to remove nasofrontal angle bone is shown in "before" and "after" states. It must be emphasized that in many patients there is a practical limit to the amount of deepening that can be realistically achieved in this region. An attempt to take out too much bone will frequently give rise to a webbing of soft tissue across the depression, obviating the correction.

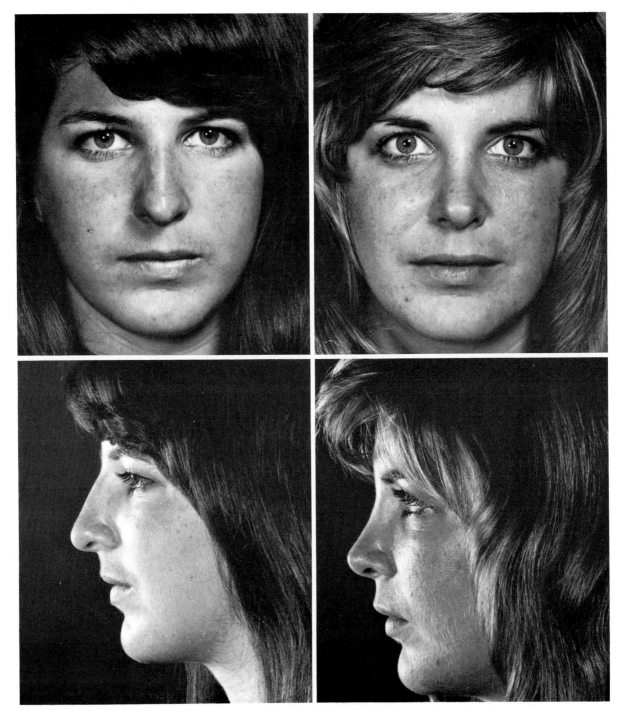

Figure 8–24.   This patient demonstrates the results that can be expected in forming a nasofrontal angle using the technique illustrated in Figure 8–23.

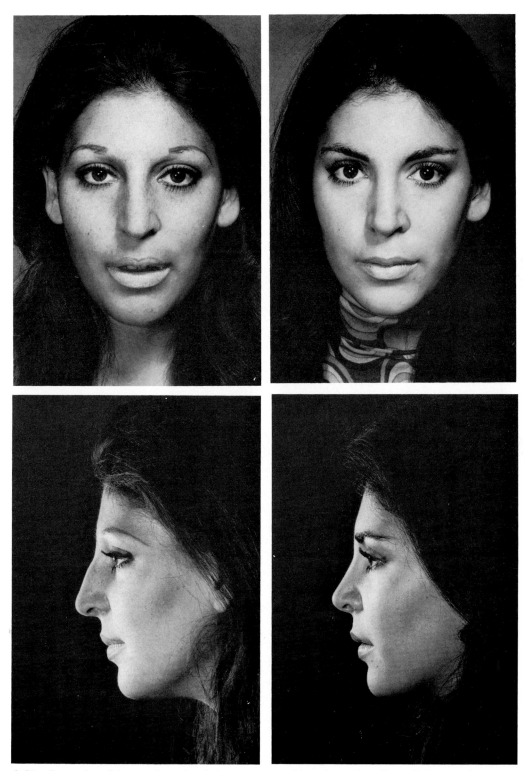

Figure 8–25. Deepening of the nasofrontal angle by osteotome excision of a portion of bone. Such corrections are usually minimal.

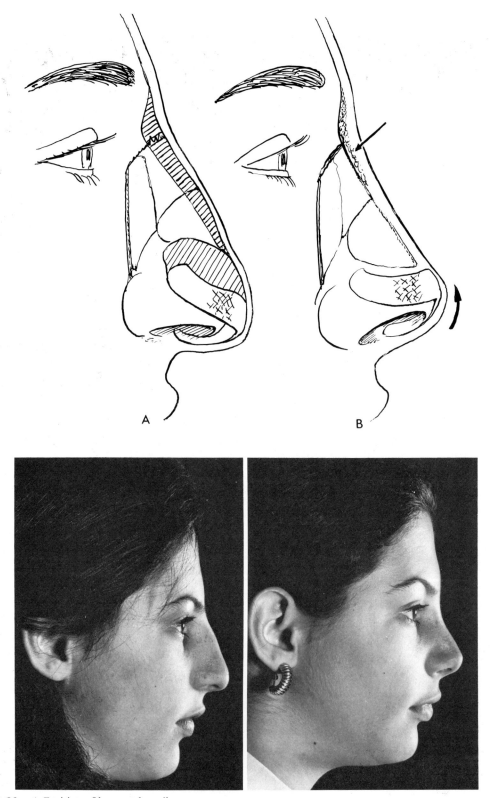

Figure 8–26. *A*, Excision of bone and cartilage.

B, Although muscle and subcutaneous tissue have been removed from the nasofrontal angle, the angle is still partially concealed by the looseness of excess skin (and the receding forehead).

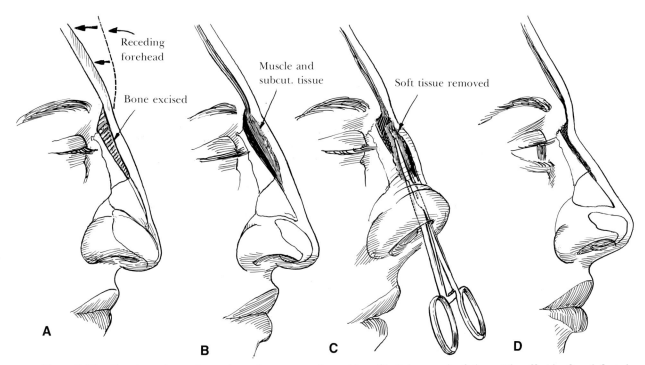

Figure 8–27. Creating a depression at the nasion may require excision of both bone and soft tissue. The effect is often defeated by lack of frontal bossing and by a sloping forehead.

A–D, The surgical steps required to gouge out a nasofrontal depression. It is also helpful to change the patient's hairstyle in order to disguise the receding forehead. A limited result was achieved in this patient because of the anatomic problems discussed. The forehead is flat and receding. Bone, muscle, and soft tissue were all resected to improve the profile.

8–22), the Skoog technique of hump removal and replacement was used to shift the hump to a lower level of the dorsum in order to correct an old traumatic saddle deformity. The hump was removed with an osteotome of the McIndoe type, trimmed to size and stripped of all periosteum, and replaced into the dorsum at a site just inferior to its original one.

The Nasofrontal Angle

Figures 8–23 through 8–27 demonstrate the importance of the nasofrontal angle in achieving a pleasing facial contour.

LATERAL OSTEOTOMY AND INFRACTURE

Lateral osteotomy along the frontal process of the maxilla and successful infracture is usually the final operative step in rhinoplasty (Figures 8–28 through 8–32). It is important because it provides the final graceful line of the nose and converts the nasal pyramid into a delicate shape. In very few instances, it is the only step in the operation, and in a large number of patients, it is the most important step. It converts a wide, somewhat gross structure into a narrow and more delicate one. Lateral osteotomy and infracture is also fraught with minor technical difficulties no matter how carefully the osteotomy is performed, since it is not always possible to control the superior fracture line exactly. Comminution can occur, and the fragments may require considerable manipulation for positioning so that no postoperative deformities result.

The osteotomy line should be as complete as possible so that pressure on the bones toward the midline result in a Greenstick fracture with narrowing of the pyramid at the base with minimal disruption of the dorsal remnants, particularly when minimal hump removal was performed and the dorsum at the root of the nose is more or less undisturbed.

In most patients, the lateral osteotomy fracture line should be made in the thick portion of the frontal process, not through the thin nasal bones; otherwise, a stair-step deformity can result (Figure 8–34). In the non-Caucasian nose, lateral osteotomy and thinning infracture are exceedingly important not only to reduce the width of the nose but to elevate the dorsal profile.

After completion of a well-directed lateral osteotomy, medial pressure applied with the opera-

Text continued on page 164.

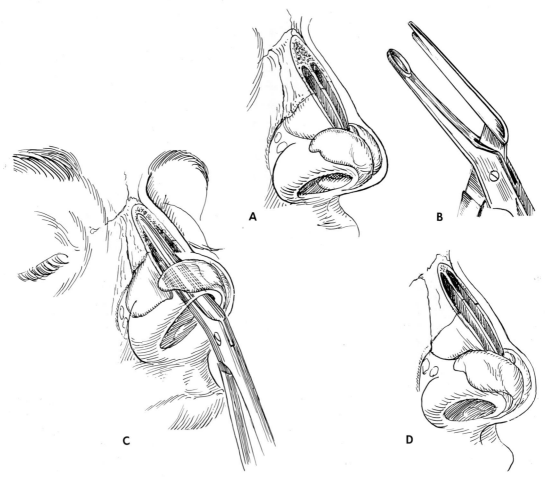

Figure 8–28. In many patients a web of bone in the nasal root region remains after the dorsum is modified. If this bone is left intact, it will prevent the complete narrowing of the nose in the upper third. The web may be removed with osteotomes or, as illustrated, with nasal root forceps.

A, A heavy nasal root web whose presence will impede the infracturing of the nasal bones and result in an excessively broad nasal septum with gaps between the nasal bones and the nasal septum.

B, The Converse (-Kazanjian) nasal root forceps, a heavy and specially designed style of rongeur, is available in broad and narrow shapes, the latter being more generally useful.

C, The nasal root forceps are inserted to the region of the web, which is encompassed by their tips. The forceps must be in good condition and they must be completely closed before removing nasal root bone. Failure to observe these two points will not infrequently result in total evulsion of the nasal bone, a calamity to be studiously avoided. Any resistance to removal of the forceps is to be regarded with suspicion, and the forceps should be reapplied and reclosed in such situations.

D, There is now no barrier to good infracture.

It is appropriate to point out that it is rarely necessary or even desirable to attempt such narrowing of the upper nose. In fact, excessive narrowing of the nose at the level of the inner canthi is to be avoided in most cases since the nose assumes a most unnatural look. The tip and lower nose frequently appear inordinately wide when the bony pyramid is narrowed too much. As in many ancillary techniques in rhinoplasty, this technique is presented for use in highly selected patients. It is by no means put forward as a routine component of the rhinoplasty procedure.

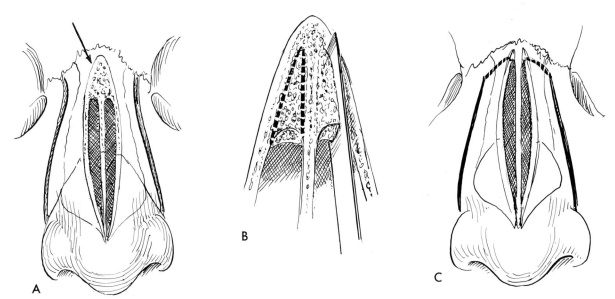

Figure 8–29.   *A,* Sufficient narrowing of the bony nose requires complete fracture and, in addition, room for the fractured bones to move medially. *B,* Removal of a medial wedge of bone at the root of the nose may be necessary to achieve this medial movement. *C,* The complete lateral osteotomies and the clean superior fracture that are necessary for success.

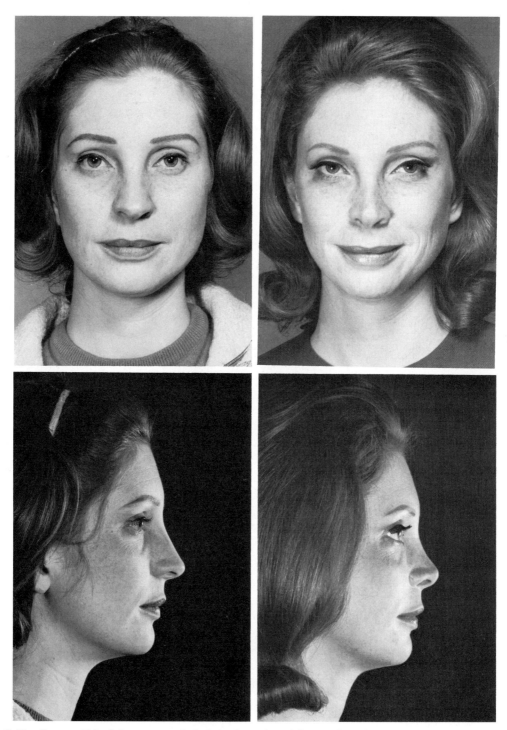

Figure 8–30.   Excess width of the nose, particularly in the region of the nasofrontal angle, was corrected by minimal dorsal excision, removal of excess bone tissue in the region of the nasal root by Converse forceps, and lateral osteotomies.

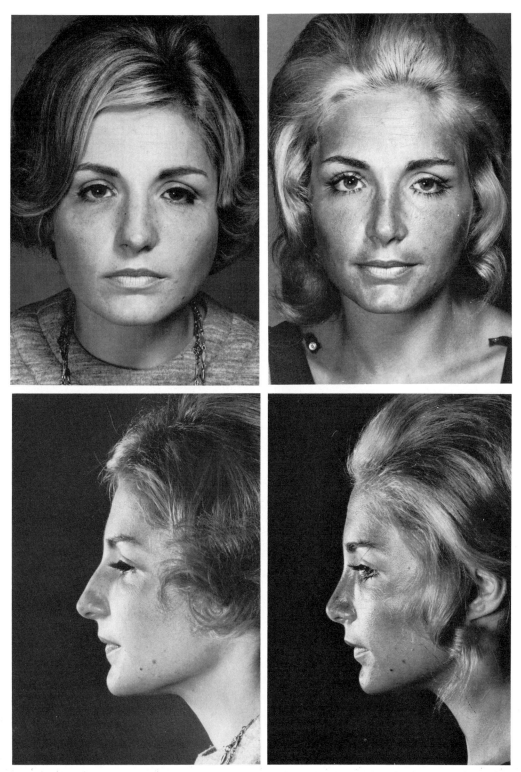

Figure 8–31.   In this patient the dorsal profile was reduced by rasping and a minimal tip reduction was performed, but notice the salutary effect on the final front-face result achieved by the narrowing osteotomy, which extended to the root of the nose. A small web of bone was excised by the osteotome technique demonstrated in Figure 8–12.

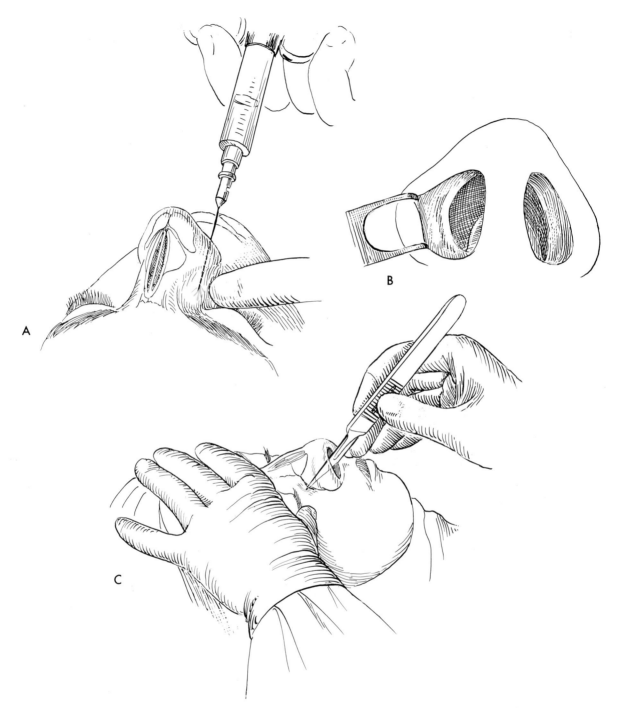

Figure 8–32. *A*, Through a point in the pyriform aperture shown at *B*, 2 to 3 ml. of anesthetic solution is injected along the line of osteotomy. The needle is directed to the immediate precanthal region; it is important that too much anterior inclination of the needle be avoided.

C, An incision is made in the pyriform aperture through the lining skin and soft tissues, to and through the periosteum overlying the maxilla. The pyriform aperture may be conveniently thrown into prominence by retraction laterally of the thumb on the adjacent cheek tissues, or with a nasal speculum.

Illustration continued on the opposite page.

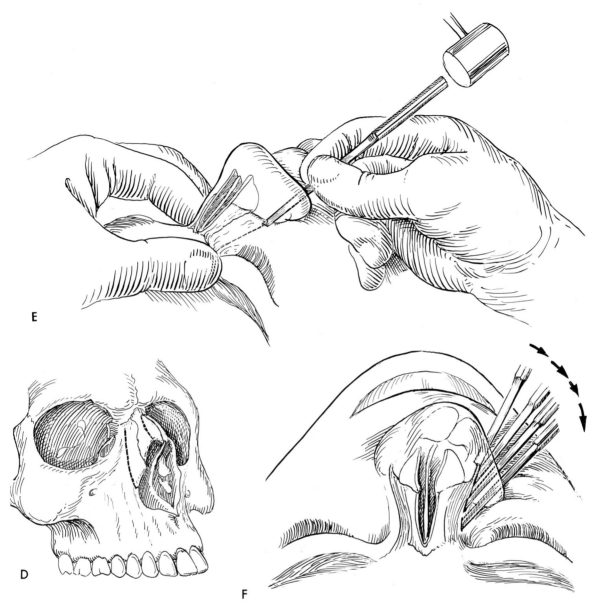

Figure 8–32 *Continued.*   *D,* A desirable line of osteotomy, emphasizing that it lies on the nasal process of the maxilla rather than in the nasal bone proper.

E, The narrow osteotome (2 or 3 mm.) is inserted along the previously formed subperiosteal tract.

F, A series of osteotome perforations of the nasal process is made; usually four or five of these will suffice. As the osteotomy is continued upward, it is necessary to rotate the osteotome progressively laterally.

G, Infracture is accomplished by compression of the nasal dorsum between the thumb and forefinger. No "waggling" motion should be imparted, and the pressure is applied equally from both sides. Any twisting motion at this time creates a definite risk of fracture of the nasal septum.

Every precaution must be taken to insure that the bones are in the desired position at the end of the procedure; the surgeon should not hesitate to make as many cuts as necessary with the osteotome in order to obtain complete fractures. Comminuted fractures, or incomplete fractures with spicules of bone remaining attached to the frontal bones, may occur. Comminution, while worrisome to the novice, is not important provided the bones are in the proper position.

Up to this point, it is not wise to separate the periosteum or soft tissue completely from the nasal bones. One of the main reasons is that if comminution does occur, the periosteum provides a sling or anchorage for the fragments.

Illustration continued on the following page.

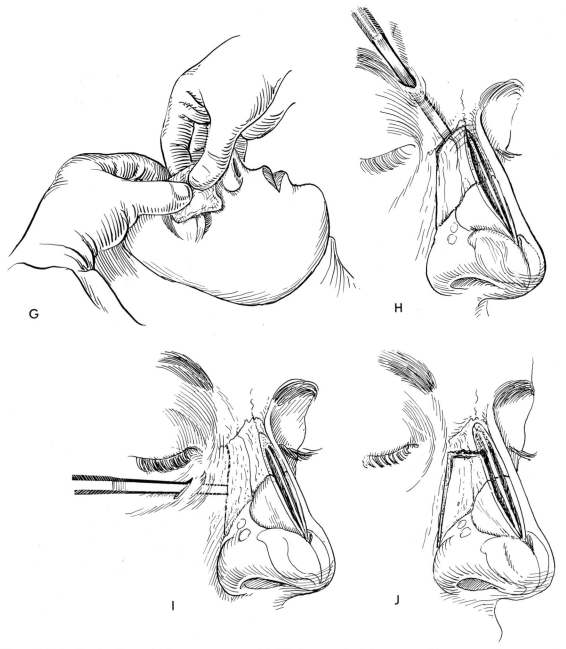

Figure 8–32 *Continued.*   Greenstick fractures are acceptable if the bones are in their correct position. It cannot be overemphasized that if they are not, no amount of postoperative splinting, clamping, or other forms of pushing and pulling will put a bone into position. What the surgeon achieves at the operating table is the final result.

H, When infracture is difficult or impossible in the standard manner, it may be accomplished by passing a 2-mm. osteotome through a stab incision in the medial aspect of the eyebrow. The osteotome perforates the nasal bone in two or three places in the region of its junction with the nasal process of the frontal bone.

I, Lateral osteotomy may also be accomplished through a stab incision in the skin of the lower eyelid, but this technique will frequently give rise to considerable ecchymosis.

J and *K,* When excessive nasal root bone webbing is present, the superior osteotomy may be undesirably low. This will require removal of the nasal web tissue as shown in Figures 8–28 and 8–29.

Immediately following infracture, it is advisable to visually check and palpate the dorsum to make sure that no irregularities or projections of bone or cartilage exist. If they are present, they are rasped or resected. This last-minute nasal "toilet" is very important and can prevent much aggravation to the patient and surgeon in months to come. It is disconcerting to both parties to have to schedule a second operation simply to rasp down a small spicule of bone or trim a small protrusion of upper lateral cartilage.

Illustration continued on the opposite page.

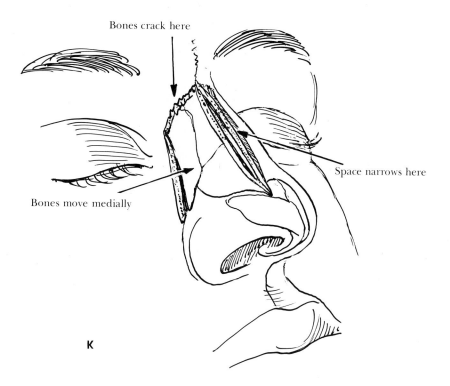

Bones crack here

Space narrows here

Bones move medially

K

Figure 8–32 *Continued.*

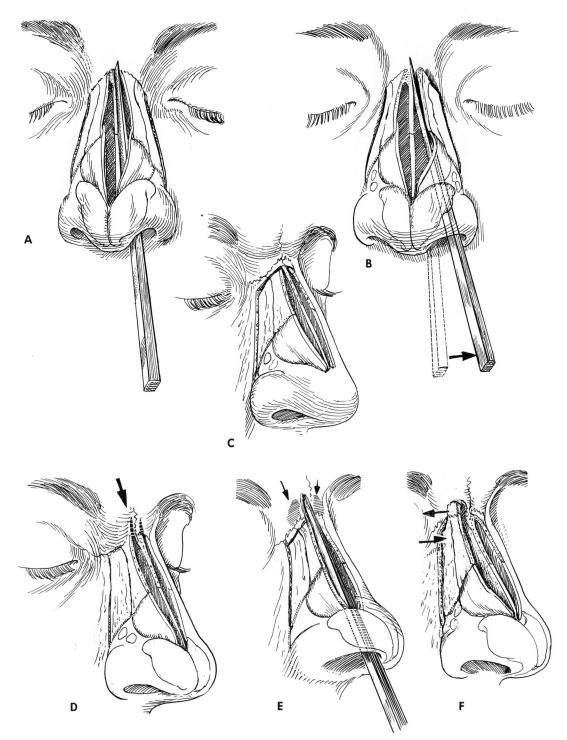

Figure 8–33. *A,* An osteotome is gently guided along the bony septum and driven firmly into the nasal process of the frontal bone.

B, Pivoting on the nasal process, the osteotome is pressed laterally, with resultant outfracturing of the nasofrontal bone junction.

C, A satisfactory outfracture.

D, The usual limits of the osteotomy for outfracture.

E, Excessive passage of the osteotome into the nasal process of the frontal bone, resulting in a weakening of the bone laterally and its widening in this region.

F, The outfracture may be accompanied by a relative protrusion of an attached segment of the nasal process of the frontal bone (the "rocker effect of Becker"), which will require modification by rasping or comminution.

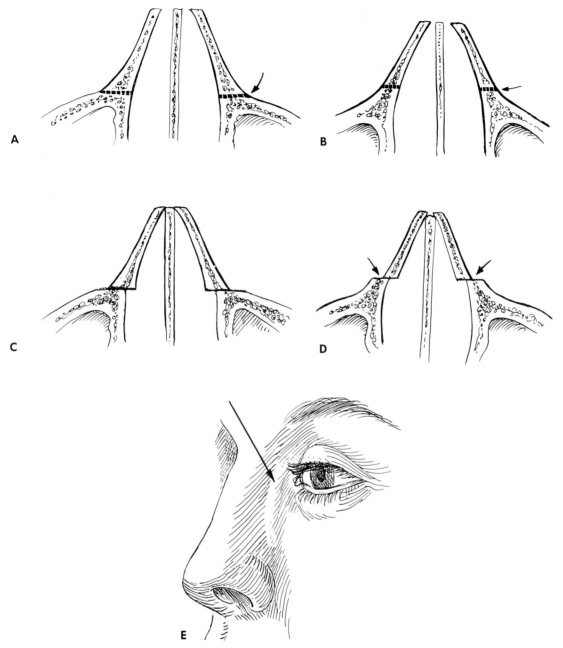

Figure 8–34. A common stigma of rhinoplasty is a visible ridge that can result from a lateral osteotomy at too high a level. The osteotomy must be made through the thick portion of the nasal process of the maxilla in order to prevent this "stair-step" deformity. Osteotomy at this level by a surgeon inexpert in the use of a saw will be tedious and difficult, and an osteotome will be easier to use.

A, The desirable lines of osteotomy. *B,* An osteotomy made too high on the bony vault. *C,* Ideal lines of osteotomy following infracture. *D,* Lines of osteotomy that will result in a typical "stair-step" deformity (*E*).

(From Rees, T. D., Krupp, S., and Wood-Smith, D.: Plast. Reconstr. Surg. 46:332, 1970. Reproduced with permission.)

tor's thumb usually suffices to obtain an infracture because the superior fracture line occurs at the weakest point, which also happens to be the desirable level just below the nasal root. A Greenstick fracture then occurs at the superior fracture line, and the bones move medially (Figs. 8–32, *K* and 8–42). In some instances, the superior fracture occurs at undesirable levels, either too high or too inferiorly, or it may fracture unevenly and leave small jagged edges of bone near the root of the nose. Such irregularities should be cut with an osteotome or rasped.

Medial osteotomy is usually not necessary in operative narrowing of the nose, but occasionally the bones do not fracture satisfactorily along the nasofrontal suture. In such cases, they may be outfractured with an osteotome, or an osteotomy along the nasofrontal suture may be done with a 2-mm osteotome (Figs. 8–32, *H* and 8–36, *B*).

Instead of risking a Greenstick fracture, which may or may not break along predetermined lines, or relying on a percutaneous osteotomy with a fine osteotome, some surgeons prefer to control the fracture line superiorly with a curved osteotome that continues the lateral osteotomy forward to the nasal dorsum just caudal to where the nasal bones become thickened in the nasal root (Figure 8–35). Such a planned bone cut prevents rocker formation because it is completed. As shown in Figure 8–35, any bone spicules remaining after the oste-

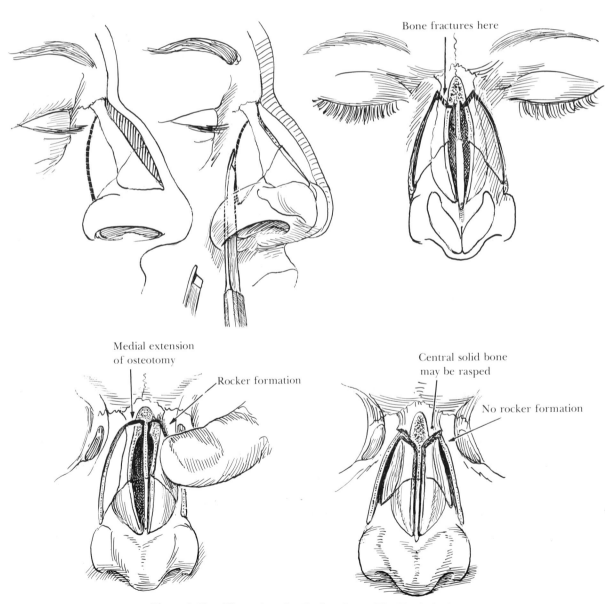

Figure 8–35. (Illustration after Becker, Surg. Clin. North Am.)

otomy and infracture can be filed or rasped. The integrity of the natural width of the nose at the level of the canthi is preserved.

It is necessary to obtain and secure an anatomic infracture at the time of operation. No amount of postoperative splinting will correct a drifting tendency of the bones.

It is not important whether the lateral osteotomy is done with saws or chisels, but the osteotome is preferred for its ease of use and for the fact that it creates a less complete osteotomy, preserving periosteum as a sling. The osteotome also cuts without dust, is more easily controlled than a saw, and is much less fatiguing to use.

The patient in Figure 8–37 has a minimal external deviation of the nose to the right and a wide bony pyramid with deceptively thick nasal bones. Despite every effort made to keep the lateral osteotomy fracture line as low as possible, a slight stair-step deformity resulted, which is visible in the front view. Notice also that because of comminution of the bones at the root of the nose that occurred during infracture, there is an indentation visible opposite the canthi. Such minor problems are sometimes difficult to avoid. The surgeon should strive to angle the osteotome during lateral osteotomy as deeply as possible to avoid stair-stepping. About the only structure that could be injured is the lacrimal duct, which actually lies far posteriorly, and it is well protected from injury because of this deep anatomic location from all but excessive posterior angulation of the osteotome.

The saw technique of lateral osteotomy, shown in Figures 8–38 and 8–39, is similar to hump removal but more difficult to control, and stair-stepping is more apt to occur.

Narrowing or infracture of the bony pyramid may be all that is required in some patients, or it may be the focal point of the operation — tip plasty and other modifications being incidental. In such patients, it is often not even necessary to remove any cartilage or bone from the dorsum of the nose. Despite this fact, it is possible to perform a lateral osteotomy with small osteotomes introduced through pyriform incisions or transcutaneously through the cheek skin and to cut the bone along the nasomaxillary groove. Pressure on the side wall of the nose will then cause infracture and narrowing. It is particularly important that the lateral osteotomy extend superiorly to the level of the inner canthus or above (Figures 8–40 and 8–41).

A lateral osteotomy and Greenstick fracture was accomplished in the patient in Figure 8–42 without difficulty by thumb pressure; however,

Text continued on page 172.

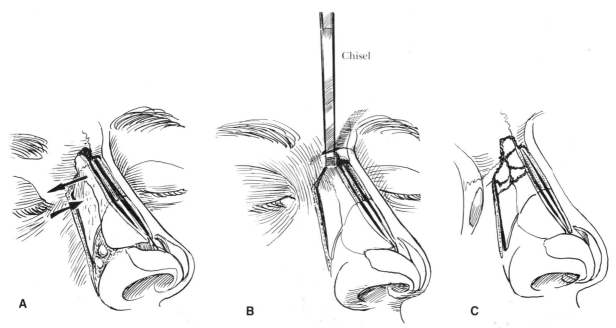

Figure 8–36. *A,* With a superior fracture line that is too high or connected to a piece of thick bone from the root of the nose, there is a tendency for the dorsal margin of the bone to spring laterally, even though the main bone plate fractures medially.

B, A direct approach with a 2-mm. osteotome or chisel through a direct percutaneous puncture in the dorsal skin is required to recut the bone at the desired level to permit a stable infracture.

C, It may be necessary to purposefully comminute the bones. Comminution often occurs in older patients or in post-traumatic deformities at the time of infracture. Comminution does not pose a problem unless support is lost, or the periosteum has been stripped, in which case the pieces can fall into the nasal aperture.

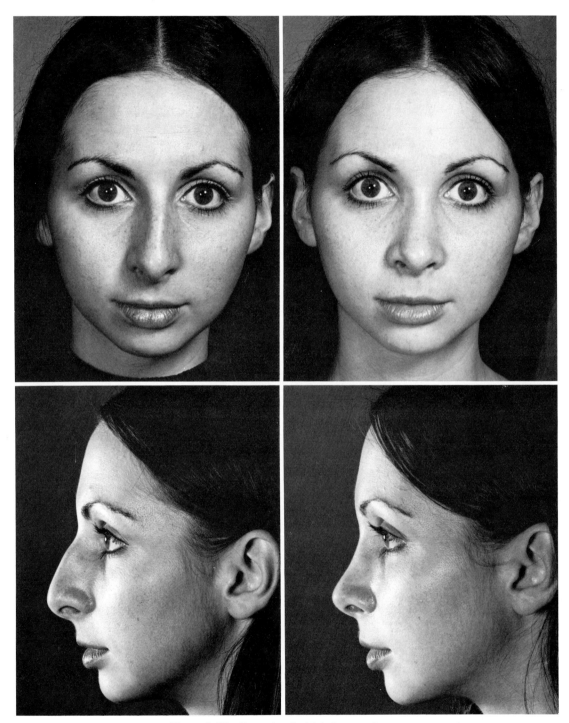

Figure 8–37. Example of a high fracture line.

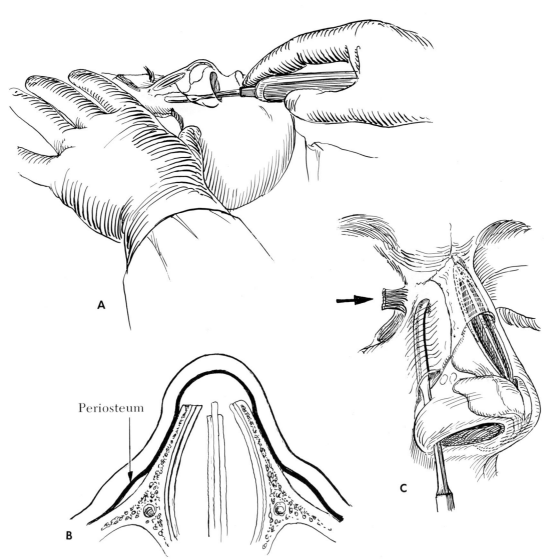

Figure 8–38.   The saw technique illustrated on these pages requires that a tunnel of periosteum be raised first.

A, The periosteal elevator is placed through the incision and directed to the immediate precanthal region by a straight push. Excessive lifting of the periosteum in this region is to be avoided, as only a narrow tract is needed.

B, The line of elevation should be made to lie on the anterior aspect of the maxilla at the beginning of the nasal process. This is important to prevent the formation of a step in this region following osteotomy and infracture.

C, The elevator is pushed far upward to lie immediately in front of the anterior slip of the medial canthal ligament. The novice operator is frequently afraid of injuring this structure, but even in the most expert hands this has proved to be a difficult feat to accomplish.

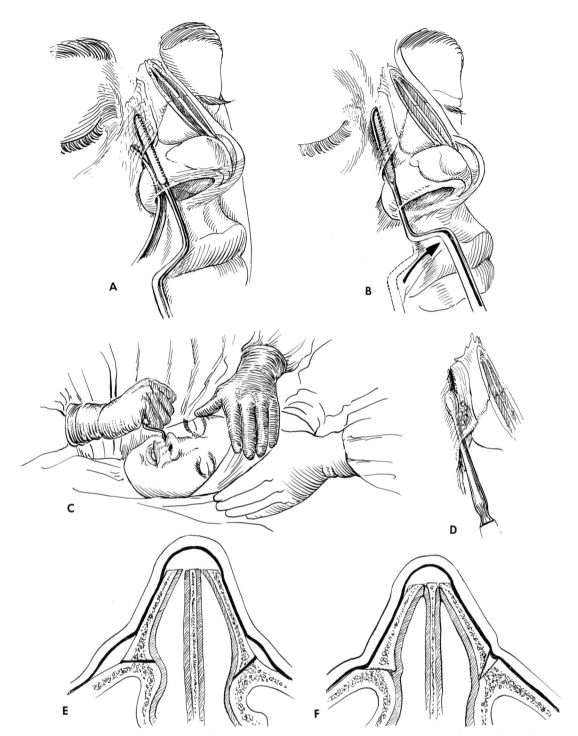

Figure 8–39. *A,* Following the formation of a subperiosteal passage, the nasal saw guide is inserted through the stab incision and the nasal saw is passed along the tunnel. This procedure is facilitated by keeping the saw teeth against the underlying nasal bone until the saw is in position.

B, The saw is turned so that it will pass directly across the face. The tip must be maintained in contact with the nasal bones to prevent entanglement with overlying soft tissues and the consequent production of ecchymosis. Correct use of the saw requires that a minimum of force be employed. Too much pressure jams the teeth and slows the cutting.

C, The patient's head is steadied between the two hands of the assistant during the entire sawing procedure. The operator's comfort and ease of working are aided by lowering the table and turning the patient's head to the side.

D, Bone dust and spicules are removed from the osteotomy site by a curette, frequently called a "nasal sweeper."

E, A correct osteotomy, passing straight across the face, contrasted to an incorrectly angled osteotomy.

F, Following infracture the natural shape is mimicked on the side of correct osteotomy.

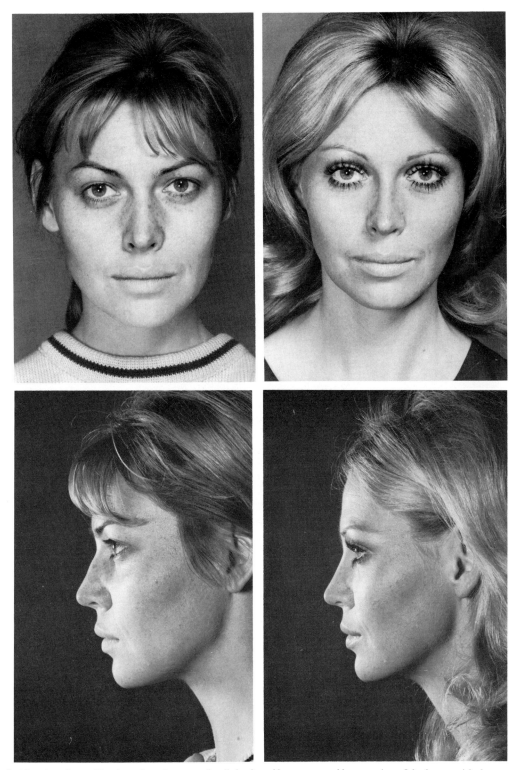

Figure 8–40. A patient with a broadened nose and a slight dorsal hump treated by resection of the hump with the osteotome and lateral osteotomies with infracture.

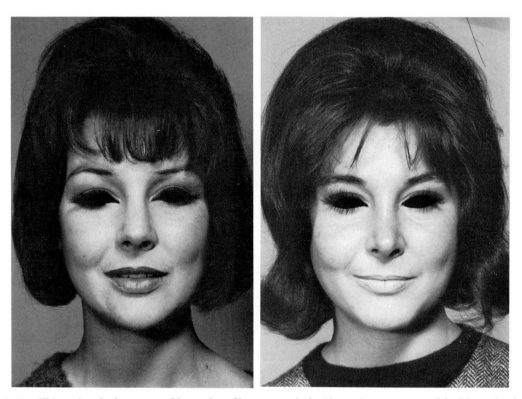

Figure 8–41.   This patient had an acceptable nasal profile preoperatively. Narrowing was accomplished by a simple lateral osteotomy and infracture.

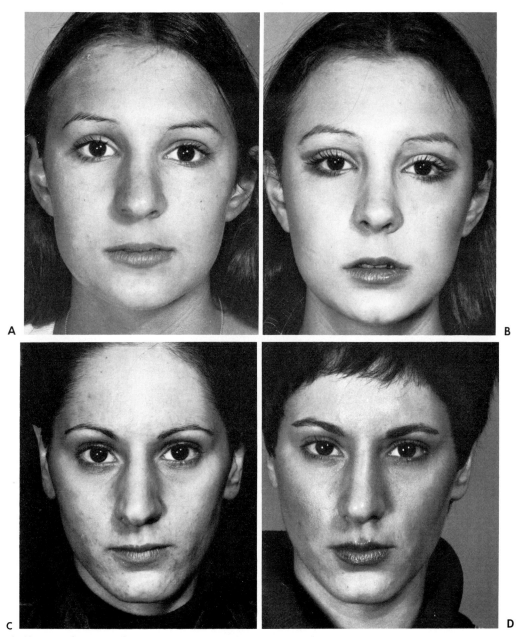

Figure 8–42. *A* and *B,* Lateral osteotomy with unstable Greenstick infracture. Immediately following surgery, the nose was considerably narrower than indicated in the postoperative photograph. The Greenstick fracture in this patient was unstable, and the nasal bones drifted slightly laterally in the postoperative period. The surgeon must be satisfied that the infracture is complete and stabilized at surgery.

C and *D,* This patient had a satisfactory and stable Greenstick infracture.

note that the thickness of the bone at the root of the nose and the upper dorsum militated against further narrowing in this region. The initial hump was minimal and the rasp was used. Deeper hump removal would have resulted in a saddle effect. Further narrowing could be achieved with root forceps or an osteotome removal of a bone web; however, such techniques carry the risk of excessive sacrifice of bone from the root and unnatural narrowing. The surgeon must sometimes make a choice based on aesthetic judgment as to whether extra efforts should be made to achieve narrowing of the root of the nose in a given patient or whether the natural width of the nose at this level is more pleasing.

The slight but clearly noticeable depression seen on the right side of the nose just inferior to the nasion in the patient in Figure 8–43 resulted from a fracture line that developed slightly too low and from an excessive infracture of the nasal bones. Such a minor deformity is sometimes unavoidable even in the best hands; however, great care in executing the fracture at exactly the right level can minimize the problem.

If such a depression is too obvious, it can be improved by elevating the nasal bones laterally or purposely comminuting them caudally to narrow the root of the nose.

The patient in Figure 8–44 underwent rhinoplasty during which the surgeon removed a dorsal hump but did not do a lateral osteotomy or infracture. The result is a flattened nose that appears "splayed out." The most important step in correcting this deformity in a secondary operation was a simple lateral osteotomy with 3-mm osteotomes and an infracture. A dorsal graft was not required, since the infracture elevated the dorsum to acceptable levels.

Many surgeons are under the mistaken impression that lateral osteotomy and infracture of the nasal bones significantly diminishes the nasal airway by "crowding" the inner vault. A study of coronal sections through the nose shows the fallacy of such thinking. The major airways lie well below the nasal bone region, so that the *volume* of inspired air is disturbed very little (Figure 8–45). If the anatomy of the all-important internal valve (the relationship of the upper lateral cartilages and

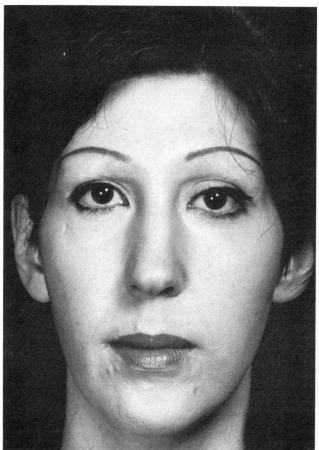
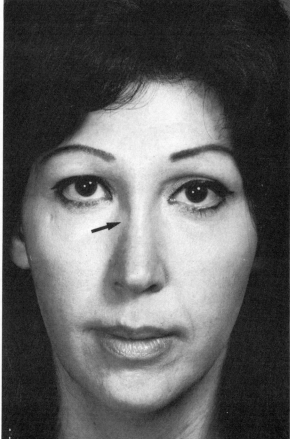

Figure 8–43.

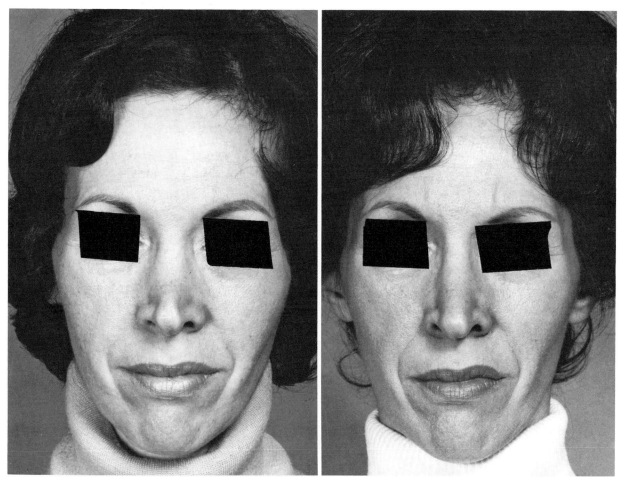

Figure 8–44.

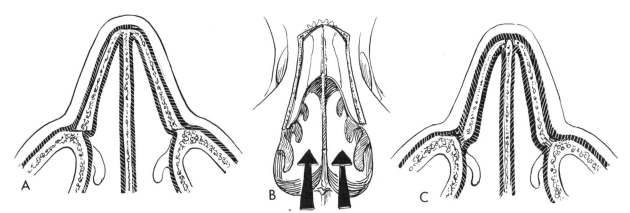

Figure 8–45. *A,* Schematic representation of the usual infracture.

B, Infracture does not interfere with the volume of inspired air.

C, Most infractures probably result in almost complete medial displacement of the bones, which are, however, still supported by their soft tissue attachments.

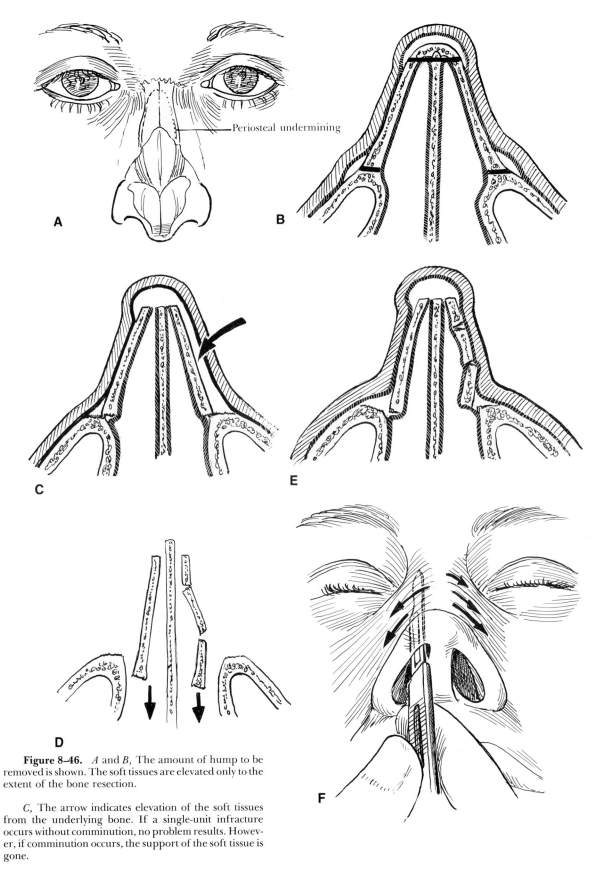

Figure 8–46. *A* and *B,* The amount of hump to be removed is shown. The soft tissues are elevated only to the extent of the bone resection.

C, The arrow indicates elevation of the soft tissues from the underlying bone. If a single-unit infracture occurs without comminution, no problem results. However, if comminution occurs, the support of the soft tissue is gone.

D, With stripping of the soft tissue, the bone fragments are unsupported and can slip into the pyriform aperture.

E, Soft tissue attachments with periosteum intact help support the bony fragments.

F, After the fractured bones are stabilized in their new position, redraping of the skin can be accomplished without fear of loss of support.

174

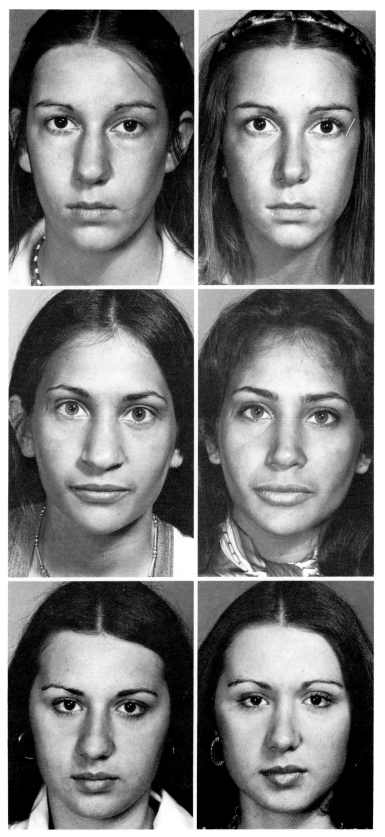

Figure 8–47.

the septum) is upset, nasal respiration is disturbed because of loss of perception of the air eddies in this region.

The importance of maintaining the intact relationship between the periosteal attachments of the soft tissue flaps and the lateral surfaces of the nasal bones throughout the procedure cannot be overemphasized. Initially, the soft tissue should be raised only over the area of proposed hump removal. After removal of the hump and infracture, the soft tissues can be redraped if necessary (Figure 8–46).

The patients in Figure 8–47 show very clearly the importance of the lateral osteotomy and infracture in the final result of rhinoplasty. All the steps are interrelated: reducing the dorsum, remodelling the tip, restructuring the caudal septum and columella-lip complex, repairing the septum, and finally, narrowing the osteotomy. In the overwhelming majority of patients, all these steps must be performed but moderated according to the needs of the individual. It is exceedingly rare that lateral osteotomy with infracture is not required, although the surgeon may begin the operation with the belief that this step will not be necessary. It is therefore unwise for the surgeon to promise the patient that "breaking the bones" won't be required.

(For references, see pages 450 to 453.)

Chapter 9

Surgical Approaches to the Tip

THOMAS D. REES, M.D., F.A.C.S.

CORRECTION OF THE LOBULE AND LOWER NOSE

Since it is the aim of this book to describe rhinoplasty and its variations in chronologic order as a series of steps that more or less follow one another, this section will deal with corrections of deformities of the tip, caudal septum, columella, lip, and nasal spine complex. These anatomic structures are dealt with after the nasal dorsum is reduced. They will therefore be described first, before examining the septum, lateral osteotomy, and infracture.

It is difficult to separate in logical sequence the combination of technical maneuvers required to correct the lower nose, since the surgeon often must perform minor corrections on each of its structures almost simultaneously. Correction of the caudal septum, reduction of the tip, and adjustments of the nasal spine, the columella, and the upper lip must be aimed at producing a harmonious balance. The technical steps will be described separately, but it is important to realize that each has a direct aesthetic bearing on the others.

It cannot be overemphasized that the goal of modern rhinoplasty is conservative correction. This applies equally to the remodeling of the lobule and the lower nose and to the correction of deformities of the osteocartilaginous vault.

As stated previously, it is the author's usual practice to lower the cartilaginous dorsum of the nose first, and then to reduce and remodel the caudal septum, tip, columella, and lip complex. Afterward, septal corrections, infracture, and final adjustments are performed.

Prior to surgical remodeling of the alar cartilages, which most surgeons find the most challenging and difficult part of the operation, initial adjustments are made of the length and contour of

the caudal septum and the lip-columella angle. The anatomy of the nasal spine and its relationship to the caudal septum vary. The caudal margin of the septum is a gently curving convex line rather than a straight one. Trimming of the caudal margin of the septum is often only one of the several steps that must be taken to correct both the length of the nose and the lip-columella angle. Trimming should result in a caudal margin of the septum that is slightly curved rather than straight, as is the norm. Trimming of the caudal septum along with the protruding septum is shown in Figure 9–1. A pair of sharp scissors can be used. (A #11 or #15 blade are perhaps more accurate tools.) The trimming should round off the caudal margin of the septum, since this projection of the tip should not depend on the prominence of the septal angle. Care should be taken at all times to maintain as much of the membranous septum as possible, except in those patients requiring unusual readjustments of the columella to maintain normal mobility of the lower nose, as well as to aid in the physiology of respiration.

Resectioning the caudal septum and overshortening the tip with fixation at a high angle by mattress transfixion sutures may be effective in certain problems but may be disastrous when a plunging tip is a significant feature of the patient's deformity, since retraction of the columella and accentuation of the plunging angle of the tip can result. Maintaining the tip in an elevated position may require shortening of the side wall of the nose by resectioning a portion of the caudal end of each upper lateral cartilage. The lateral alar wings can be used to fill the raw defect by elevating the tip of the nose.

Generally, the trimming of the caudal septum and nasal spine should be conservative. Ambitious removal of the spine or the base of the caudal

Figure 9–1.   *A*, Short upper lip before the caudal border of the cartilaginous nasal septum is shortened.

B, When necessary, the transfixion incision is deepened posteriorly with Stevens scissors to more adequately expose the caudal border of the septum.

C, A segment of cartilage and mucosa is removed from the caudal border with a No. 15 blade. It is important that the line of resection preserve a natural curve in order to mimic the normal convexity of the columella.

D, Removal of the segment is completed by curving the line of the incision into the dorsal border. The septal angle must be curved, not sharp.

See illustration on the opposite page.

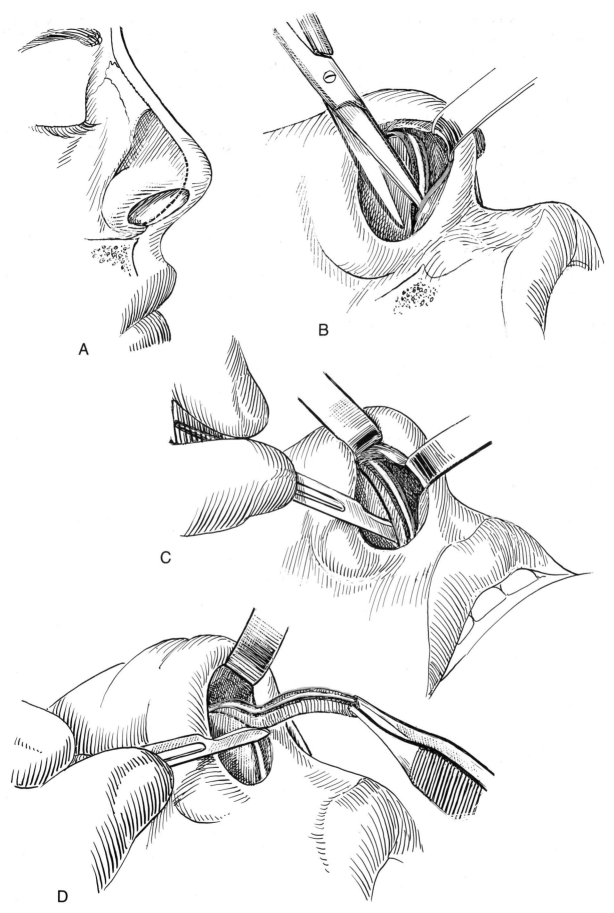

Figure 9–1. *See legend on the opposite page.*

septum can increase the plunging deformity by increasing the acuteness of the lip-columella angle. Overshortening of the nose is a common problem after incompetent surgery and is almost irreparable. The caudal margin of the septum is used as a buttress to maintain the tip in its new position. The mucosa from each side is trimmed so that the denuded septal cartilage is inserted tongue-in-groove fashion between the medial alar crura, which are held apart by scissors; mattress sutures fix the tip in position. This technique has been criticized, but when used in the proper circumstances it has been successful. Further improvement can be obtained in some instances by a retrolabial implant of bone, septal cartilage, or alloplast (Aufricht, 1969).

The changes in facial expression that occur upon animation can be of critical importance. The depressor septor nasi and the nasalis muscles are influenced by the upward pull exerted on the orbicularis by the zygomaticus. This traction depresses the tip of the nose as the patient smiles or animates, as pointed out in the section on anatomy. The dynamics of facial expression should be borne in mind during adjustments of the lower nose at operation. Overresection of the nasal spine or caudal septum without appropriate adjustments of the angle of the tip can cause the upper lip to retract and increase the plunging deformity. Overly generous excision can produce almost irreparable deformities such as an obtuse columella labial angle with retracted nostrils and flaring — the much feared "pig nose" deformity; an acute septal-labial angle with a plunging tip and retracted columella (most difficult to repair); or a flat upper lip that hangs much like a curtain. This last deformity is abhorred by patients. Inadequate excision of the caudal border of the nasal septum or spine may also result in deformities that, fortunately, are problems of omission and can be corrected at a subsequent procedure.

An excellent discussion of the role of the nasal spine in rhinoplasty was provided by Aston and Guy (1977). They quite rightly identified the problem nose as (1) projection of both the caudal border of the cartilaginous septum and the nasal spine into the columella and upper lip and (2) projection of the caudal border of the cartilaginous septum into the upper lip. There is, of course, a wide range in the size and shape of the caudal border of the septum as well as of the nasal spine.

A not infrequent problem in this region occurs when the cartilaginous caudal border of the septum has "skipped" out of its groove in the nasal spine and thus presents as a deviation with a deformity of the nostril. The answer is not always

resection of the spine; sometimes, merely freeing the septum along the floor and placing it in a new position on the opposite side of the bone works well. This maneuver often at least creates the illusion of a straight, if not perfect, septum.

Definitive correction of the columella itself by surgical remodeling of the medial crura is occasionally required. It is best undertaken after appropriate correction of the caudal septum and nasal spine and remodeling of the tip cartilages. It is described in more detail after the section on tip surgery.

OPERATIONS ON THE NASAL TIP

No one procedure is applicable for correction of all nasal tip deformities. Correction of the tip is the most challenging part of rhinoplasty, and it requires ingenuity and flexibility on the part of the surgeon.

Every surgeon should master several techniques of approach to and correction of anatomic variations of the alar cartilages in order to resolve the individual problem at hand. The author favors three basic approaches to remodeling the tip cartilages: (1) the transcartilaginous (intercartilaginous) approach, (2) the alar flap method, and (3) the retrograde eversion techniques.

The transcartilaginous approach is applicable in most cases in the author's experience (perhaps 80 percent or more). It is my technique of choice, except in patients with unusual tip deformities such as marked forward projection, unusual shape or angulation of the alar wing; bifid tip, "box tip," and excessively large, bulky tip with hypertrophic alar cartilages often associated with thickened soft tissue.

The time-honored classic operations are unquestionably useful in correction of the nasal tip. These include the hockey-stick incision and the classic operation of Joseph, among others. However, they have generally been replaced by most surgeons with the techniques to be described here, or by variations thereof.

Excellent exposure to the tip for any of the surgical incisions chosen is, of course, mandatory. Sharp, double-pronged retractors are most helpful to evert the nostril rim, and downward pressure by the operator's finger delivers the interior of the vestibule and provides excellent access to this surface of the lateral wing of the alar cartilage. The thimble, double-pronged retractor of Millard has been found to be a useful instrument in gaining such exposure (Figure 9–2).

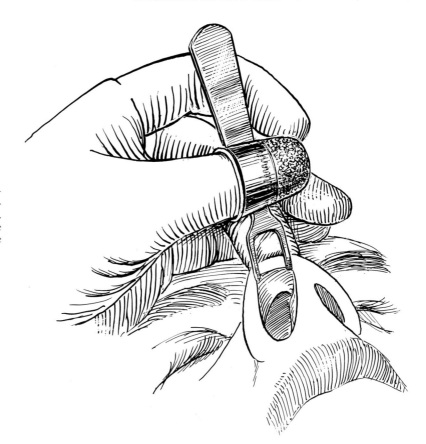

Figure 9–2. The thimble double-pronged retractor of Millard is a most useful instrument in surgery of the nasal tip. It facilitates accurate control of the alae during surgery and finger palpation of the external skin during cartilage excision.

ANESTHESIA FOR TIP SURGERY

If the nose has been properly blocked at the beginning of the operation, there is actually little or no need for additional anesthesia in most instances. Occasionally, complete anesthesia of the alar cartilage region has not been obtained by regional block and must be supplemented by further injections prior to dissection of the cartilages.

Perhaps the best case for further injection is its aid in subperichondrial dissection, provided by the "hydraulic dissection" effect of injecting the subperichondrial plane with local solution using a 30- or 27-gauge needle (Figure 9–3). (Injection points are demonstrated by the numerals 1, 2, and 3.) As in submucous resection, it is important to inject in exactly the right plane in order to lift the perichondrium from the underlying cartilages. Accurate injection helps avoid irritating tears and lacerations of the vestibular lining, which can easily occur from traction with skin hooks during the tip procedure.

THE INTERCARTILAGINOUS TECHNIQUE

Figure 9–4 illustrates the steps in the intercartilaginous technique.

Dangers. Certain pitfalls should be guarded against when using the intercartilaginous approach. When the alar cartilages are quite wide, particularly with increased width in the medial dome area, a two-thirds resection of the cartilage will usually suffice. Settling and shrinking occurs with the passage of time, when the finer architectural details become evident (Figure 9–5, *A, B, C*).

With a narrow lateral wing and narrow dome, as it approaches the transition area with the medial crus, the typical intercartilaginous type of excision could thin out the transition area and result in a tip that is unduly narrow (Figure 9–5, *D, E, F*).

If the lateral wing is wide and/or flat but narrows considerably where it joins the medial crus at the dome transition area, great care must be taken not to transect this very narrow junction because sharp cartilaginous points can appear several months after surgery. Many surgeons fail to grasp the anatomic fact that even when the lateral crura are very wide or hypertrophic, they often narrow down to only 3 or 4 mm at their transition (juncture) with the medial crus (Figure 9–5, *G, H, I*).

With a wide wing and narrow dome, it is easy to excise too much cartilage in the dome area, resulting in unsightly sharpness or "knuckling" in the final result (Figure 9–5, *J, K*).

In summary, the intercartilaginous tip resection is the most conservative technique available

Text continued on page 185

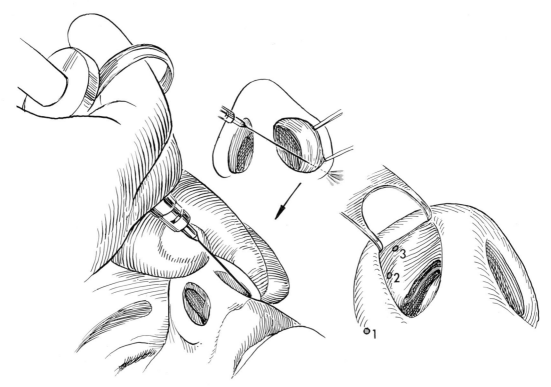

Figure 9–3. Injection of local anesthetic solution into the subperichondrial plane.

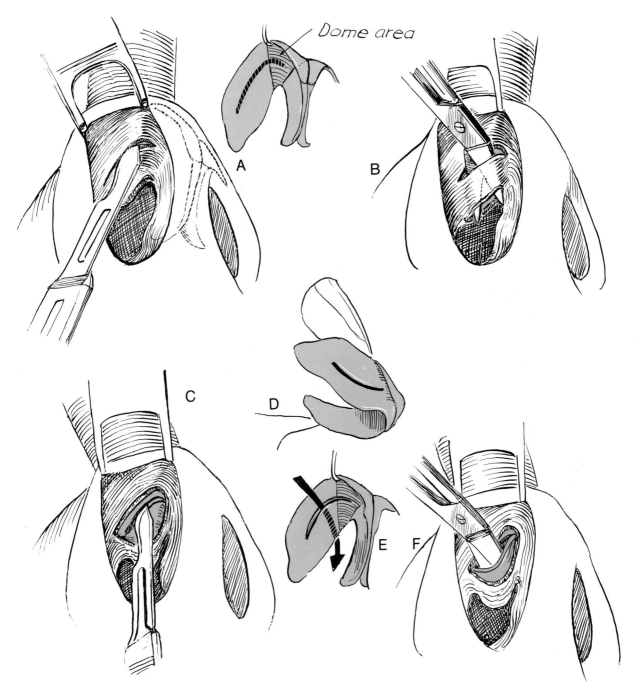

Figure 9–4.   *A*, The proposed line of cartilaginous excision in the lateral crus extending to the junction of the medial crus.

B, The incision in the vestibular lining is made with a #15 blade along a line estimated by the surgeon to be approximately where the cartilage-splitting incision in the lateral crus will subsequently be made.

C, The vestibular lining is elevated in the subperichondrial plane by small, sharp, angulated scissors.

D, Variations in the shape of the alar cartilage, the position of the dome, and the transition area must be noted before designing the incision.

E, The incision through the cartilage is made with a #15 blade.

F, The direction of subcutaneous elevation on the external surface of the cartilage to be accomplished by the dissecting scissors is indicated.

Illustration continued on the following page

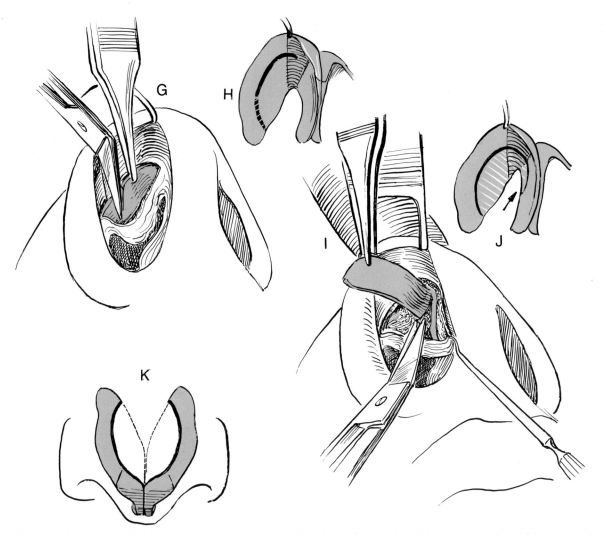

Figure 9–4 *Continued.   G,* Scissors are used to complete the dissection and separation of the external surface of the alar cartilage from the skin and subcutaneous tissue.

H, The proposed line of excision is indicated by the stippled line. The lateral and superior portion of the cartilage is preserved for support.

I, The incised cartilage is grasped with tooth forceps and the lateral incision is made with the scissors.

J. The extension of the incision around to the medial crus is indicated.

K, The redundant cartilage is finally incised along the line extending into the medial crus indicated in *J.*

The amount of excision of the lateral crura in most cases is indicated by the dark line. Note that in the intercartilaginous technique, sufficient inferior rim of the alar cartilages along with a lateral "flange" is maintained intact without interruption of the integrity of the cartilaginous spring.

Support and shape to the tip is thereby maintained. Only the redundant (excess) portions of the alar cartilage are removed. Finally, the incision in the vestibular lining can be sutured with two or three fine catgut sutures if desired.

and is applicable in most cases, but it requires careful anatomic study by the surgeon to guard against overresection and to insure that the basic integrity of the "spring" of the alar cartilage is maintained by preserving at least 3 or 4 mm of the tip intact. It is rarely necessary to resect more than two thirds of the cephalic portion of the lateral crura.

It is important to maintain whenever possible the most lateral and cephalic flange of the lateral crus, since maintenance of this plate of semirigid structure for support just above the alar rim mitigates against the formation of a deep groove extending from the nasolabial fold around the base of the ala and curving toward the dorsum of the

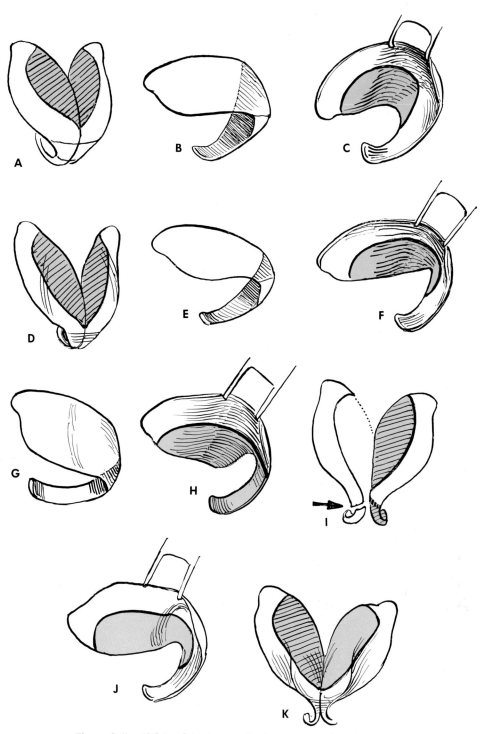

Figure 9–5. Pitfalls of the intercartilaginous approach to tip surgery.

nose — an unsightly and recognizable stigmata of postoperative rhinoplasty. In some patients, such a groove occurs normally, but it can be grossly accentuated by excision of this lateral plate of cartilage.

The Alar Crease. Typically, in the nose with a thick tip, there is no extension of the natural alar crease. It is then aesthetically desirable to create one.

This can be accomplished by extending the intercartilaginous incision laterally and slightly superiorly and resecting the cephalic excess of cartilage along with its overlying subcutaneous tissue (Figure 9–6). Here, too, it is important to maintain

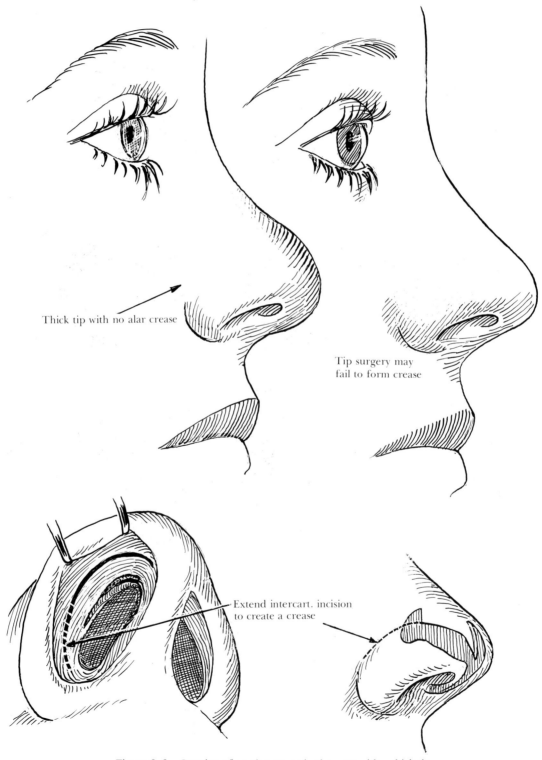

Thick tip with no alar crease

Tip surgery may fail to form crease

Extend intercart. incision to create a crease

Figure 9–6. Creation of an alar crease in the nose with a thick tip.

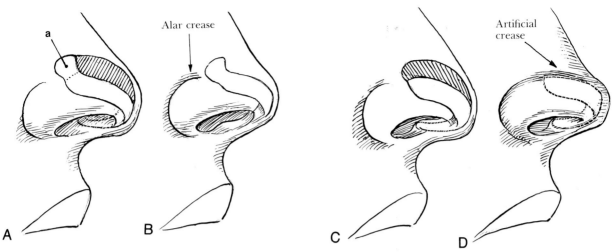

Figure 9–7.

a small lateral flange of cartilage to prevent the crease from developing into a deep groove.

In patients who have a deep pre-existing alar groove extending medially from the nasolabial line, preservation of a cephalic extension (flange) of cartilage at the lateralmost angle of the lateral crus (Figure 9–7, *A*) guards against the formation of a continuous crease extending from the nasolabial line to the dorsum of the nose — an obvious stigma of a rhinoplasty.

Results. Figures 9–8 and 9–9 are preoperative and postoperative photographs of patients that demonstrate results that can be expected from the intercartilaginous tip-remodeling technique. Tip problems range from minimal to moderate hypertrophy of the alar cartilages. When the cartilages are huge or the angle formed between the medial and lateral crura is more obtuse or box-like, the author prefers the alar flap or eversion technique for correction. These will be discussed subsequently. However, the intracartilaginous approach suffices in the great majority of patients.

The Hockey-Stick Incision

The hockey-stick incision is a variation of the intercartilaginous technique. It is applicable in patients with excessive cartilaginous domes or when recession or resection of the projecting transition area where the crura meet is required (Figure 9–10).

The Joseph Tip Plasty

The classical Joseph tip plasty (Figure 9–11) is included here for historical reasons, although this operation is apt to result in sharp points of the cut ends of the medial or lateral crus, which may be-

come obvious only after edema has completely subsided — weeks or sometimes months after primary surgery. Pinching of the tip also may occur after this technique. Figure 9–12 shows preoperative and postoperative views of a patient who underwent a modified Joseph technique. Sharp cartilage points can, of course, result after any tip procedure that transects the entire width of the alar cartilage spring (Figure 9–13).

The rule in tip plasty is to be conservative, since there is nothing harder to repair than an overoperated nasal tip. If too much cartilage or lining has been sacrificed, little can be done to salvage the situation (Figure 9–30). Some surgeons have claimed that all the lateral crus can be resected without impairing the tip, either cosmetically or functionally. Although this may be true in patients with thick, rigid skin and subcutaneous tissue, or in secondary operations in which considerable scar tissue is present, it is not true in the average patient with more delicate tip cartilage and skin. Alar collapse can and does occur, and it is always preferable to leave a small margin of the cartilage to act as a spring. It is also better not to break this spring, although in fact this is often necessary, particularly at the domes. Dicing or morseling the cartilage so that it can be shaped or molded is a reasonable alternative. This is discussed subsequently.

THE ALAR FLAP TECHNIQUE

It is axiomatic that the key to good surgical technique is obtaining adequate exposure to the structural elements. Unusual configuration in the size or shape of the alar cartilage demands careful and exact sculpting. Full exposure of almost the entire lateral crus, the dome, the transition area,

Text continued on page 199

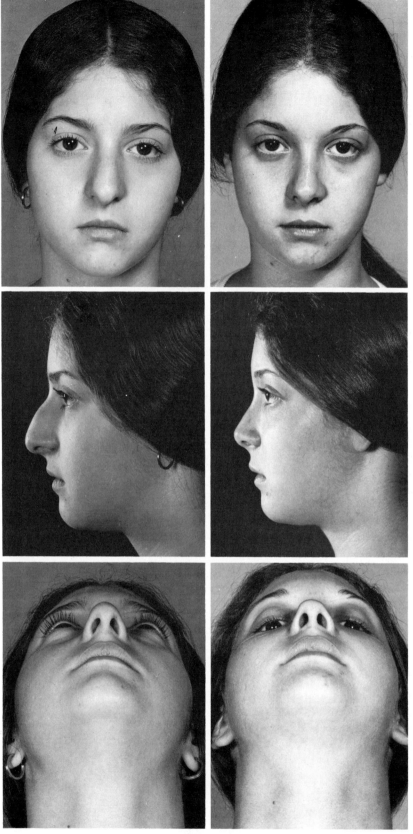

Figure 9–8.

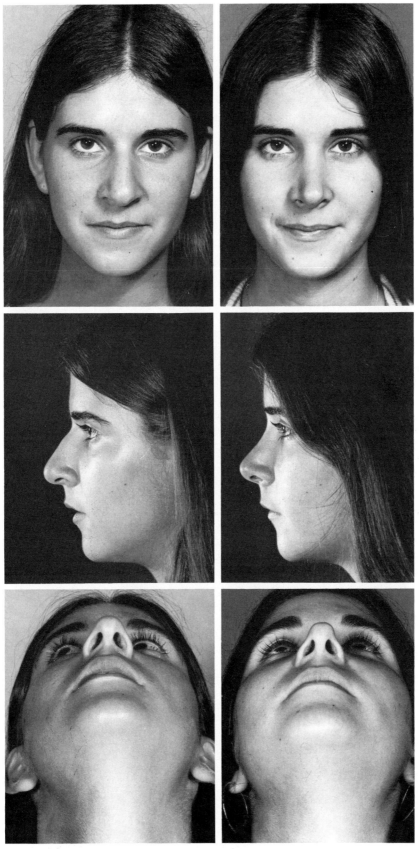

Figure 9–9.

Figure 9–10. *A,* The nostril rim is everted after block anesthesia of the alar base is obtained. The vestibular lining may be elevated from the lateral crus by injection with local anesthetic, using a very fine needle. This infiltration aids the dissection by defining the subperichondrial plane.

B, A hockey-stick–shaped incision begins medially at a point corresponding to the mark representing the alar dome on the external skin. The incision parallels the rim, extending from the apex of the dome laterally for a variable distance, usually about 1.5 cm. A slight medial or lateral shifting of the point where this incision is started will result in a corresponding diminution or increase in nasal tip width in this region.

C, Using the nasal tip scissors and spreading them widely, the surgeon raises the nasal lining from the underlying lateral crus of the alar cartilage.

D, Another incision of the same shape is made through the lateral crus. The incision leaves intact a margin of at least 3 mm. of alar cartilage, so that approximately two thirds or three fourths of the cephalic portion of the crus will be resected in the average patient.

See illustration on the opposite page

"HOCKEY STICK" INCISION

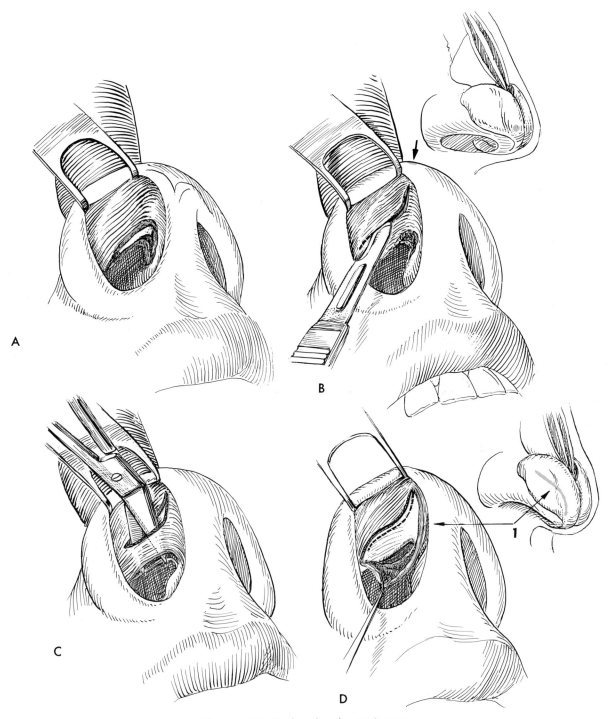

Figure 9–10. *See legend on the opposite page.*

Illustration continued on the following page.

Figure 9–10 *Continued.*   *E,* The incision is made down to but not through the cartilage, and the lining is elevated subperichondrially with nasal tip scissors.

F, The cartilage is carefully incised and dissected free from the subcutaneous tissue. When traction is applied, the cartilage is transected laterally. Resection does not extend for the entire lateral width of the cartilage, for grooving of the overlying skin is apt to occur if this is done.

G, The redundant cartilage is raised medially with forceps and resected to the dome, where it narrows markedly in width. The dome is not interfered with unless this is necessary for a contour change. The surgeon should endeavor to accomplish this third cut with a single movement so as to minimize the chance of leaving a small spicule of cartilage that may later become evident as healing progresses.

H, A few interrupted plain catgut sutures may be used to close the incision. They are not necessary, but they facilitate healing and flap apposition.

I, The cartilage resection from below.

J, The resection viewed from above.

See illustration on the opposite page

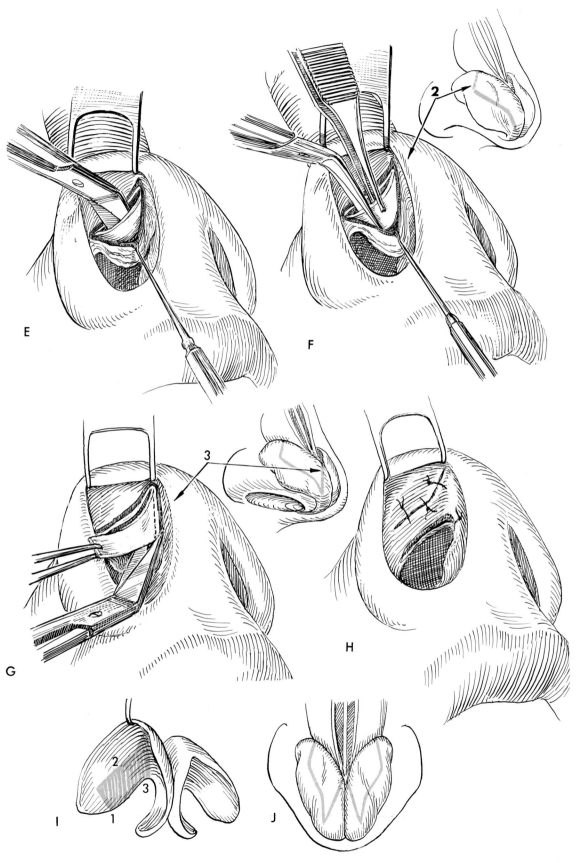

Figure 9–10 *Continued. See legend on the opposite page*

Figure 9–11.   *A*, A transverse incision is made laterally from the point of junction of the medial and lateral crura. The incision may be made through both skin and underlying alar cartilage and is usually at the junction of the middle and lower thirds of that cartilage so as to straddle the region of the alar dome.

B, A similar but shorter transverse incision 1 to 2 mm. from the inferior border of the alar cartilage straddles the region of the alar dome.

C, With the nasal tip scissors, the lining nasal skin and overlying soft tissues are removed from both aspects of the lateral crus of the alar cartilage.

D, The segment to be removed is transected, both medially and laterally.

E, The area of cartilage excision.

See illustration on the opposite page

THE JOSEPH TIP PLASTY

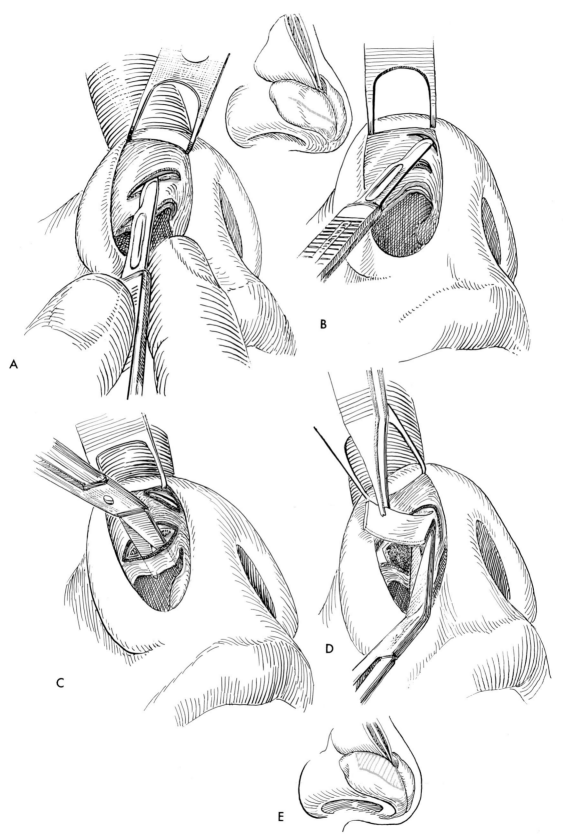

Figure 9–11. *See legend on the opposite page.*

Illustration continued on the following page.

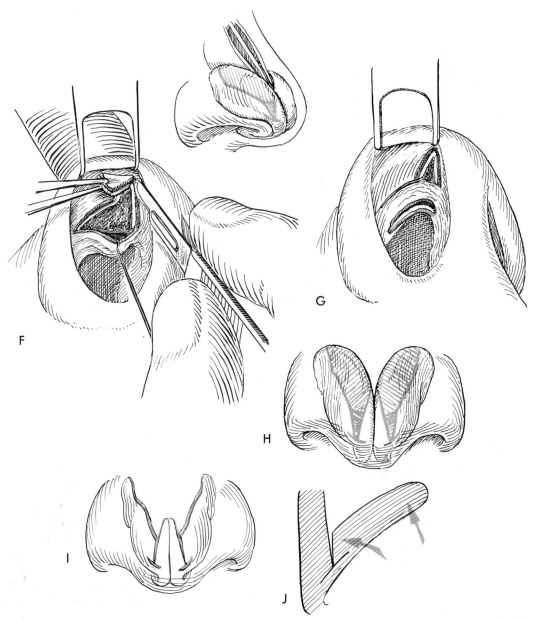

Figure 9–11 *Continued.* *F,* A triangular segment of nasal lining skin and the underlying adherent alar cartilage is removed. The apex of this triangle lies at the alar dome.

G, The resection is completed.

H, The areas of cartilage to be resected.

I, Closure of the triangular defect by superior and medial rotation of the lateral crura of the alar cartilage.

J, A schematic diagram of the rotation: the intact narrow strip of cartilage at the alar border serves to soften the angle formed by this resection and produces a more rounded tip than does, for example, the hockey-stick resection procedure.

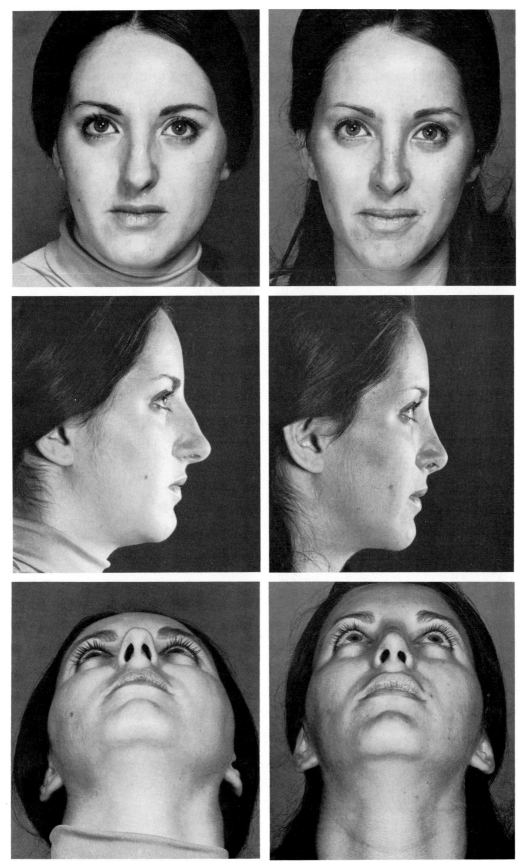

Figure 9–12. Correction of a nasal tip deformity by the modified Joseph technique.

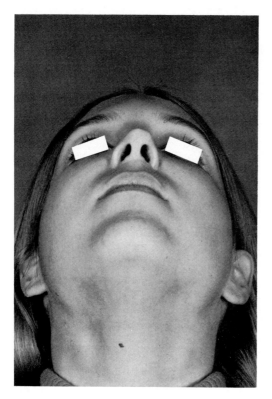

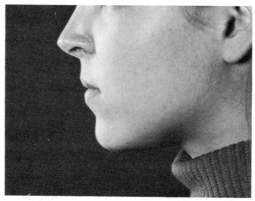

Figure 9–13. A complete breaking of the continuity of the alar cartilage may result in a small spicule of cartilage distorting the nasal tip skin, as in the postoperative view of this patient.

and even a good portion of the medial crus may be required. A bipedicle or unipedicle flap consisting of the cartilage attached to its vestibular lining can be fashioned to provide such exposure.

An alar flap requires careful dissection and separation of the cartilage from the external skin and subcutaneous tissue. Exposure is gained by a para-rim incision extending around the inferior and caudal margin of the lateral crus, carefully following the border of the cartilage as the lateral crus rounds the tip and becomes continuous with the medial crus. It must be extended as far down into the columella as necessary to obtain the exposure desired. It is emphasized that this is a para- or marginal rim incision and not a true rim incision. It is important not to violate the "soft triangle" of skin in order to prevent scarring or notching of the nostrils. Upon completion of this dissection and delivery of the bipedicle flap attached to its lining, a unilateral flap can be created by dividing the flap across the medial crus below the transition — a laterally based flap. Likewise, a medially based flap is fashioned by dividing the lateral crus. The alar cartilage can then be appropriately shaped, resected, transected, weakened, or morcellized as required. Various contributions to this technique have been made over the years by Eitner (1932), Safian (1935, 1970), Aufricht (1943, 1971), Goldman (1957), Dufourmentel (1959), Lipsett (1959), Fomon (1960), Gordon and Baker (1977), and others.

The author reserves the use of the alar flap technique for unusual configurations of the alar cartilages in which the more or less standard transcartilaginous approach would fall short of the mark in obtaining sufficient exposure and repositioning. When the alar flap technique is utilized, it is of considerable importance that an accurate and meticulous repair of the lining be done after suitable remodeling of the cartilages. Care must also be exercised in molding the tip postoperatively, and it is perhaps following such techniques in which the cartilage has to be completely incised or transected that cross-tape stripping of the tip at the end of the procedure becomes important to maintain the repositioned cartilaginous elements in their proper position until fibrous union has occurred.

THE SAFIAN TECHNIQUE

The laterally based single alar pedicle flap was championed by Safian (1935, 1970) (Figure 9–14). Many of Safian's students have followed this technique successfully over the years. The author

hopes that Dr. Safian's technique is represented accurately in every detail.

The broad, flat tip can be improved by the laterally based single pedicle alar flap, provided the skin and subcutaneous tissue are not too thick to prevent molding. The single pedical alar flap was used to improve the tip in the patient shown in Figure 9–15.

It is reemphasized that precise approximation of the edges of the alar flaps is important. Suturing is best done with 4–0 plain or chromic catgut sutures.

THE BIPEDICLE ALAR FLAP

The cartilage in the bipedicle flap can be weakened in several ways if it is desirable to remodel the tip, particularly in patients whose cartilage is thick and unyielding. Weakening of the alar cartilages can be compared with weakening and reshaping the cartilage of the ear. The final shape attained depends upon remolding of the weakened cartilage and fibrous union and fixation of the fragments.

The bipedicle alar flap technique lends itself well to remodeling of the alar cartilages, particularly in those deformities with a broad, flat, or box tip (Figure 9–16).

It cannot be overemphasized that the incision is made along the free inferior margin of the alar cartilages around the dome and hugs the caudal margin of the medial crus. The incision is *not* made through the soft tissue of the nostril margin or the soft triangle; otherwise, postoperative deformities may result. Cartilage can be weakened by superficial incisions, as shown in Figure 9–17.

The bipedicle alar flap can also be used advantageously in the reduction of the projecting tip. In remodeling of the nasal tip using the bipedicle alar flap technique with resection of the redundant cephalic portions of the lateral crura, the rims are maintained intact. This is an alternative method to the standard intracartilaginous technique previously described (Figure 9–18). Complete excision of a major portion of the alar domes (bipedicle flap technique) with careful maintenance of an intact lining and realignment of the transected cartilaginous borders and remodeling of the cartilage is shown in Figure 9–18, *D* through *J*. Some surgeons such as Safian and others feel strongly that redundant mucosa such as indicated in *J* should be removed along with the cartilage, whereas others emphasize preservation of the lining at all times.

The alar flap technique (either bipedicle or single pedicle) is useful in remodeling the alar car-

Text continued on page 207

Figure 9–14.   *A,* A bipedicle flap is developed with a para-rim incision similar to that described previously.

B, C, and *D,* The greater portion of the lateral wing and the dome and a portion of the medial crus of the alar cartilage are delivered as a unipedicle flap after transecting the medial crus. Care is taken to maintain the lining attached to the cartilage as it is dissected free from its external covering.

E, F, and *G,* The cartilage is dissected as far laterally as required. The cephalic excess of alar cartilage and its lining are excised. Several variations are possible in the shape and amount of cartilage and mucosa to be excised, depending on the presenting deformity.

H, Safian emphasized the importance of resecting lining, contrary to the preservation of it, as shown in Figure 9–11, to reduce the tip size and to provide alignment of the cartilage and mucosal edges. Provided the excision is accurate and the incisions are well approximated, healing without scar or cartilage distortion occurs. When the cartilage is completely transected or a strip is excised, the lateral wings move medially (arrows).

I, A minimal rim of cephalic cartilage is excised (a) in the bipedicle flap technique. In performing the various surgical maneuvers indicated here on the alar cartilages, it is important to maintain the maximum width of cartilage to prevent distortion leading to secondary deformity.

J, K, and *L,* Sometimes, a resection of a small triangle from the inferior margin of the ala is required to reset the angle of the tip or to reshape the nostril edge.

See illustration on the opposite page

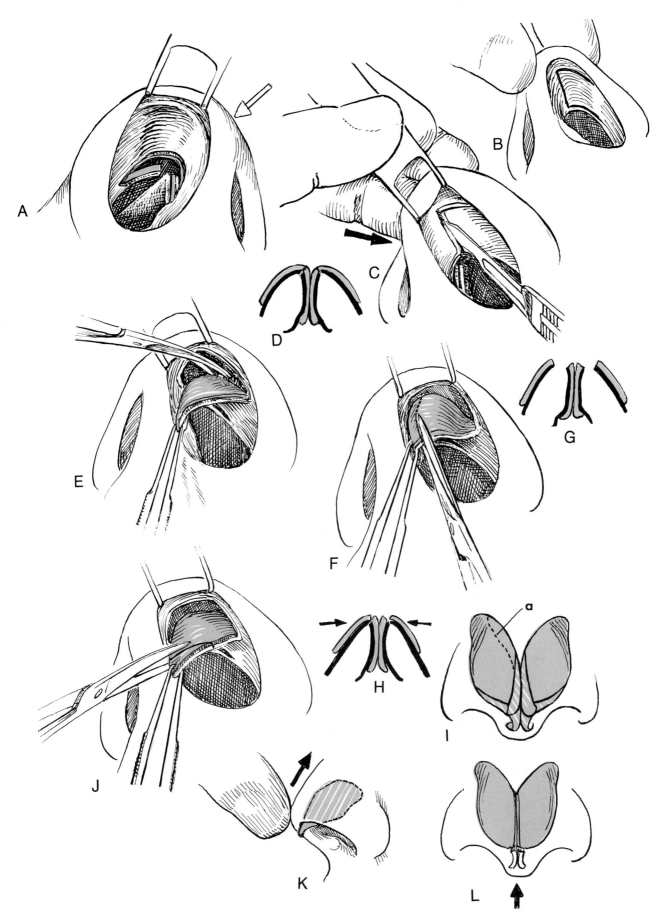

Figure 9-14. *See legend on the opposite page.*

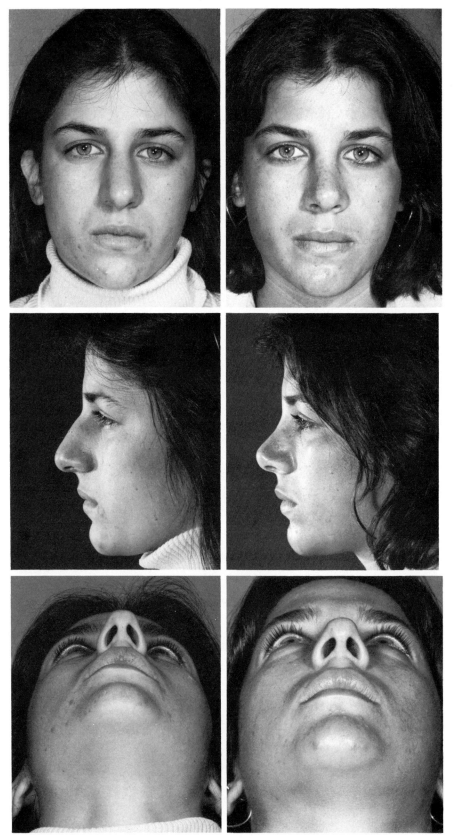

Figure 9–15.   Broad, flat tip improved by pedicle alar flap technique.

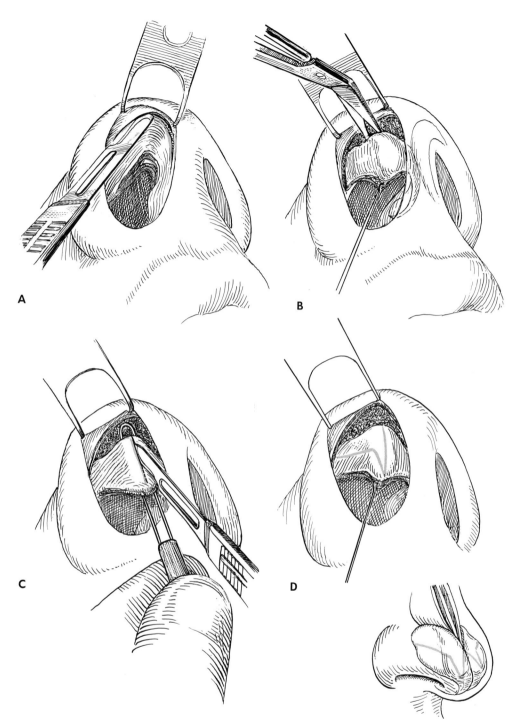

Figure 9–16. *The Bipedicle Alar Flap.*

A, A para-rim incision is made extending as far laterally and medially as necessary, with care taken to preserve the "soft triangle."

B, The double-edged nasal tip scissors are useful in completely freeing the cartilage from its external soft tissue attachments of skin and subcutaneous tissue. Its attachment to the underlying vestibular lining is, however, maintained intact. This is important to maintain blood supply to the cartilage.

C, Illustration of the cartilage being incised across its widest portion. Such an incision can be used as a weakening incision or to effect whatever design of remodeling the surgeon desires.

D, A useful variation is the hockey-stick–shaped incision. Some of the rim can be maintained intact depending on the individual problem. The nasal vestibular lining is protected from damage whenever possible.

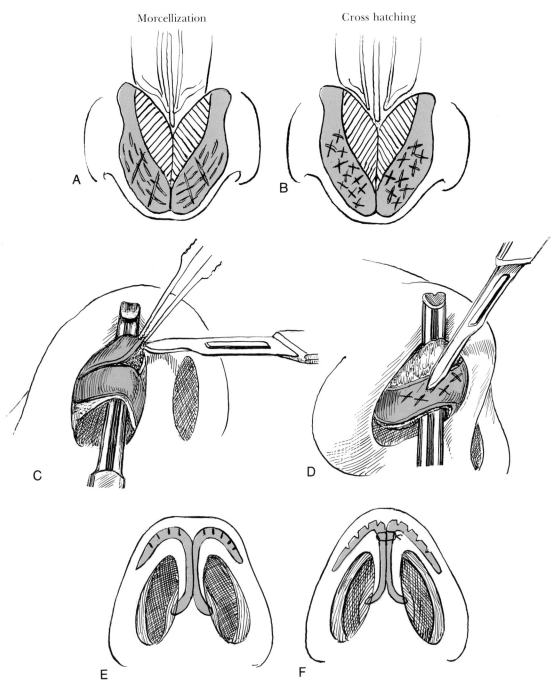

Figure 9–17. *A* and *B*, Cartilage can be weakened by superficial incisions, with care being taken to preserve its attachment to the vestibular lining.

C, A curved hemostat or Neivert retractor is useful for delivering the bipedicle flap.

D, A #15 blade can be used to crosshatch or weaken the remaining cartilage superficially.

E and *F*, The weakened cartilage can then be molded into shape, and a more acute dome angle is achieved.

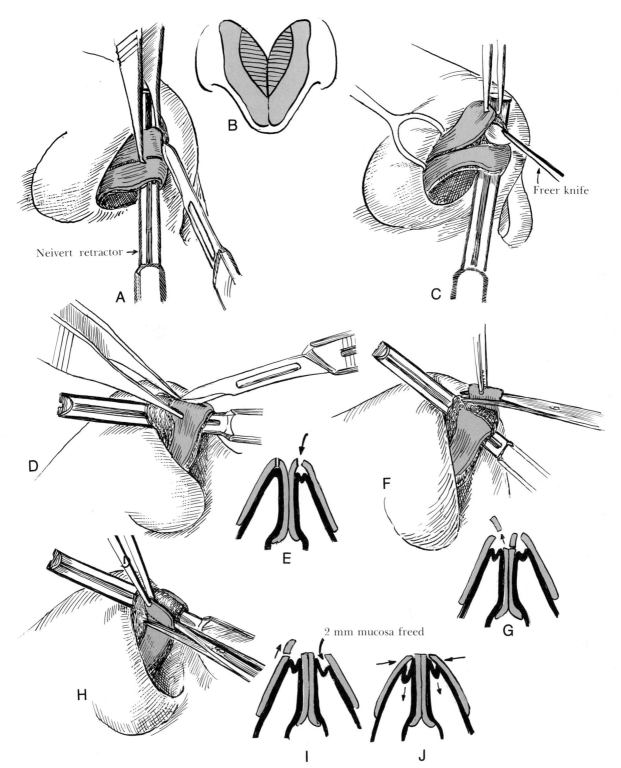

Figure 9–18.   Resection of the protruding tip by bipedicle alar flap technique.

A and *B*, Hump removal should be conservative in order to avoid accentuating the tip projection.

C and *D*, Resection of the domes with complete transection through the cartilaginous rim, with measured portions removed from each side.

E–I, Simple resection of the redundant cephalic lateral crura and conservative trimming of the dorsum.

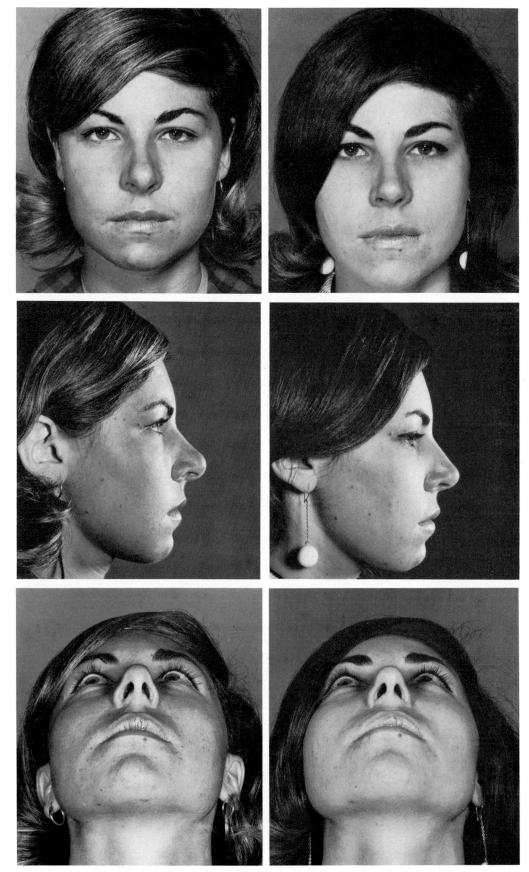

Figure 9–19. Correction of a tip deformity by the modified alar flap technique. Note the maintenance of the natural alar base following the resection.

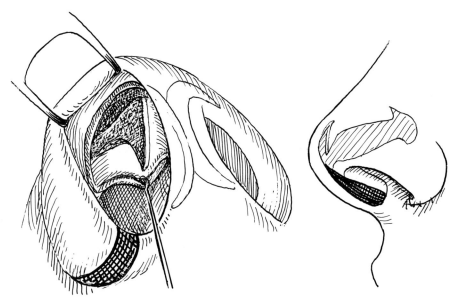

Figure 9–20. A modification of the alar flap and rim technique with preservation of the continuity of the alar rim, and alar base resection combined with a modification of the caudal border of the medial crura.

tilage when moderate forward projection is the chief problem. In such cases, the dorsum is reduced very little or not at all.

A bipedicle alar flap with resection of most of the dome and transition area was used in the patient in Figure 9–19, according to the technique shown in Figure 9–20.

RESECTION OF THE PROTRUDING TIP

Excessive protrusion of the lobule (tip) is often referred to as the "Pinocchio" nose. In such a deformity, the medial and lateral crura are excessively long; therefore, the length of the nostrils as well as that of the columella is increased, and the nostrils are often stretched out. Nostril size is not only excessive but appears even more so because it is literally stretched out. In addition, the alar cartilages may or may not be hypertrophied. Such noses constitute a most challenging problem for the surgeon. The results are imperfect, and thus many surgeons prefer not to attempt correction. Good results for the patient, however, can often be achieved by a series of operative corrections that must be suited to the individual case.

Total resections of the transitional area or domes between the medial and lateral crura may be required, particularly if the tip angle plunges downward (Figure 9–21). Any hump removal should be most conservative in order to avoid accentuating the tip projection. Resection of the domes with complete transection through the cartilaginous rim must be done accurately, with meas-

ured portions removed from each side. In many patients, simple resection of the redundant cephalic lateral crura and conservative trimming of the dorsum suffice.

In addition to resection of alar cartilage redundancy, trimming of the dorsum and/or total resection of the domes, alar base resection to set back the tip, and removal of the feet of the medial crura in the base of the columella may also be required to reduce the projection further.

Another method of reducing forward projection is resection of a segment of the medial crus as well as weakening of the domes, or resection of the domes and feet of the medial crus. Resection of the medial crus is often performed in the single pedicle alar flap technique and in the Pollet (1976) procedure (Figure 9–23).

A simple method of setting back the forward projection of the tip in lesser degrees of the "Pinocchio" nose is to reduce the large alar cartilage when it is this structure that is hypertrophied and largely responsible for the projecting tip. The steps required to reduce the huge lateral crus, leaving only a small inferior rim of cartilage, are shown in Figure 9–24. This is often combined with resection of the feet of the medial crus at the base of the columella, and sometimes with an alar base resection.

Figure 9–25 shows all combinations described here that may be required to achieve correction of the "Pinocchio" nose. Note that alar base resection in this deformity extends along the line of the ala. It is designed so as to reduce the ala in its forward projection rather than to correct flaring; however,

Text continued on page 213

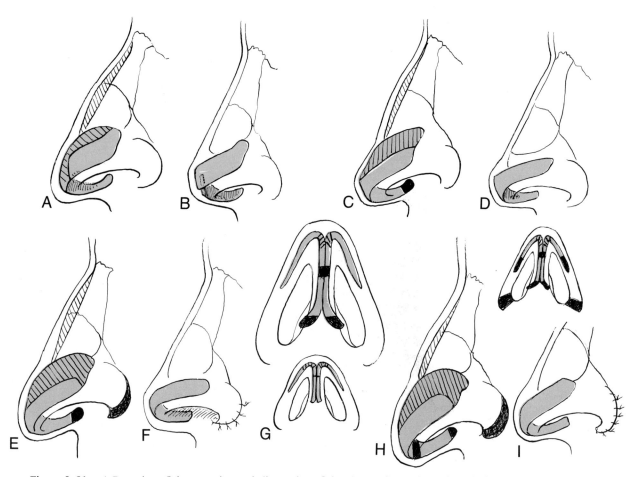

Figure 9–21. *A*, Resection of the excessive cephalic portion of the alar cartilages, including the full thickness of the junction of the medial and lateral crura, is indicated by the crosshatching. This resection of the domes allows for recession of the protruding tip. Modest dorsal reduction is indicated by crosshatching.

B, Resection of the domes or transition area through the entire width of the cartilage results in medial and lateral plates of cartilage which form a new junction that is reduced by the amount resected.

C and *D*, Resection of the redundant cephalic cartilage from the lateral crus and the foot of the medial crus on both sides can also recess the tip projection.

E and *F*, The procedure shown in *C* and *D* in combination with an alar base resection is required in some cases.

G, Recession of the tip can also be achieved by removing an appropriately sized section from the medial crura in the mid or forward portion of the cartilage plates.

H and *I*, A combination of all of the above steps may be used in correcting the markedly protruding tip.

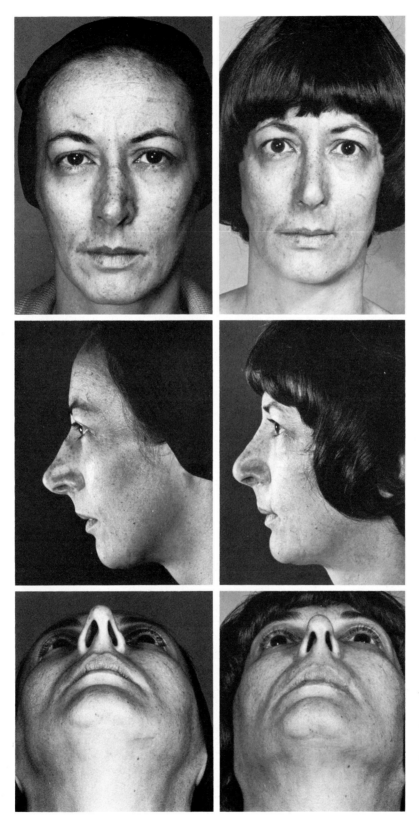

Figure 9–22.   Example of reduction of the projecting "Pinocchio" tip by resection of the alar domes.

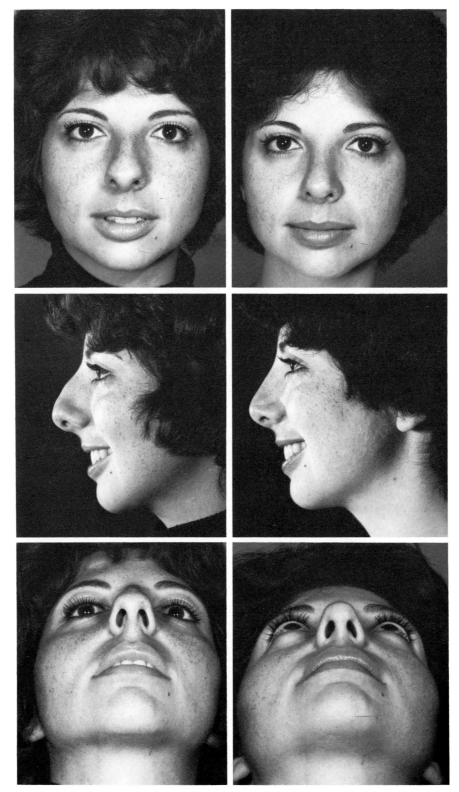

Figure 9–23.   Example of the Pollet technique of tip correction. (See Figure 9–39.)

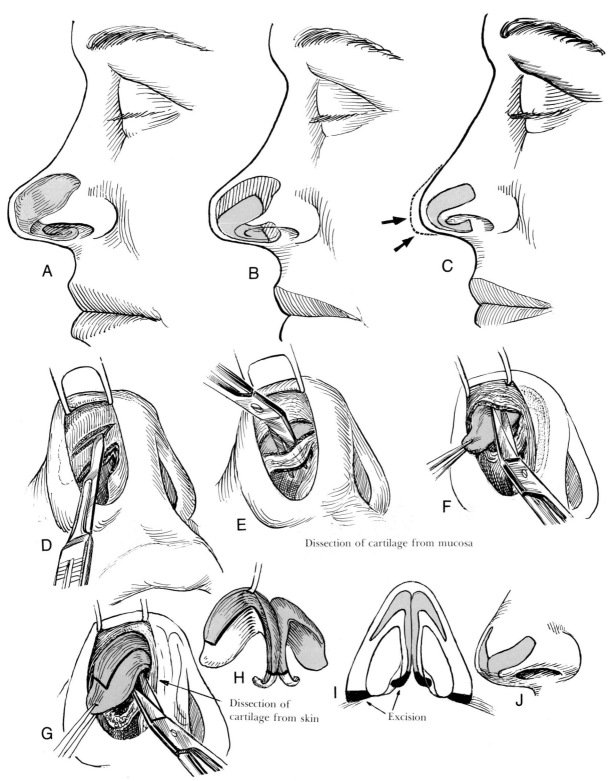

Dissection of cartilage from mucosa

Dissection of
cartilage from skin

Excision

Figure 9–24.

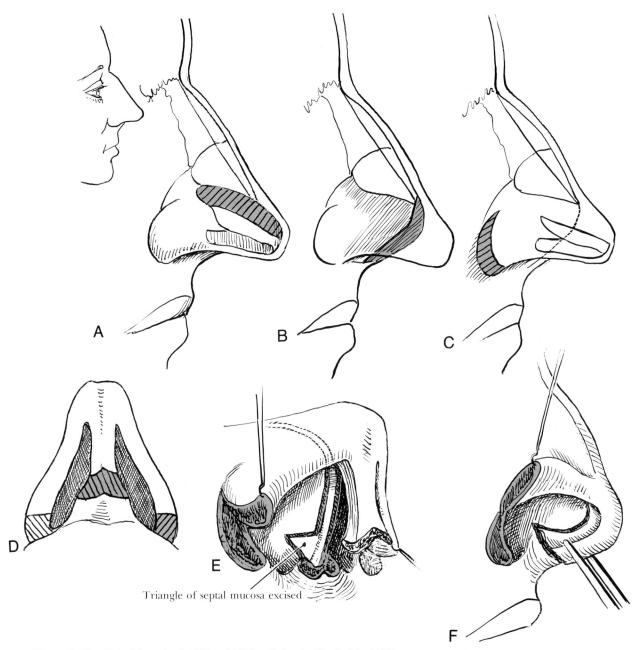

Triangle of septal mucosa excised

Figure 9–25. *Tripod Resection for "Pinocchio" Nose Deformity* (Fredericks 1972).

A, Reduction of projection by standard resection of the cephalic portion of the alar cartilages and conservative trim of a dorsal profile (if required).

B, Trim of the caudal septum and septal angle if required. This step must be *very* conservative, and it is preferably done after tip reduction, otherwise, overreduction of the septum may lead to drooping of the tip in these exaggerated cases.

C, Standard alar base resection further helps.

D, Tripod resection of the alar bases and base of the columella just above the flap is illustrated.

E, Resections of the tripod elements completed. The transfixion incision is complete.

F, The columella is fitted into position first.

Illustration continued on the opposite page

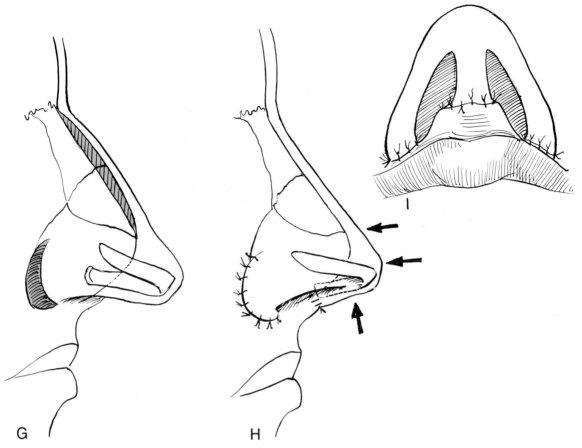

Figure 9–25 *Continued.   G, H,* and *I,* Incisions are sutured with the tip in its recessed position.

once the projecting tip is reduced, flaring of the nostrils may occur.

THE LIPSETT TECHNIQUE

Although strictly speaking it is a variation of the alar flap method, the technique proposed by Lipsett (1959) is of sufficient importance to warrant separate consideration. Lipsett extends the marginal incision down along the anterior border of the medial crus to the point of junction of the middle and anterior thirds (Figure 9–26). At this point, he incises through skin and medial crus back to join the transfixion incision; the cartilages are separated from each other and from the overlying skin but remain attached to the vestibular lining skin and are prolapsed into the nostrils. The cartilages are then reshaped by a series of vertically directed incisions that spare the vestibular skin, and any excess of cartilage is removed from the medial crus. The new dome is remodeled with the now easily malleable cartilage.

The Lipsett technique has been criticized by some surgeons who believe that the extensive dis-

section and cross-hatching of the alar cartilage lends itself to postoperative deformities such as pinching, "knuckling," or asymmetry of the tip. Yet, in complicated nasal tip deformities, the Lipsett procedure shows great versatility in reshaping the nasal cartilages (Figure 9–27).

Certainly, the Lipsett procedure is technically applicable only to certain deformities. It must be executed with precision, like any tip operation that delivers the entire ala. However, such extensive dissection is more prone to difficulties. Accurate anatomic repair of all incisions indicated are mandatory. Postoperative taping and splinting are also important in such patients.

The original Lipsett technique has been modified to provide greater safety. It was altered primarily to avoid pinching and "knuckling" yet retain the desirable feature of cartilage weakening in order to permit remodeling and recession of the tip (Figure 9–28). The technique consists of partial instead of complete cross-sectioning of the alar cartilage with a series of parallel cuts extending through the cartilage but not the lining. The cuts are staggered so as to allow a continuity of the cartilages to remain throughout the flap. In this

Text continued on page 221

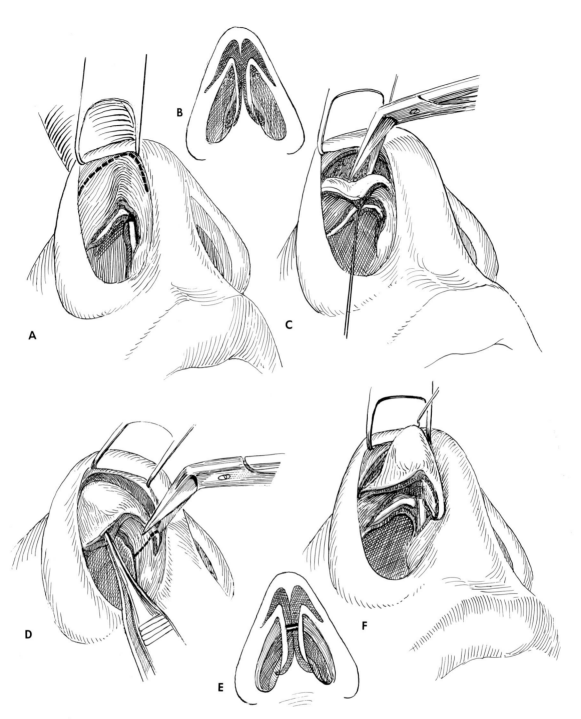

Figure 9–26. *The Lipsett Technique.*

A, A rim incision carefully preserves the soft triangle.

B, A phantom view of the cartilages from below.

C, The alar cartilages are freed from their attachment to the overlying nasal skin.

D, The alar cartilages and their attached nasal lining skin are pulled laterally, and the medial crus of the alar cartilage is transected at its approximate midpoint.

E, Transection of the medial crura.

F, The alar cartilage is prolapsed inferiorly.

Illustration continued on the opposite page

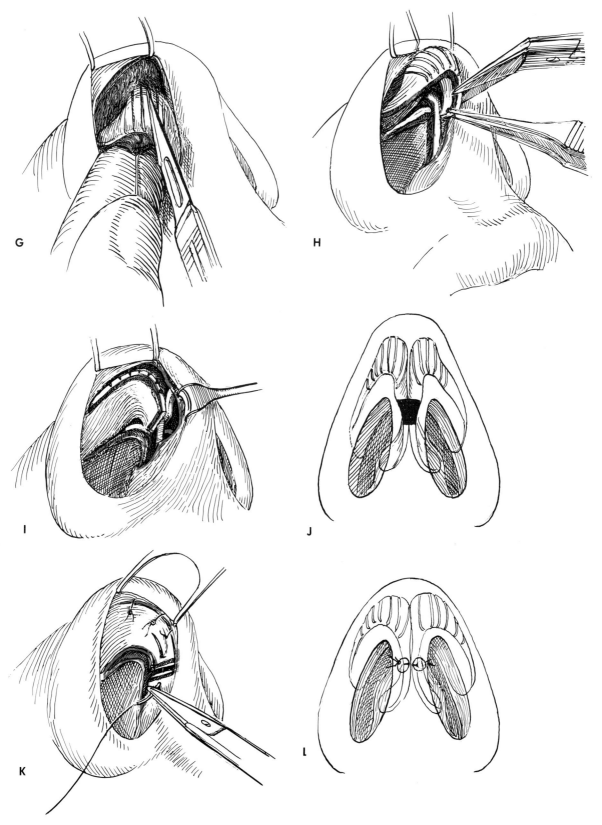

Figure 9–26 *Continued.* *G,* Anteroposterior cuts are made through the alar cartilage, preserving the nasal lining skin.

H, After the new nasal tip contour is formed, the excess length of medial crus is estimated and resected with its attached nasal lining skin.

I, The area of resection.

J, Phantom view of the nasal cartilages, showing the lines of incision and the area of resection.

K, Repair by 4–0 plain catgut sutures.

L, The completed procedure in phantom view.

215

Figure 9–27.   In complicated nasal tip deformities, the Lipsett procedure shows great versatility in reshaping of the nasal cartilages.

A, The lines of incision and resection of the standard Lipsett procedure.

B, The Lipsett procedure combined with resection of a deformed, enlarged lateral crus.

C, The same procedure, this time combined with modification of the inferior border of the medial and lateral crus.

D, Elevation of the nasal tip achieved by this technique.

See illustration on the opposite page.

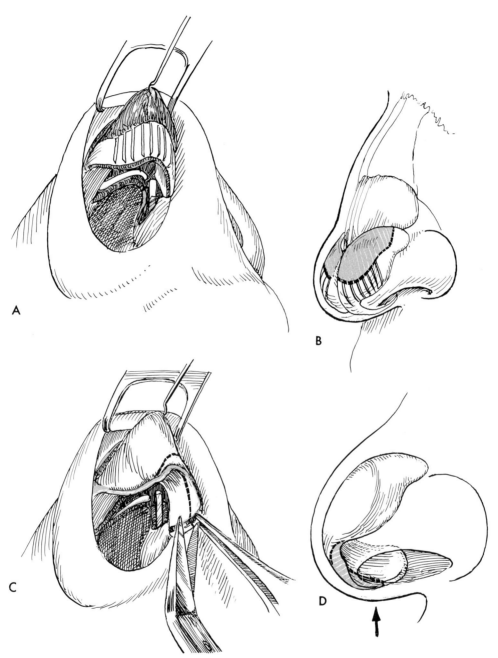

Figure 9–27. *See legend on the opposite page.*

Figure 9–28.   *The Modified Lipsett Technique.*

A and *B,* A pedicle alar flap is developed.

C, The excess cephalic portion is excised.

D, The medial crus is incised.

E, Staggered cross cuts are made through the width of the cartilage. These cuts are incomplete.

F, A portion of the medial crus is excised (indicated by the darkened area).

G, The resection and weakening incisions viewed from above. The cartilage bends to form the desired shape.

H, The area of excision of the medial crus to recess the tip.

I and *J,* The defect is carefully repaired by suturing. Suturing of the mucous lining is important to prevent synechia.

See illustration on the opposite page.

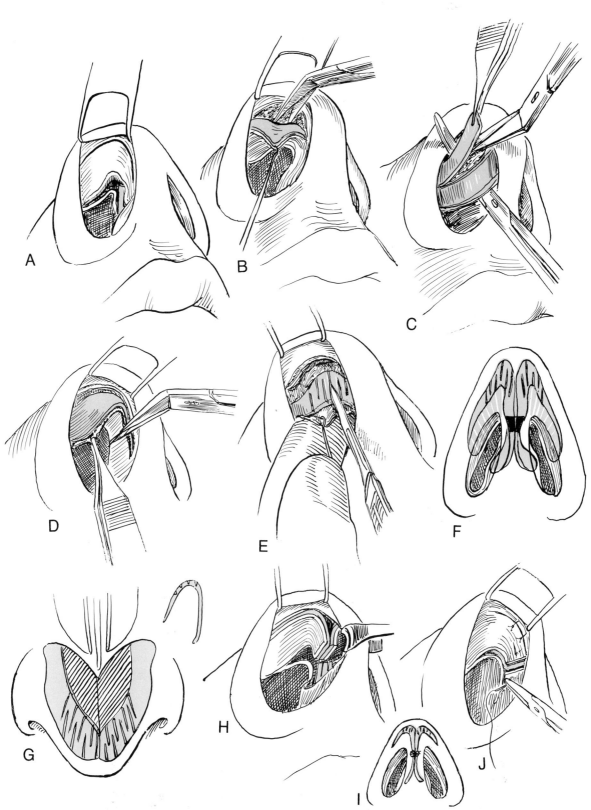

Figure 9–28. *See legend on the opposite page.*

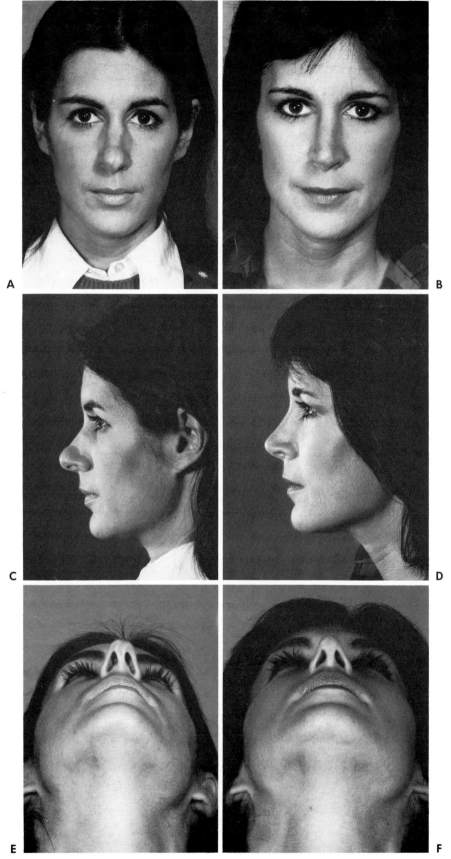

Figure 9–29. Repair of the nasal tip by the Lipsett procedure.

way, sharp points of cartilage that would become visible postoperatively are avoided, and "knuckling" is minimized.

Recession of the prominent tip is obtained by resecting a portion of the medial crus with its lining, as in the original Lipsett procedure.

Figures 9–29 and 9–30 demonstrate very well the use of the modified Lipsett technique to correct the strong and forward-projecting tip and considerable bulbous quality of the alar cartilage. Meticulous repair of the soft tissue incisions and postoperative tape splinting of the remodeled cartilage

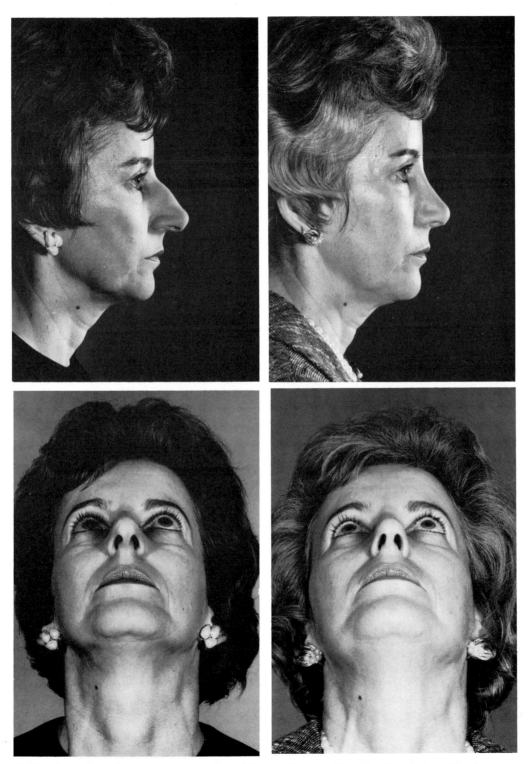

Figure 9–30. Correction of a complicated nasal tip deformity by a modified Lipsett technique. The technique employed resection of the alar base, of the lateral crus of the alar cartilage, and of a portion of the rim in the dome region.

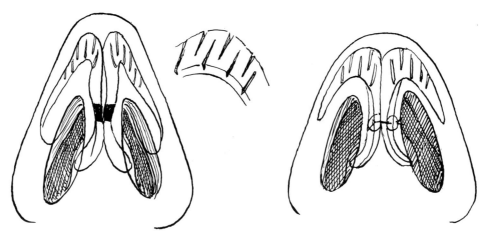

Figure 9–31. Reformed alar cartilage in modified Lipsett technique.

prevent kinking and knuckling or visible sharp cartilage points. Figure 9–31 shows the reformed alar cartilage.

A method has been formulated for the correction of postoperative knuckling of cartilaginous elements of the tip that may occur after the classic Lipsett technique (Williams, 1977) (Figure 9–32). The procedure essentially recreates the original defect and then repairs it according to sound surgical principles. Splinting is required for about two weeks. The splint can be replaced after a daily cleansing.

The results of many surgical techniques depend on the degree of skill with which they are executed. Sometimes it is the surgeon — not the technique — who determines success or failure. To obtain the required results in different types of deformities, the surgeon must have mastery of several different techniques in his armamentarium. Surgeons must avoid becoming slavishly devoted to any one procedure.

THE EVERSION TECHNIQUE

The eversion technique is useful for correcting very bulky, thick tips. The prime object is to reduce the size of the tip and to reshape it within the possible limits. A maximal reduction of cartilage and soft tissues, including subcutaneous fat as well as an appropriate amount of lining, is required (Figure 9–33). In such tips, the eversion technique has proven highly useful. Safian and others have shown that lining can be sacrificed, provided the repair is accurate, the amount of excision is carefully measured, and the raw surface is covered (Figure 9–34).

The main difference between the eversion technique and others is that the dissection is retro-

grade. This method was favored by Rode (1938), Brown and McDowell (1965), and McIndoe (1955), and it is still advocated by many surgeons today, including Gordon and Baker (1977). Eversion facilitates direct access to the cartilage and, as with the alar flap technique, wide surgical exposure of the alar cartilage is gained. It is sometimes difficult for the novice surgeon to understand the anatomic orientation and to become aware that he is approaching the cartilage from above.

Figures 9–35 through 9–38 show patients who underwent surgery by the eversion technique. The Pollet technique of tip dissection is shown in Figure 9–39.

MODIFICATION OF THE SQUARE (BOX) AND BIFID TIP DEFORMITIES

Correction of the square (box) tip deformity (Figure 9–40) depends on what proportion of the deformity consists of cartilaginous framework or is caused by redundant soft tissue. When the skin and subcutaneous tissue are excessively thick, the results are limited. However, when the squareness of the tip is mostly the result of an open angle between the medial and lateral crura of the alar cartilage, much can be done to reconstruct a more acute angulation of the alar cartilages by transecting and reshaping the cartilages. Various techniques such as the alar flap, a combination of the alar flap and multiple cross-cuts (Lipsett), and weakening of the cartilage by morcellation or multiple cross-hatching can be used to mold a more acute angle. The Pollet (1976) method of medial crus resection is also an excellent technique for correction of the box tip.

When bifidity is moderate, it is usually associated with diastasis of the alar cartilages in varying

Text continued on page 231

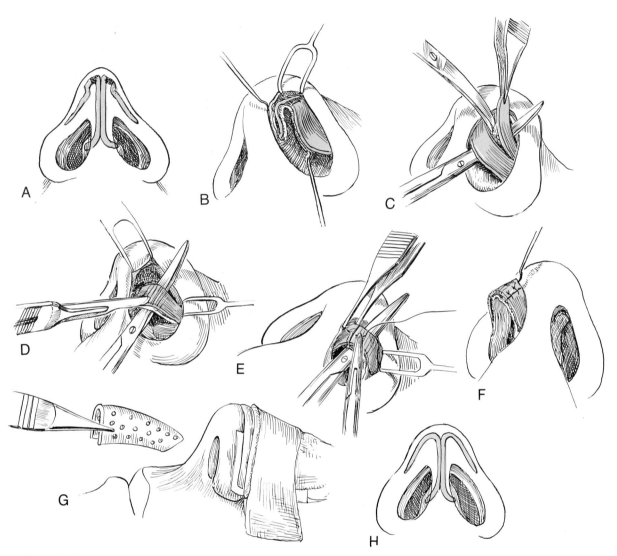

Figure 9–32. *A*, The deformity.

B, The alar flap is refashioned as a bipedicle flap.

C, If there is an excess of cartilage, a portion of the cephalic edge of the lateral crus is removed.

D, The cartilage is scored as in the original procedure.

E, After weakening the cartilage and excising the offending sharp edges, the medial and lateral crura are sutured together.

F, The re-created and sutured dome is illustrated.

G, A splint is inserted until fibrous union occurs.

H, The desired result.

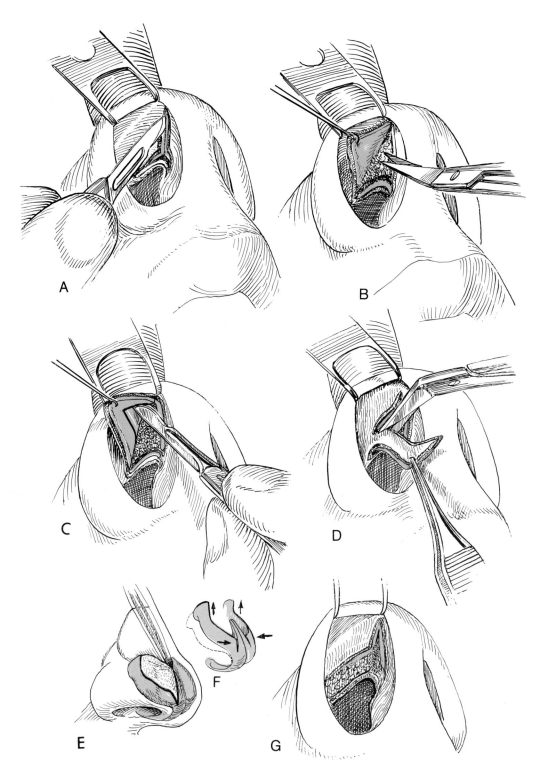

Figure 9-33. *A*, A vertical incision that splits the mucosa and cartilage along the junction of the medial lateral crura with the dome is helpful but optional in the eversion technique. It does facilitate dissection of the external side of the cartilaginous plate and its delivery as an eversion flap. When this cartilage-splitting incision is made, it may or may not extend completely through the tip.

B, The nasal tip scissors dissect the cartilage from the skin and subcutaneous tissue. Eversion traction is exerted by a skin hook.

C, The desired portion of lining and cartilage to be excised is designed according to the surgeon's judgment.

D, The redundant cartilage can then be dissected with or without its vestibular lining.

E, The usual portion of cartilage to be resected is indicated by the stippled area.

F, The arrows indicate the medial rotation of the lateral crura remnants that occurs following the excision. Further narrowing of the tip is facilitated by excision of the lining in very bulky defects.

G, The completed excision is indicated. Closure of the vertical incision with fine, plain catgut sutures is optional.

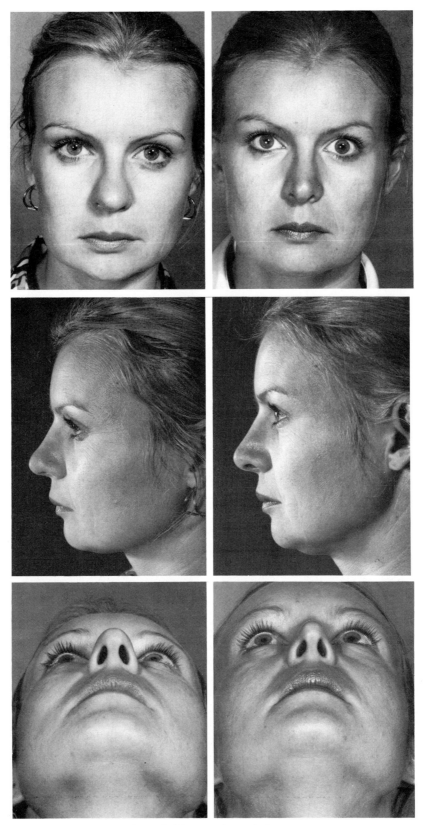

Figure 9–34. Eversion technique.

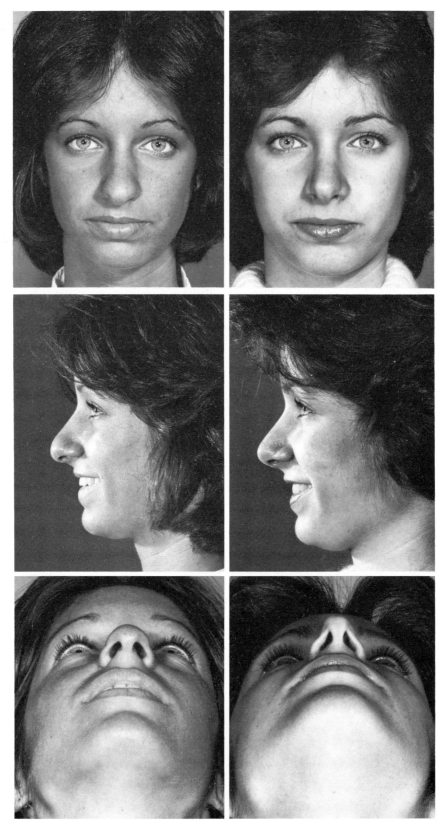

Figure 9–35.   Eversion technique on the flat box-tip nose.

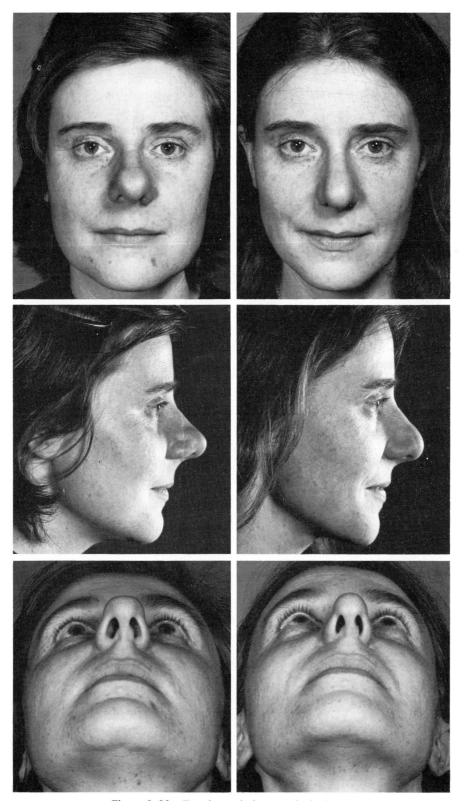

Figure 9–36. Eversion technique on the bulky tip.

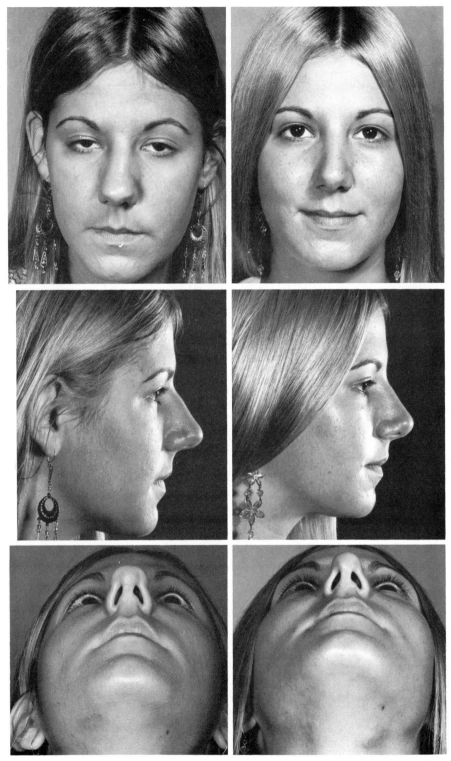

Figure 9–37.   Eversion technique for correction of marked hypertrophy of the alar cartilage.

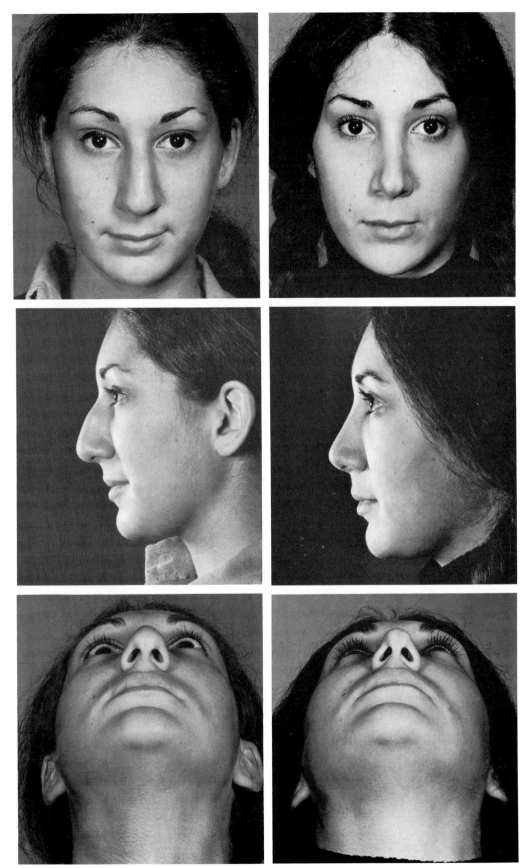

Figure 9–38. Correction of a thick nasal tip by the eversion technique. The postoperative result, although satisfactory, shows that limitations were imposed on the operator by the thick skin. Note the sharp cartilage in the tip that can occur if the dome is not transected on the medial side through the medial crus.

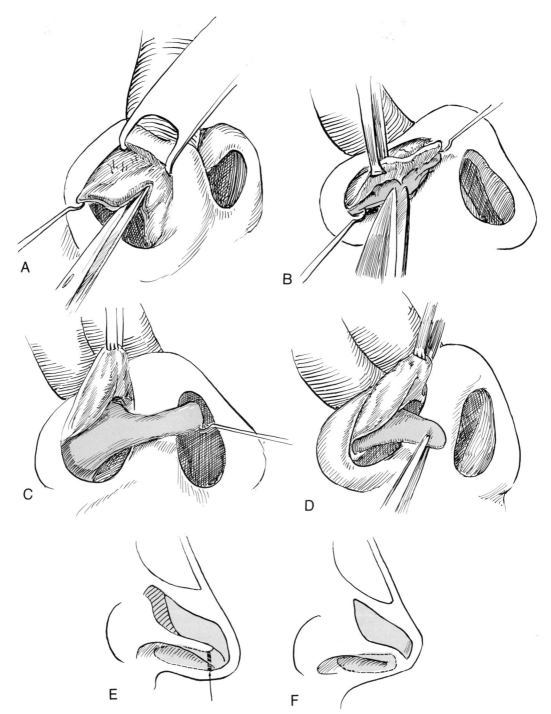

Figure 9–39. *The Pollet Technique of Tip Dissection.* (See also Figure 9–23.) The Pollet technique is a useful method of setting back the very strong or projecting tip. In many ways, it resembles the eversion technique. The cartilage is completely transected and the dome portion excised, leaving the lateral crural plates as support for the tip.

A, A para-rim incision is made extending around the dome down the caudal margin of the medial crus.

B, The caudal margin of the alar cartilage is dissected free of lining, and it is transected through the medial crus well around the dome.

C, The freed end of the cartilage is then dissected free of all soft tissue and unfolded. The excess is excised.

D, The remaining cartilage is seen to be a lateral pillar of support consisting of a plate of the caudal portion of the lateral crus.

E, The line of incision through the medial crus is indicated by the small arrow. Further recession of the tip can be achieved by excising the superolateral end of the lateral crus.

F, The tip is supported by the lateral crura.

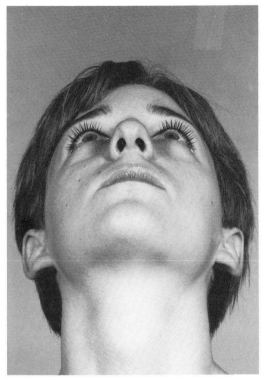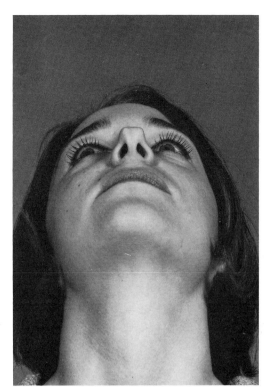

Figure 9–40. Development of a "boxed" tip after nasal tip plasty in which bifidity was not corrected and the alar "spring" was broken.

degrees. Moderate bifidity is often correctable by breaking up the soft tissues between the domes (Figure 9–41). Separating the alar cartilages from the skin with double-edged scissors and resecting the connective tissue between the crura may suffice. The Le Garde maneuver may be all that is required (Figure 9–42). Continuity of the nasal lining and its attachment to the alar cartilages should not be violated.

Direct approximating sutures between the medial crura help to eliminate the potential space between these structures, enhance the results, and insure against recurrence of the deformity. Other methods of correcting the box tip include the hockey stick incision and a complete sectioning of the tip through the medial edge of the dome, similar to the Joseph tip plasty. Pollet transected the cartilage on the medial side of the junction of the lateral and medial crus. He routinely resected a portion of the medial crus.

There may be some question as to the anatomic accuracy of the ligament of Pitanguy; however, there is often an identifiable thickening of the subdermal tissues in the tip and supratip region that resembles a connective tissue ligament. Trimming such redundant tissue unquestionably aids in minimizing the tip deformity in such problem cases — especially in the non-Caucasian nose. Figure 9–43

shows other methods of reducing the wide or box tip.

Often, a wide tip that is a result of box-like cartilages and highly vaulted domes can be improved by resection of the redundant cephalic portions of the cartilages, leaving the transition zone between the medial and lateral crura narrow so that a natural weakening of the cartilage occurs at the juncture (Figure 9–43, *A, B, C*). The effects of wound contracture close the open angle between the medial and lateral crura and result in the formation of a more acute angulation, indicated by the arrows in *C*.

When the alar cartilages are thick and resilient as well as redundant, multiple cross-hatchings may help to weaken the cartilage so that an acute angle is achieved (Figure 9–43, *D, E, F*). Cross-hatching can be done with a sharp #15 blade or more roughly with crushing forceps (morcellation).

Another technique that must be performed very accurately is excision of a strip of cartilage at the junction of the medial and lateral crura so that total rupture of the cartilaginous spring occurs (Figure 9–43, *G, H, I*). The strip excision must be at exactly the same level on either side to prevent asymmetry and projecting cartilage points following healing.

Correction of bifidity and forward projection

Text continued on page 242

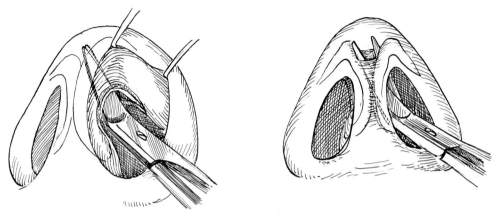

Figure 9–41.   Moderate widening of the interdome proportion may be reduced by breaking up the fibro-areolar tissue in this region. Resulting scar contraction will pull the domes together. This technique is facilitated by resection of the supratip ligament (Pitanguy, 1965).

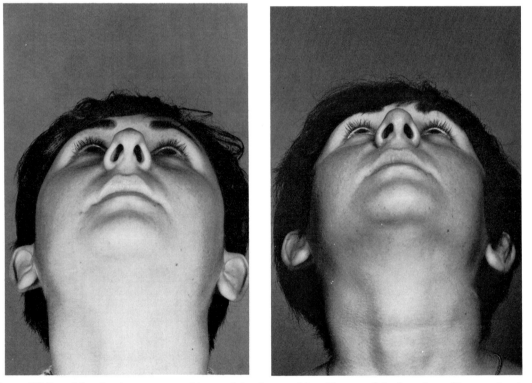

Moderate bifidity of the alar domes corrected by nasal tip plasty and breaking up of the interdome fibro-areolar tissues.

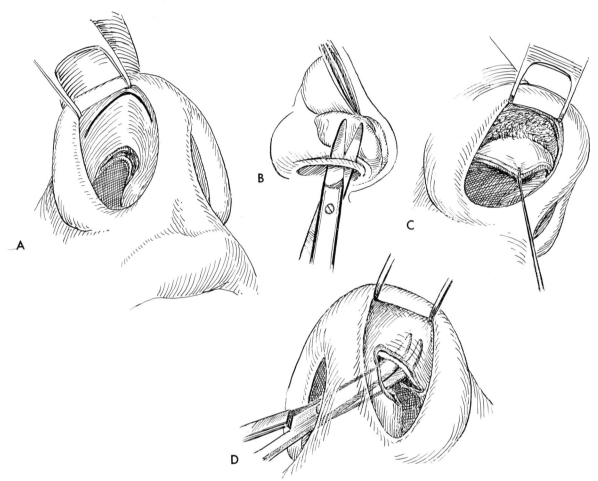

Figure 9–42. The LeGarde maneuver for modification of the nasal tip contour with or without cartilaginous resection.

A, A standard rim incision is made.

B, The nasal tip scissors are passed through the rim incision and the external aspect of the lateral crura of the alar cartilages to free these from their attachment to overlying skin.

C, The freed cartilages permit redraping of the skin.

D, Following a routine nasal tip plasty, the redraping is aided by freeing remaining alar cartilage remnants from the overlying skin.

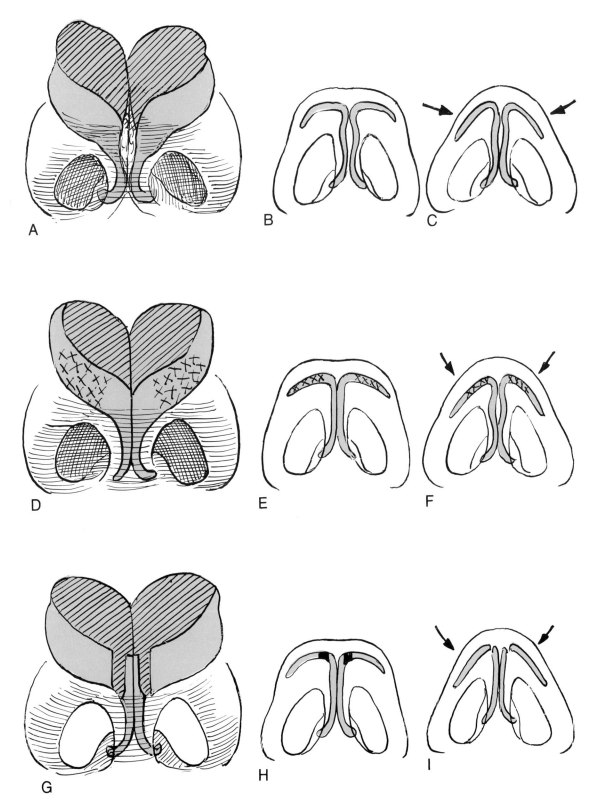

Figure 9–43.   Reducing the wide or box-like tip.

A, B, and *C,* Resection of the redundant cephalic portions of the cartilages.

D, E, and *F,* Multiple crosshatchings of thick, resilient alar cartilages.

G, H, and *I,* Excision of cartilage strip at junction of medial and lateral crura.

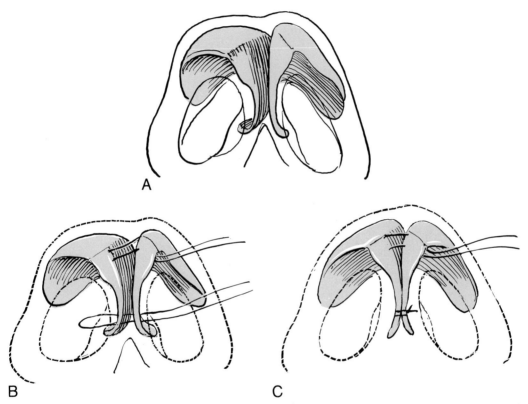

Figure 9–44. *A*, The left alar cartilage is drawn in a normal position in the wide tip nose and the right alar cartilage is shown to be rotated.

B and *C*, Correction of the rotation of the medial crus should and probably does aid in correction of the broad and flat tip in many instances.

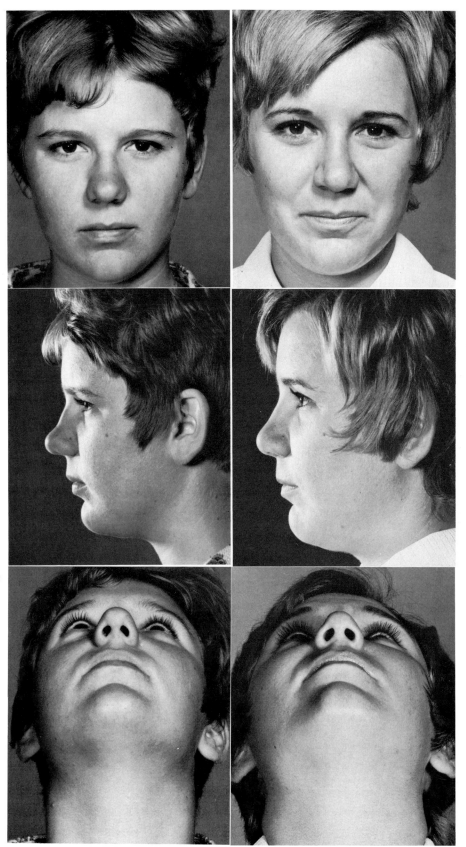

Figure 9–45. Correction of the thick or "beefy" tip is severely limited by the morphology of the problem, and both patient and surgeon must be prepared to accept limited improvement. If the patient and family do not seem to comprehend that only a *relative* improvement can result, surgery is best postponed or cancelled.

The principal limiting factor is the skin and subcutaneous tissue, which is usually quite unmanageable. Cartilage and bone can be reshaped, but not skin. Sometimes excessive subcutaneous fat can be resected, but the procedure is hazardous and can cause unsightly scar depressions and contour irregularities. Focal skin loss can occur. The alar eversion approach is often helpful, because as a rule some nasal lining can be spared, but excision of the lining must still be minimal.

In this patient, the tip was improved by complete removal of the lateral crura, including the alar domes.

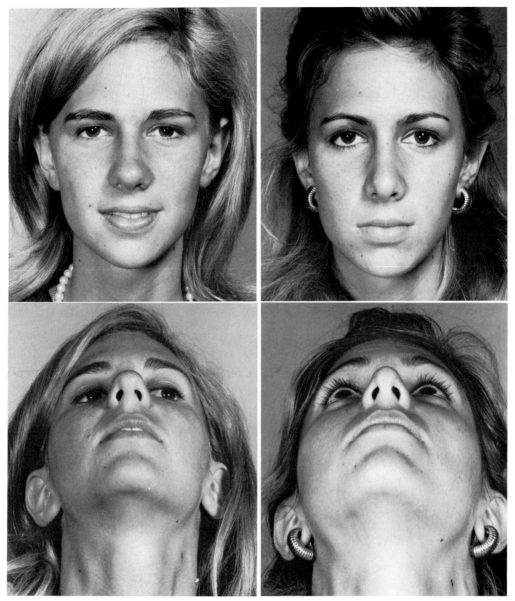

Figure 9-46.   Thickened nostril rims in a patient with thick, oily skin and an ample pad of subcutaneous tissue. Some improvement was obtained by the eversion technique and nostril rim excision.

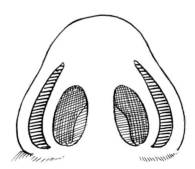

Figure 9-47.   Modification of the nostril border.

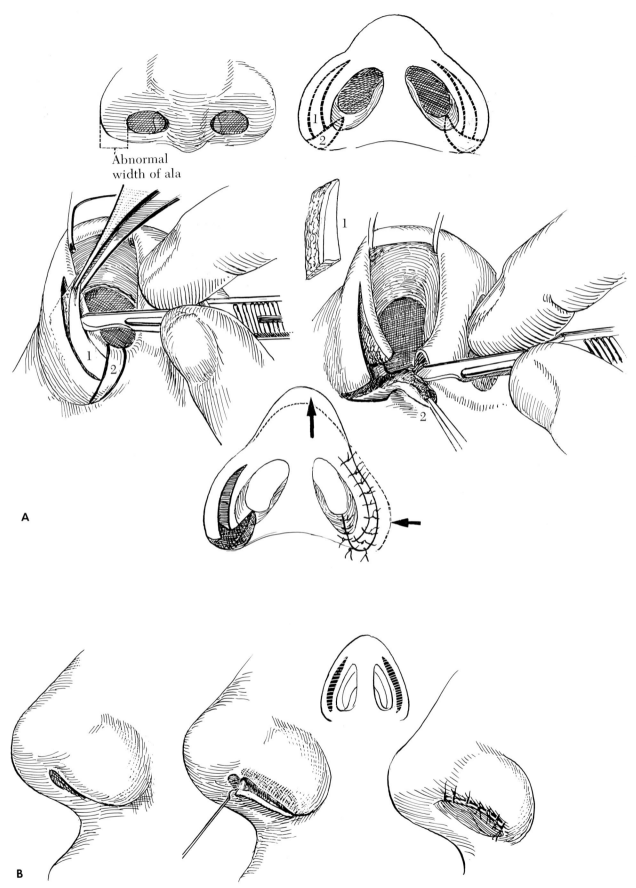

Abnormal width of ala

A

B

Figure 9–48.   Thinning of the nostrils by the "piece-of-pie" excision technique can be combined with various designs of alar base resections advocated by Millard as shown here (*A*). The "hanging" nostril margin can be improved by the technique shown in *B*.

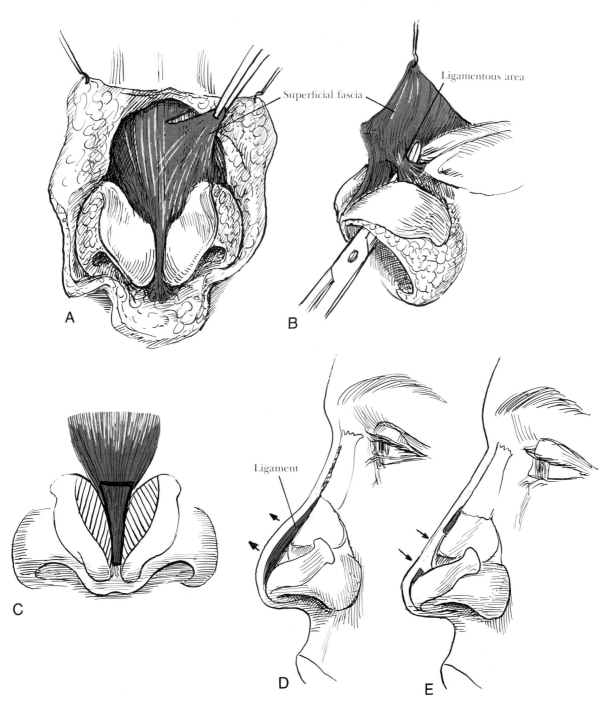

Figure 9–49. *A* and *B*, The ligament is demonstrated in this simulated cadaver dissection.

C, The caudal midline portion of the ligament to be resected (according to Pitanguy) is shown. The point of transection of the ligament across the dorsum is represented by a dark line.

D and *E*, A sagittal view showing the line of resection.

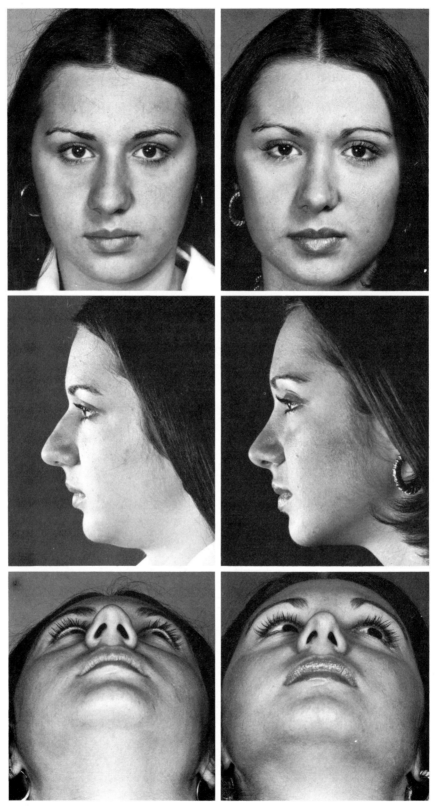

Figure 9–50.   Excision of subcutaneous tissue and excision technique for treatment of alar cartilages.

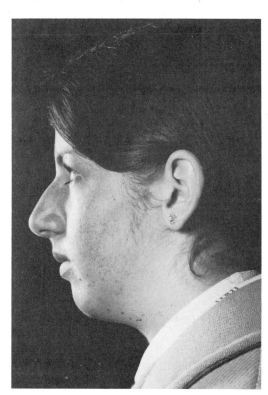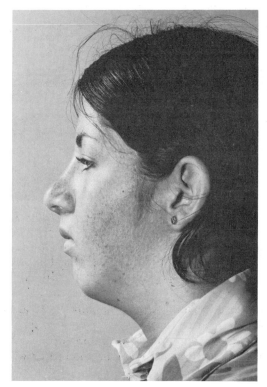

Figure 9–51.   The result of an injudicious excision of subcutaneous tissues and damage to the overlying dermis. Note the depressed scar over the left alar dome area.

of the tip along with increased angulation between the medial and lateral crura can also be achieved when the alar cartilages are thin and pliable by approximating the medial crura with simple mattress sutures (Figure 9–44).

Further reduction of the wide (beefy) tip (Figure 9–45) requires excision of redundant soft tissue. Many patients with this deformity have an excess of subcutaneous fat as well as thickening of the skin. The skin, of course, cannot be sacrificed. However, removal of all extraneous subcutaneous fat along with the excision of excess portions of alar cartilage often accomplishes surprising results (Figure 9–46).

Access to the subcutaneous fat is easily obtainable by any of the standard approaches to the alar cartilages, but it is facilitated by the alar flap technique or the intracartilaginous incision.

REDUCTION OF THE NOSTRILS

Direct surgical approach to reduction of the hanging, bulky nostril is indicated less often than excision of soft tissue and fat of the subcutaneous area of the tip. The surgical plan involves removal of a wedge-shaped section of tissue (Millard, 1960). The incision is best accomplished with a #11 blade inserted directly into the nostril rim and the excision of a long, vertical "piece of pie," designed to achieve the desired modification of the nostril border (Figure 9–47). The nostril border can be sutured in such a way as to be arched, thereby overcoming the drooping or overhanging nostrils. Nostril rim excision is frequently combined with an alar base resection to reduce the forward projection of the tip or the flaring of the nostril (Figure 9–48, A). The hanging nostril is a most unattractive deformity, since it obscures the natural curve of the columella. It is well to remember that the nostril rim is composed of skin and connective tissue and *not* alar cartilage, except anteriorly (Figure 9–48, B).

When such external incisions are used about the nares, it is important to obtain the best possible scar and to eliminate the only visible evidence of surgery. Tension from suture lines is relieved with chronic catgut sutures. Skin sutures should be a very fine 6–0 or 5–0 nylon and removed early in the postoperative course (usually on the third or fourth postoperative day).

We use such thinning incisions only rarely, and only in those patients in whom no other approach is possible. Scars along the nostril rim heal quite well in most instances and are surprisingly inconspicuous, but the novice surgeon would be wise to proceed with care.

Pitanguy, in describing the technique required to correct the thickened nose often found in non-caucasions, described a dermatocartilaginous ligament lying on the dorsum of the nose and extending from the alar cartilages cephalically (1965). He recommended resection of this ligament and considered it important not only in reducing the bulbous nose but in preventing postoperative supratip swelling (Figure 9–49).

On occasion, the author has resected subcutaneous tissue in the thick, bulbous nose (Figure 9–50). Sometimes, a definite plane of tissue resembling a ligament seems to exist, and it can be separated by blunt or sharp dissection from the dermis. Great care must be exercised, however, to avoid injuring the dermis during such procedures; otherwise, a scar deformity similar to the one shown in Figure 9–51 will result.

(For references, see pages 450 to 453.)

Chapter 10

The Lip-Tip-Columella Complex and the Alar Base

THOMAS D. REES, M.D., F.A.C.S.

THE LIP-TIP-COLUMELLA COMPLEX

The relationship of the lip to the nose is important to facial contour (Figure 10–1). Lip posture depends on several factors but primarily on the shape of the maxilla and the upper dental arch and on the configuration of the nose. Rhinoplasty usually affects the lip to some degree, and sometimes the procedure must include some dissection of the lip's attachments to the maxilla.

The angle formed between the columella and the lip has been the subject of much discussion in the literature of nasal plastic surgery. The most pleasing angle is said to be 100 degrees, and nu-

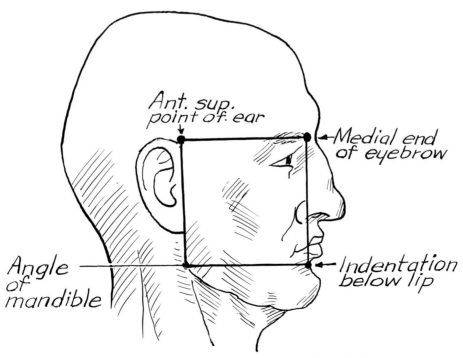

Figure 10–1. Leonardo's square for assessing relationships of facial structures.

243

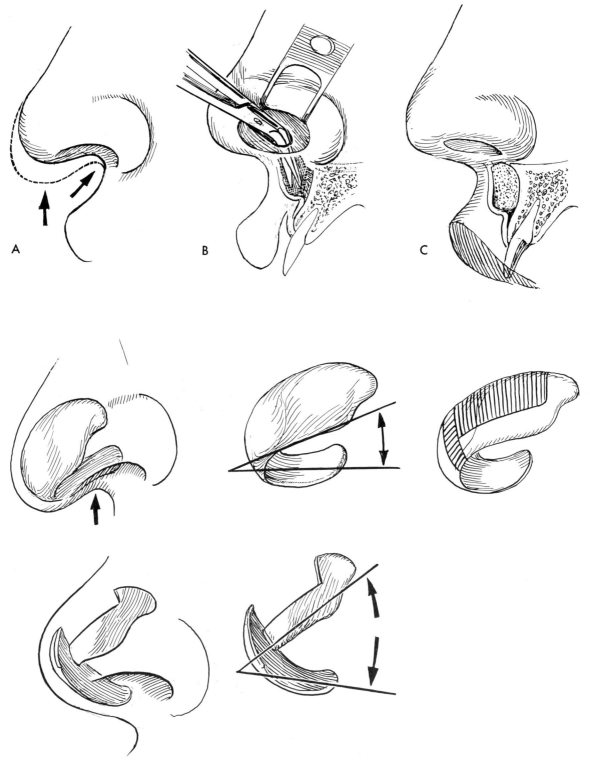

Figure 10–2. Correction of an acute nasolabial angle by an implant of bone, cartilage, or alloplastic material, according to the technique of Aufricht.

A, The prolapsed nasal tip.

B, Formation of a pocket in the region of the nasal spine.

C, The implant in place and correction achieved.

The lower series of drawings demonstrate the necessity of remodeling the nasal tip by breaking through the alae at the level of the domes in order to change the angle between the medial and lateral crura in some patients with plunging tips, which are the result of such an anatomical angulation of the alar cartilages.

merous gadgets have been devised to measure the angle and to aid the surgeon in achieving the putative ideal — often easier said than done.

The lip-nose angle depends on the posture of the septum, the nasal spine, the columella, and the lip. The nasal spine is the most important element. Resection of this structure can result in retraction of the base of the columella and consequent overhanging or "plunging" of the tip. In many patients, the nasal spine is poorly or not at all developed. the tip of the nose of such a patient often hangs down, and the nasolabial angle is acute. Aufricht (1969) recommended implantation of cartilage or an alloplast to simulate the normally developed nasal spine, and his results are impressive (Figure 10–2). However, I have resorted to this procedure on very few occasions because it produces a stiffness of the lip, of which the patient is quite conscious, and sometimes a loss of normal animation.

Excessive shortening of the nose, with removal of a large piece of the caudal margin of the septum, can relax the lip, sometimes to an extreme degree so that it hangs almost like a curtain over the upper teeth and appears overly long. The length of the lip as well as the shape of the upper dental arch should be thoroughly studied preoperatively in each patient. The surgeon should project in advance what the effect of the total operation will be on the lip. Often, a judicious trimming of the lower nose and particularly the nasal spine is indicated in order to maintain a natural looking upper lip. An excellent alternative to removing the nasal spine is simply to fracture it and allow it to remain in place.

If, on the other hand, a dropped or plunging tip is a part of the nasal deformity, which is the case in a high percentage of patients, other adjustments in technique are required (Fig. 10–2). In some instances, the dropped tip can be improved only partially without such excessive surgery that the secondary deformity would be more unattractive than the original. Such a result would certainly have all the stigmata of a "nose job."

Anatomic features contributing to the plunging tip are (1) the shape of the alar cartilages, (2) the relation of the septal angle to the alar cartilages, (3) the height of the nasal dorsum, (4) the shape of the caudal margins of the septum and the nasal spine, (5) the action of muscular attachments of the alae, (6) the length and shape of the maxilla and teeth, and (7) the shape of the upper lip.

Resection of the caudal septum and "overshortening" of the tip with fixation at a high angle by mattress transfixion sutures may be effective when a small correction is required, but it can be disastrous when a plunging tip is a significant fea-

ture of the patient's deformity. Maintaining the tip in an elevated position may require shortening of the side wall of the nose, which involves resection of a large part of the caudal end of each upper lateral cartilage. The lateral alar wings can be elevated to fill the raw defect when they are fixed in their new position.

Generally, the trimming of the caudal septum and nasal spine should be conservative. Ambitious removal of the spine or the base of the caudal septum can increase the plunging deformity by increasing the acuteness of the lip-columella angle. Overshortening of the nose is a common problem after incompetent surgery and is an almost irreparable defect. The caudal margin of the septum is used as a buttress to maintain the tip in its new position. The mucosa from each side is trimmed so that the denuded septal cartilage is inserted tongue-in-groove fashion between the medial alar crura, which are held apart by scissors; mattress sutures fix the tip in position. This technique has been criticized, but when used in the proper circumstances, it has been successful.

THE NASAL SPINE

The anatomic variations found in the nasal spine and the relationship of the nasal spine to the cartilaginous caudal border of the septum are key structural factors in the columella-lip-nose complex. These must be modified occasionally to produce a harmonious result. Surgical approach to the caudal septum and the nasal spine is, however, based on ultraconservatism, since overresection of these structures results in overshortening of the nose and frequently in retraction of the columella, accentuating the dropped tip deformity. They should be trimmed only after correction of the dorsal profile and preferably after tip surgery. The anatomic variants of the spine and caudal septum that deserve the surgeon's attention are illustrated in Figure 10–3.

The bony nasal spine is rarely the culprit in lip-nose deformities. In fact, resection of the spine is the exception rather than the rule. The spine should never be resected until all other adjustments have been made, including correction of the dorsum, tip, and soft tissues of the lip (freeing from the maxilla) and finally trimming of the redundant caudal margin. Then and only then should consideration be given to resecting the spine. Some surgeons (e.g., Aufricht) make the point of implanting cartilage and bone into the lip-columella angle to restore the slight natural obliquity of this angle. Resection of the spine unneces-

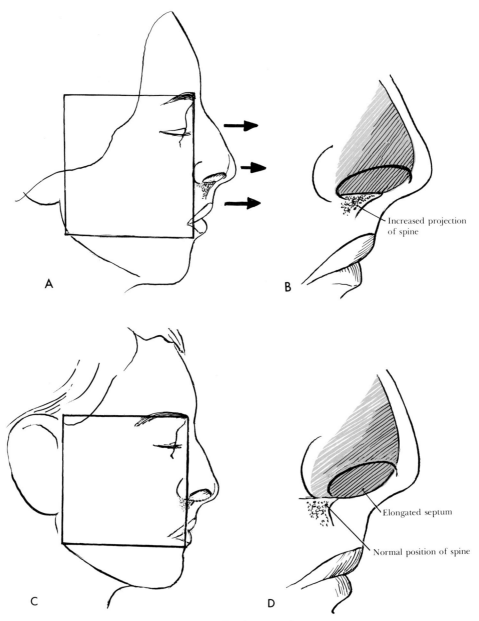

Figure 10–3. *A* and *B*, The nose appears to "precede" the face because of the prominent caudal septal border and nasal spine. The upper lip appears shortened. It also may be tethered. *C* and *D*, An obtuse labiocolumellar angle is produced by a prominent caudal septal border. The spine may be normal. The lip also appears to be shortened.

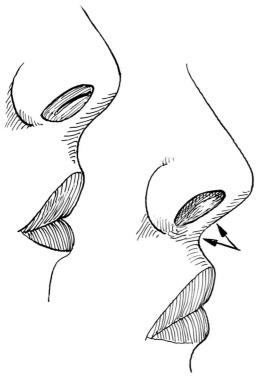

Figure 10–4. Judicious sculpting of the caudal septum and nasal spine effectively elongates the upper lip and creates a pleasing nasolabial angle.

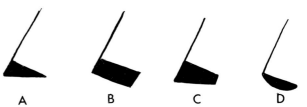

Figure 10–6. Designs for resection of the caudal septum. *A,* Tilts tip in a cephalic direction. *B,* Shortens nose (provided the tip does not droop). *C,* Tilts tip and shortens nose. *D,* Helps reduce the effect of the hanging columella.

figuration of the face and particularly on the shape of the nose. Different designs of resection of the caudal septum are diagrammed in Figure 10–6. These varying shapes can produce, at least theoretically, different results in the configuration of the final result; however, this is overly simplistic since the final result depends on combination of many surgical steps.

Steps for correction of the caudal border of the septum and nasal spine are shown in Figure 10–7.

Figure 10–8 shows a patient with a surgically repaired nasal spine.

THE TETHERED LIP

The tethered foreshortened upper lip is usually associated with a hump nose deformity and a prominent nasal spine-caudal-septum complex. The lip assumes an "open posture" when the face is not animated, and when animation occurs in speaking, eating, or especially smiling, the soft tissues curl upward and accentuate the deformity. It is often possible to soften the effect or to overcome it altogether by a series of surgical maneuvers.

Anatomically, the upper lip is often fixed to the alveolus at a high level so that there is a lack of coverage of the upper incisors. The deformity and its correction are illustrated in Figures 10–9 through 10–11.

Exposure of the upper incisors infers a "Bugs Bunny" look. Patients with this problem are forced to purse their lips muscularly and thus assume an unattractive facial attitude. Figure 10–11 shows a patient in whom a more relaxed expression was obtained by minimal resection of the dorsal profile, trimming of the nasal spine, and subperiosteal release of the upper lip.

THE COLUMELLA

The columella is an important aesthetic component of the nose. It provides much of the grace

sarily results in an acute angulation and retraction of the columella in many instances. Careful study will confirm that the fullness of this angle is usually the result of soft tissue and the bulging caudal margin of the septum, and a pleasing nasolabial and columella-alar angle can be adjusted to a large extent during rhinoplasty (Figure 10–4).

The "normal" angles are illustrated in Figure 10–5. The columella hangs lower than the alar bases and the nasolabial angle is roughly 90 degrees. There are many minor variations, of course, that are acceptable, depending on the overall con-

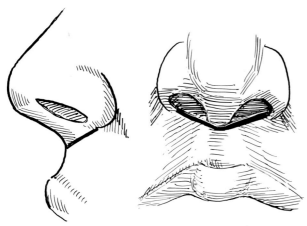

Figure 10–5. Normal columella-alar angles.

Text continued on page 255

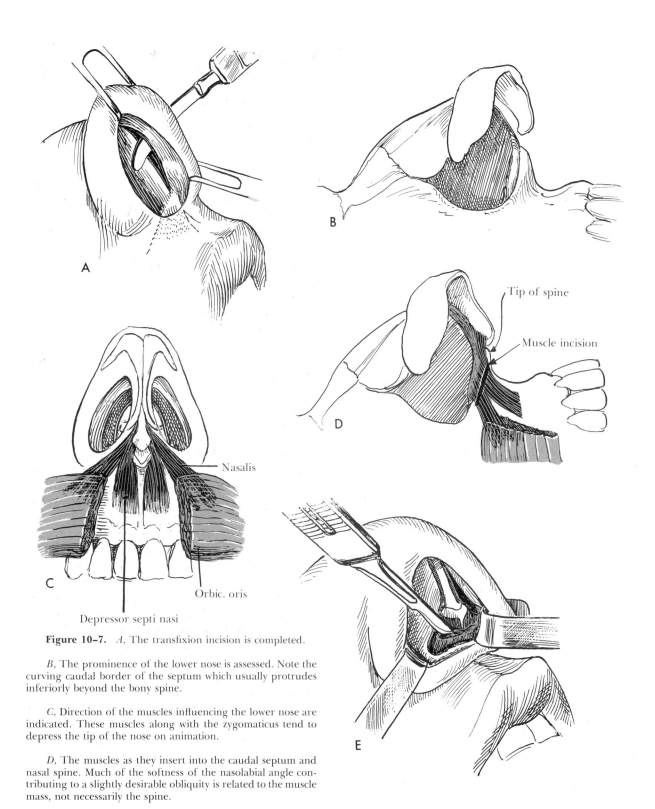

Nasalis

Orbic. oris

Depressor septi nasi

Tip of spine

Muscle incision

Figure 10–7. *A*, The transfixion incision is completed.

B, The prominence of the lower nose is assessed. Note the curving caudal border of the septum which usually protrudes inferiorly beyond the bony spine.

C, Direction of the muscles influencing the lower nose are indicated. These muscles along with the zygomaticus tend to depress the tip of the nose on animation.

D, The muscles as they insert into the caudal septum and nasal spine. Much of the softness of the nasolabial angle contributing to a slightly desirable obliquity is related to the muscle mass, not necessarily the spine.

E, An incision is made into the muscle, clearing it from the spine. This step helps eliminate plunging on animation and provides access to the caudal septum and spine for appropriate trimming as required.

Illustration continued on the opposite page.

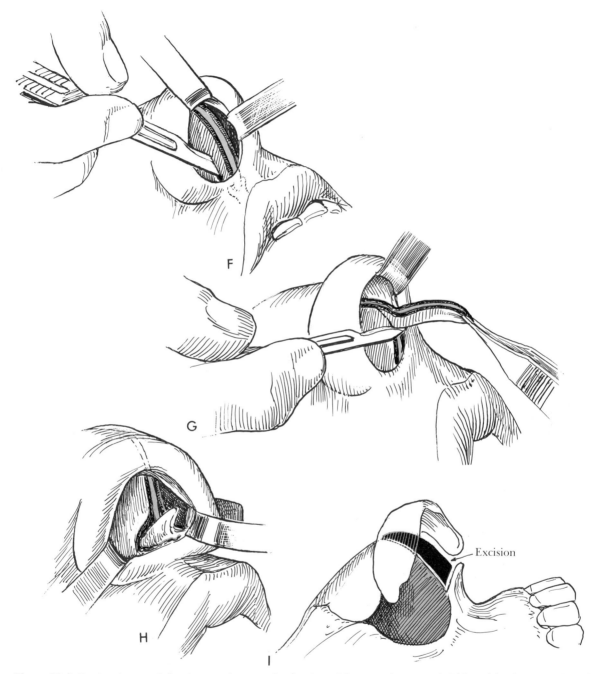

Figure 10–7 *Continued.* *F* and *G*, The prominent (redundant) caudal septum is removed. This excision is usually done first just prior to tip surgery. It should always be very conservative, since more can be removed later in the operation as required. It is very important not to overshorten the nose. The incision in the caudal septum is slightly curving, and the septal angle is rounded off. No straight lines exist in nature.

H and *I*, With trimming of the cartilaginous septum, the nasal spine is brought into bas relief. More accurate assessment as to whether it is excessive in width or length can then be made. Excision may or may not be required.

Illustration continued on the following page.

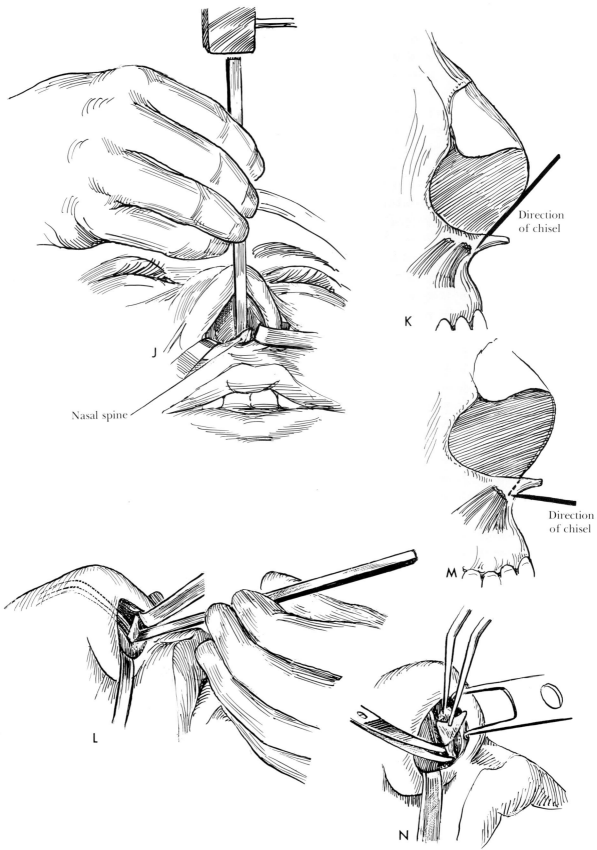

Nasal spine

Direction
of chisel

Direction
of chisel

Figure 10–7 *Continued.*

J–N, A small 5- or 7-mm. sharp osteotome or chisel is an effective instrument for removing the offending spine. A double-action rongeur is also excellent for this purpose. It is usually necessary to clean the small piece of bone free of soft tissue and periosteal attachments.

It is emphasized again that the foregoing must be carefully assessed in each patient. It is frequently necessary to reduce the caudal margin of the septum. It is *rarely* necessary to remove bony nasal spine. Either step must be done cautiously to prevent retraction of the columella or overshortening of the nose.

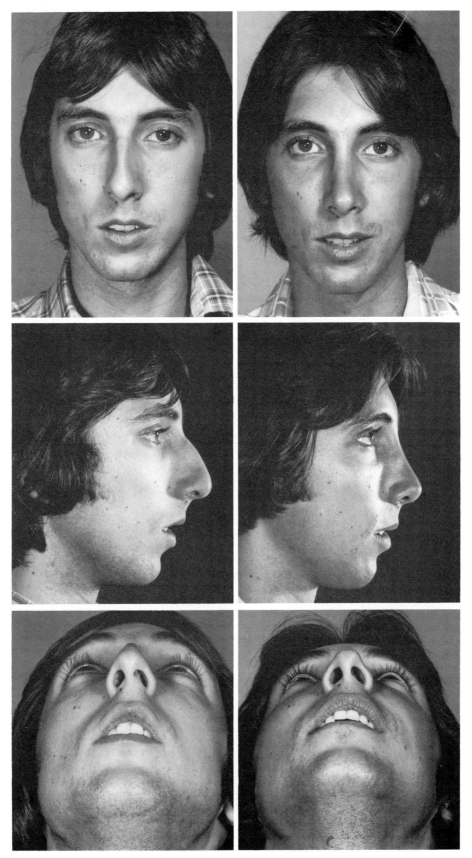

Figure 10–8.   Surgically repaired nasal spine.

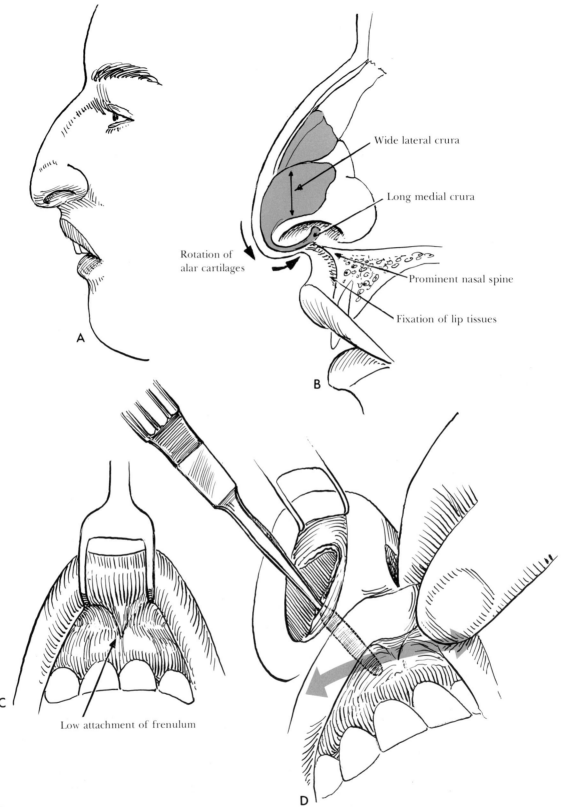

Figure 10–9.   *A,* The "tethered lip."

B and *C,* The anatomic characteristics of the deformity are indicated. Note the low attachment of the frenulum and the caudal rotation of the alar cartilages.

D, An elevator (Joseph) is inserted through the base of the transfixion incision. The soft tissues are elevated from the anterior surface of the alveolus at the subperiosteal level, allowing relaxation of the gingiva and a downward shift of the lip.

Illustration continued on the opposite page.

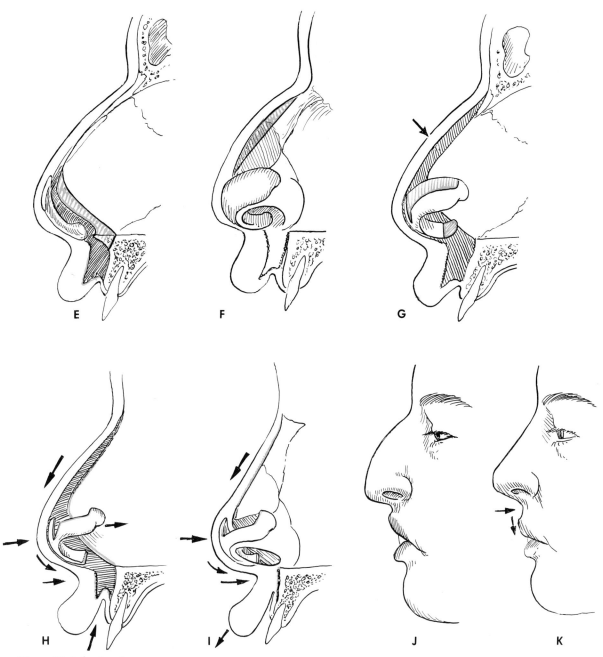

Figure 10–9 *Continued.*

E, The lip is freed, the nasal spine is resected, and the caudal border of the cartilaginous septum is resected and shortened.

F, The nasal dorsum is corrected to a new profile line.

G, The tip is remodeled by resection of the outer portion of the lateral crus on each side. Further recession and correction of the flared, widened columella base is gained by resection of the bases of the medial crura.

H, The result of these resections, and the motion they impart.

I, The procedure will allow a drooping of the tip, recession of the columella base, and release of the transverse tightness of the upper lip, combined with some degree of lengthening at the expense of both the nasal skin and the adjacent lip skin.

J and *K*, Comparison of preoperative and postoperative profiles.

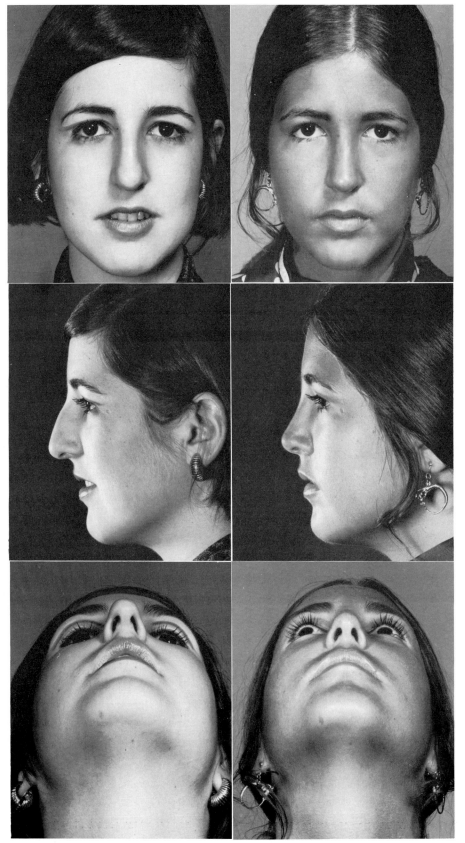

Figure 10–10.   Minimal resection of the dorsal profile is required in a deformity of this type. The relatively large nose is balanced by the strong face. The postoperative views demonstrate the result of minimal tip elevation and only slight resection of nasal dorsum. The lip was also released during the procedure.

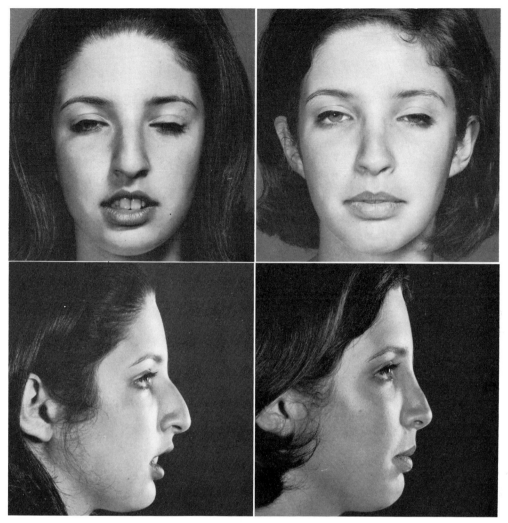

Figure 10–11.   The tethered lip can often be pleasingly relaxed by lowering the dorsum of the nasal septum and completing the transfixion incision. In this patient, the upper lip and gingiva were freed from the anterior surface of the maxilla in the region of the nasal spine.

of the lower nose and lobule. Anatomically, the columella should describe a curving line that extends slightly below the nostril margins. Such a line can be obscured by low hanging nostrils or by an unusually high columella. The base of the columella receives its shape from the "splaying" outward of the cartilaginous feet of the medial crura. This increase in width at the base of the columella is natural and attractive; however, sometimes thinning is required. This is achieved either by removing soft tissue between the base of the medial crura and suturing the crura together or by excision of the cartilaginous feet altogether (Figure 10–12). Suturing the feet together at the base of the columella is necessary in maneuvers designed to increase the length of the columella or projection of the tip (see section on non-Caucasian noses).

With his customary ingenuity, Millard reported a technique for augmenting tip projection (1971), a most difficult and challenging problem to solve. Figure 10–13 shows the technique, using three composite grafts to lengthen the columella and both ala in a young woman (Figure 10–14). The donor sites in the ears healed without difficulty and with minimal deformity. The composite grafts appeared doubtful for some time, which is not unusual, yet they were all viable and produced an excellent result.

The natural curve of the columella is exaggerated in some patients. The curve can become a rounded unattractive convexity known as the hanging columella. This deformity has two primary components and several secondary ones. The primary components are an exaggerated and prominent curving caudal margin of the septum and an exaggerated curving of the inferior (caudal) margin of the medial crus (Figure 10–15). Either or both of these excessive curves can cause

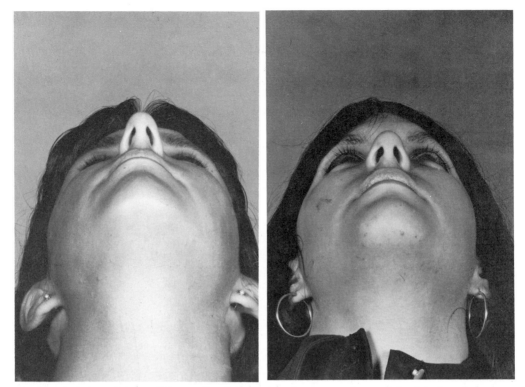

Figure 10–12. If the feet of the medial crura flare laterally to such an extent that resection is indicated to narrow the base of the columella, they can be delivered and resected through an incision similar to that described for trimming the caudal edge. Sometimes it is necessary to suture these structures when lengthening of the columella is desired. This maneuver can also increase the breathing space.

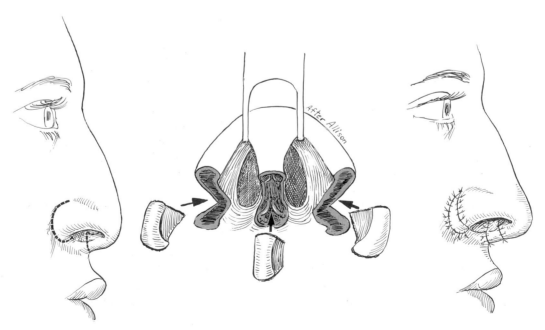

Figure 10–13. Augmentation of tip projection. (From Millard, R. D.: Plast. Reconstr. Surg. *48*:501, 1971. Reproduced with permission.)

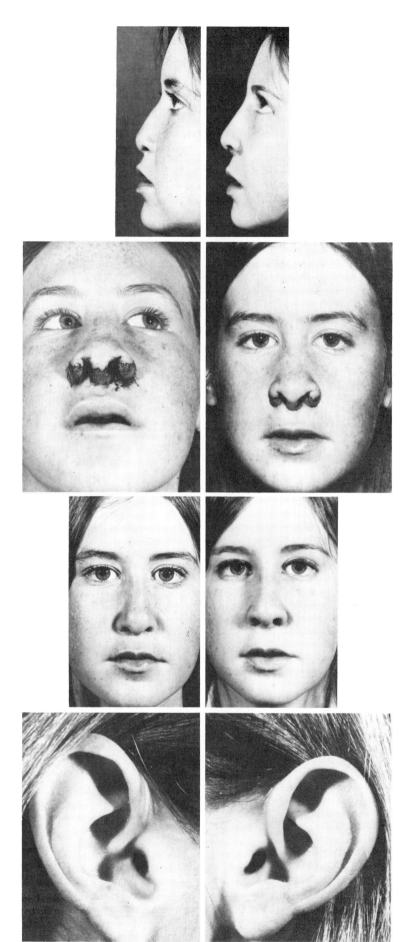

Figure 10–14. Augmentation of tip projection. (Courtesy of R. Millard.)

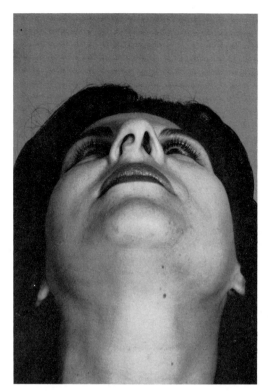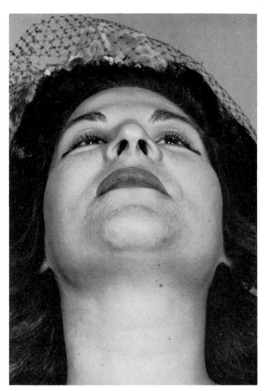

Figure 10–15.   A twisted columella can result from a developmental deformity, either of the alar cartilages or of the septum, or both. Simultaneous correction of these two structures may be necessary. These photographs demonstrate correction of a twisted medial crus, a deviated caudal septal border, and an asymmetrical tip. Improvement required nasal plasty, anterior septal plasty, and correction of the tip asymmetry by bilateral columellar rim incisions, everting the alar cartilages and correcting their points of distortion.

the problem, and trimming of one or both may be required to correct it (Figure 10–16). In most patients, trimming of the curving caudal margin of the septum is sufficient to correct the hanging columella, unless the deformity is related almost entirely to the inferior margin of the medial crus.

If the hanging columella is related to an exaggerated curvature of the medial crus, direct surgical intervention of the medial crus is required. Such exposure is often gained concomitantly with the alar flap technique, or it may be achieved independently of the remainder of the alar cartilages by a direct para-marginal columellar incision on each side of the columella (Figures 10–17 and 10–18).

The Retracted Columella

The retracted columella can occur naturally in some individuals or can be secondary to other nasal anatomic variations such as a plunging tip and high hump. It may also be ethnic as in the Mestizo nose (Ortiz-Monesterio, 1977). The retracted columella is usually, however, the result of trauma in which the caudal septum and the nasal

spine have been inadvertently or purposely destroyed or overresected.

The retracted columella deformity is distressing and not always easy to correct, since the loss of osteocartilaginous support is so frequently associated with a similar loss of soft tissue from the columella and membranous septum. If the soft tissue is not actually missing, it is frequently so scarred that it is nonelastic, thus providing very poor coverage over any type of implant whether it be autograft or alloplast.

Reconstruction of the soft tissue, and particularly of the membranous septum, is exceedingly difficult because, most often, the available soft tissue from the nose in the form of flaps from the ala (Millard) or septum is also deficient or scarred from previous surgery or trauma. Tissue grafts from other body parts for reconstruction of the soft tissue are generally unsatisfactory and technically difficult to achieve. Composite grafts from the ear and small pedicles from the nasolabial fold are possible but awkward and often unnatural.

The simplest and most natural method of correcting the retraced columella when adequate soft tissue redundancy is present is an implant to the

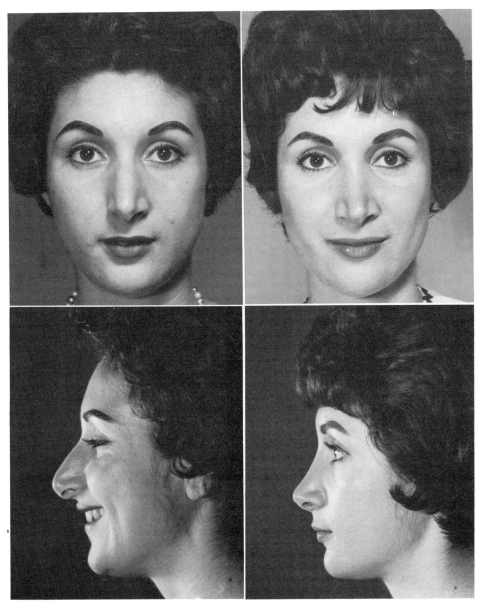

Figure 10–16. Lengthening of the upper lip was accomplished by removing the nasal spine and modifying the caudal border of the septum as well as trimming the inferior margins of the medial crura.

Figure 10–17.   Surgical intervention of the medial crus.

A, The hanging columella of the type related primarily to the caudal margin of the medial crus.

B, A para-marginal incision is made just along the caudal border of the medial crus.

C, The lining is dissected away from the medial crus.

D, The soft tissue is separated from between the medial crura.

E, With freeing of the medial crura, the extent of the anatomical problem becomes evident.

F, Slight pressure on the columella reveals the amount of caudal redundancy of the cartilage and indicates the amount to be resected.

G, The excess cartilage is trimmed. *It is frequently necessary to remove a like amount of lining.*

H, The new profile. The line should still be a slight curve, probably more curved than indicated in this illustration.

See illustration on the opposite page.

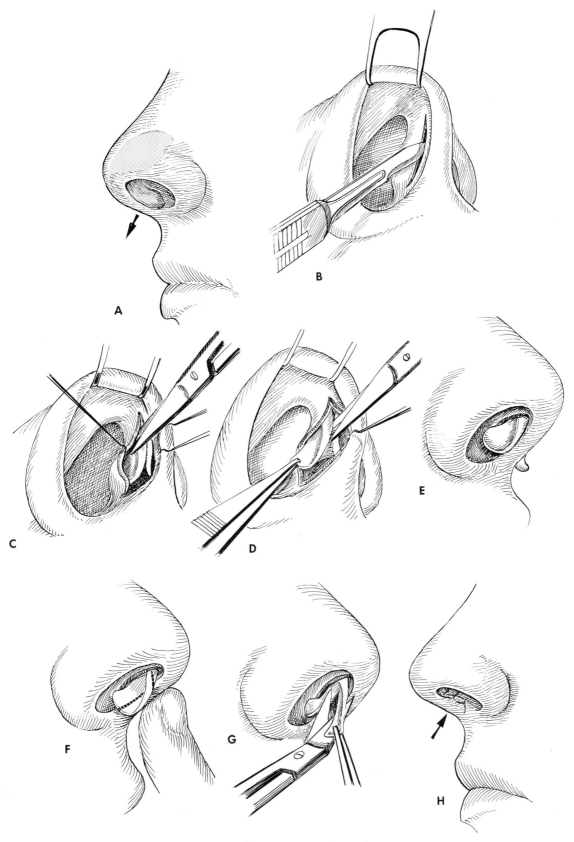

Figure 10–17. *See legend on the opposite page.*

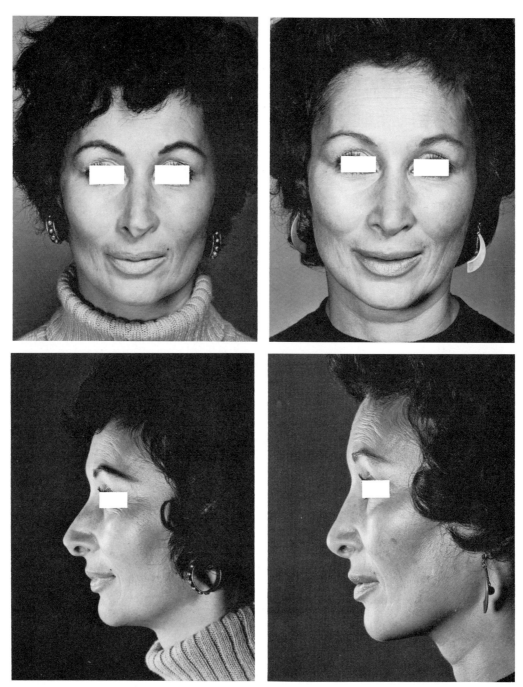

Figure 10–18. Correction of a distorted hanging columella. In addition to the cartilages themselves, it is often necessary to resect a corresponding strip of columellar skin. Marked curvature of the caudal margin of the septum can also contribute to a hanging columella and in some cases is the sole cause. The septum is easily corrected by resecting the convex portion.

columella, particularly to the base of the columella (Figure 10–19). The septum is an excellent source of such implant material, provided it has not been resected or destroyed previously. Several pieces of the cartilaginous septum and the vomer can be used to provide bulk and forward projection. Such pieces can be trimmed to the size and shape desired. Alloplastic struts are useful in "virgin" unscarred tissues such as the unoperated non-Caucasian nose, but these are generally disappointing in

the postoperative or posttraumatic nose, since their extrusion rate is high owing to the poor viability of the scarred soft tissue and the excessive pressure exerted by the implant.

The success of the implant technique depends upon the pliability and distensibility of the soft tissues. If the membranous septum has been resected or destroyed, the results of the implant are mediocre or poor. The implant material is preferably autogenous; however, carved silicone implants

Text continued on page 268

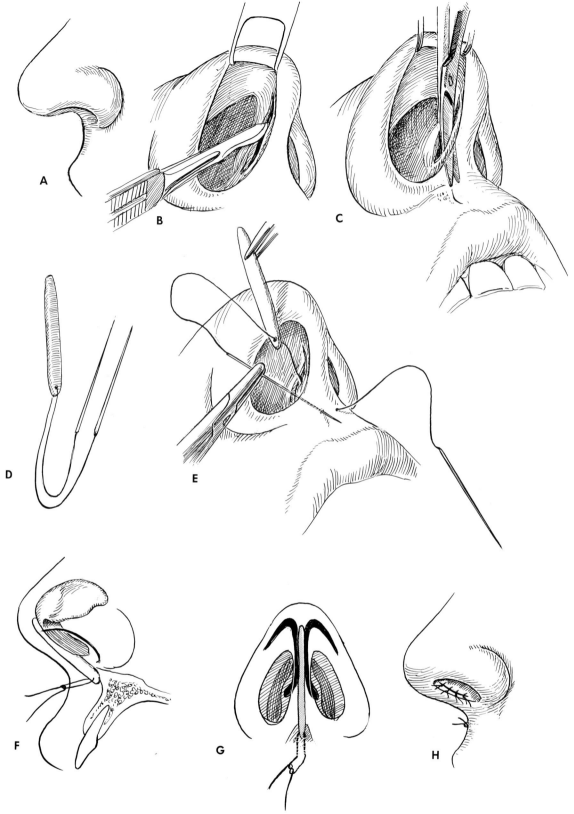

Figure 10–19. Correction of the retracted columella.

A, The retracted columella.

B and *C*, An incision is made along the caudal margin of the medial crus, and the pocket is extended to the base of the columella in the region of the nasal spine.

D, The implant strut is fashioned. A small drill hole is used to pass a double-armed suture through for fixation.

E, *F*, and *G*, The implant is placed in the pocket and fixed with the mattress suture. It is actually placed between the medial crura.

H, The columellar incision is sutured.

263

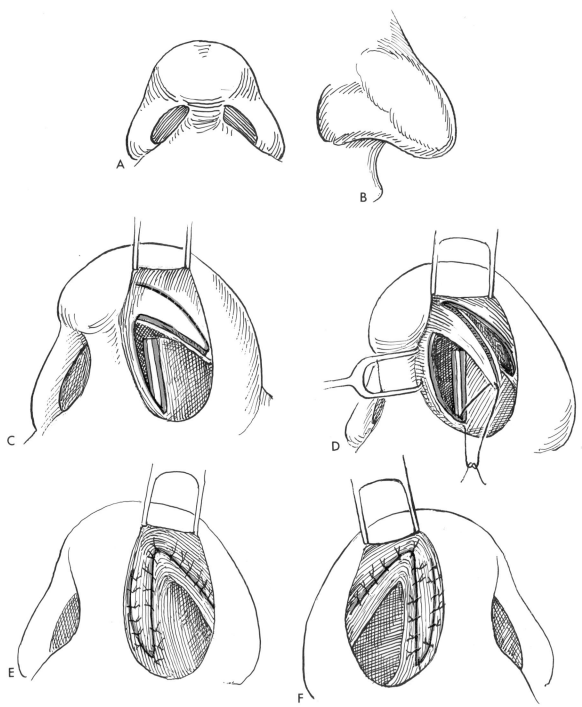

Figure 10–20.   *A* and *B*, The retracted columella with an intact alar cartilage.

C, A flap of lining and attached lateral crus is designed, based medially to rotate into the transfixion incision as an interpolation flap. It is astonishing how large this flap can be in untraumatized patients. Care should be taken to design it for the full length of the lateral crus to take advantage of as much length as possible. Length-to-width ratios are unimportant here, since the blood supply is excellent.

D, The flap is rotated into position.

E and *F*, The flap is sutured into position. (After Millard, 1972.)

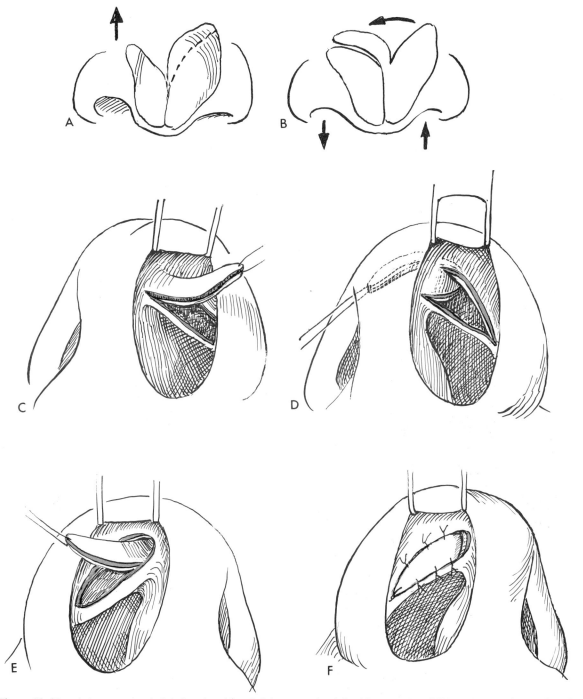

Figure 10–21. *A.* An asymmetrical deformity with a deficiency on the right side (arrow). A full lateral crus exists on the left.

B, The plan of alar flap rotation is indicated by the arrows.

C, The medially based flap is developed.

D, The flap is passed through a tunnel in the tip over the septal angle.

E, The flap is retrieved into the surgical defect on the deficient side.

F, Flap sutured in place.

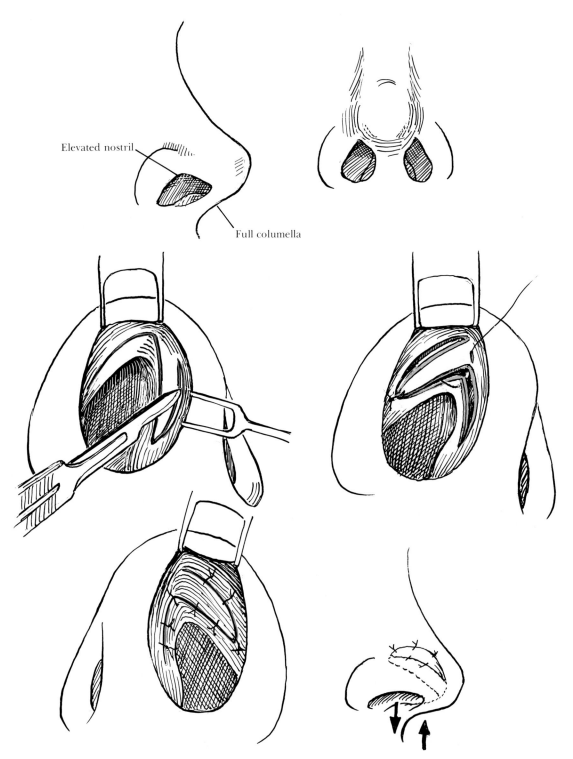

Elevated nostril

Full columella

Figure 10–22.   Millard technique for correcting asymmetry in the alar domes and lowering the retracted nostril rim.

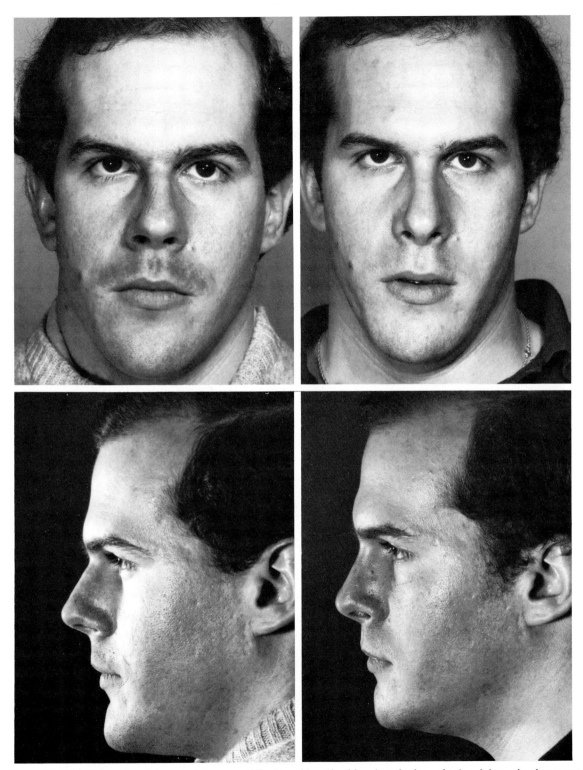

Figure 10-23.   This patient has one of the most difficult problems in rhinoplasty in the author's opinion — the short nose and recessed columella. It was developmental in this patient, but is often the result of surgery or trauma. Gaining length is difficult. Composite grafts are risky in the unscarred or traumatized nose, since the cosmetic result is uncertain. Alar turnover flaps are quite safe and provide downward projection of the columella. Although the gain was slight in this patient, the effect is significant.

can be used in selective cases, although their extrusion rate is high in the long run. Dingman and Walter (1969) described an ingenious method of reconstructing the lower septum with chondrocutaneous composite grafts from the ear.

Millard (1972) designed a very effective technique for correcting deficiencies of the columella as well as the ala with local flaps (Figure 10–20). This technique is also applicable for correcting asymmetries. The only prerequisite is that there is ample soft tissue available to form such flaps, which unfortunately is not often the case in the nose damaged by trauma or surgery. When the columella is badly retracted because of radical submucous resection, and the nasal ala are untouched, this technique is most useful (Figure 10–21). The author has used it to advantage in several patients.

Not shown in the drawing is the fact that the operation is bilateral, so that the two alar flaps are usually inserted back to back and sutured in this position with mattress sutures. Minor deformities of the nasal tip at the base of the flaps can occur, but these are easily trimmed at a second operation several weeks after the flaps have settled.

A very useful variation of the alar flap technique of Millard is for correcting asymmetry in the region of the alar domes (Figure 10–22). This trick is especially useful in correction of the cleft lip nose deformities.

A reverse application of Millard's flap is useful for repairing the deficient ala when there is abundant supply from the medial crus. Such a deformity can be present after overexuberant resection of the lateral crura and insufficient resection of the columellar structures.

The patients in Figure 10–23 demonstrate the use of Millard's alar flaps for increasing columellar show in patients with retraction of the columella or the hidden columellar deformity of the short nose.

THE PLUNGING TIP

Correction of the plunging tip requires an understanding of the mechanics of the problem and the interrelated anatomy (see section on anatomy). Remember that the strong dorsal skeleton of the humped nose acts as a fulcrum over which the tip plunges upon animation of the facial muscles. Contraction of the zygomaticus and the depressor nasi septi in particular causes the nose to plunge. A strong hump deformity of the lower nose (mostly septum), coupled with an elongated tip with a downward angulation of the domes of the alar cartilage, accentuates plunging (Figure 10–24). Such deformities are frequently associated with a shortened (tethered) upper lip. Basic corrective steps for a plunging tip are illustrated in Figure 10–25.

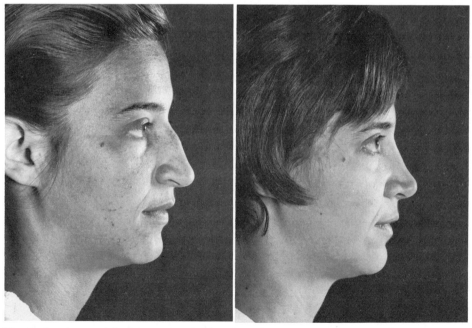

Figure 10–24.   A plunging nasal tip was accompanied by a large bony hump and flaring of the alar cartilages in this patient. The improvement shown was achieved by a quite radical shortening of the upper lateral cartilages and superior shifting of the alar cartilages to fill in the defect. The medial crura were used to embrace the caudal border of the septum and hold it in position. It should be noted that excessive resection of the caudal margin of the septum in such a patient would be disastrous and would only increase the deformity.

The patient shown in Figure 10–26 required a plunging tip operation with certain variations, which are described in Figure 10–27. Although it is not indicated in the drawing, an alar base resection was also performed in order to reduce even further the marked forward tip projection. Figure 10–28 shows another patient who required a small alar base resection for correction of a plunging tip. Of obvious importance in these procedures are the methods of suturing and splinting the tip so that it will remain in the corrected position.

ALAR BASE RESECTION

Alar base resection is frequently performed with rhinoplasty by some surgeons (Figure 10–29). Although it is a commonly done procedure, there are still subtle nuances that are important to grasp if the technique is to succeed. Noses differ greatly in their anatomic makeup; the shape of the nostril sill varies in each patient and must be given careful consideration in planning the incision and resulting scar. The surgeon must decide what he wishes to accomplish by the alar base resection. He should, in addition, utilize existing landmarks in planning the incision so that the natural roll of the nostril, particularly along the floor (the sill), is reestablished and not broken by a sharp and obvious incision line. Many patients have a natural line that breaks the sill, whereas others have a continuous unbroken line or roll.

The Nostrils and the Ala

Certain surgical corrections can be undertaken at rhinoplasty that can measurably improve the result, but overly ambitious surgery of the nostril rims or alar bases can result in later deformities that are typical stigmata of the "operated nose." The surgeon should exercise care and discretion in his approach to these structures.

Flaring of the nostrils is a racial characteristic in blacks, Asians, and Indians, but it may also occur in whites. Furthermore, flaring may result from an operative procedure when it was not apparent before; lowering of the dorsum and setting back the tip relaxes the nostril margins and creates a slight flaring at the base. Millard (1965) claims that he excises a piece of the alar base in over 90 percent of his patients for this reason, but this has not been my experience, and I average only 15 to 20 percent.

Flaring can be improved or corrected by one of the several variations of alar base resections

described classically by Weir (1892) and elaborated by Aufricht (1943) and others (Figure 10–30). It is best to maintain the scar in the natural vertical crease that is usually present in the floor of the nostril and extends slightly laterally. This is not always possible, and if significant reduction in the bulk of the ala or in the projection of the tip is required, the scar must sometimes extend laterally along the alar base. In this position, it is apt to be more noticeable, as healing is not always perfect in this skin, laden as it is with sebaceous glands.

As in all naturally curved lines, an incision that violates the curve is apt to result in a notch or depression from scar contracture. In the alar base resection, such notching can be minimized by developing a small flap at the point of juncture, much as one does in repairing the vermillion border of a cleft lip. The small flap creates a staggered line as the incision crosses the nostril sill.

Another technique that is particularly useful in reducing a projecting tip with the help of alar base resection, yet maintaining a natural roll of the nostril, is to incise the nostril on the bias, keeping the incision out of the alar crease itself and slightly cephalic to it, while maintaining the roll of the alar rim. This is useful only when large alar resections are required. Surprisingly, the incision is much less obvious than it would seem. Exact anatomic approximation of the edges and early suture removal (three days) insure an almost perfect scar.

A mattress suture of absorbable material such as chromic catgut is utilized to remove all tension from the skin sutures so that they can safely be removed in three days to obviate the possibility of pitting or cross-hatching of the alar base wound. It is *mandatory* that all skin sutures be removed by three or four days at the latest to prevent the rapid growth of epithelium along the suture tracts.

Ancillary Techniques

The alar base resection must be looked upon as an ancillary procedure because it is usually used in combination with other techniques to achieve a desired endpoint and rarely as a single definitive procedure. Such a combination of techniques is required to reduce and remodel the prominent nasal tip shown in Figure 10–31. A simple alar base resection would reduce the forward projection of this tip, but it would fall far short of the mark unless combined with other techniques. In this patient, a combination of alar base resection with generous removal of the alar and a Lipsett approach to the tip, with foreshortening of the forward projection of the tip cartilages as well as lowering of the septal angle, resulted in a more

Text continued on page 283

Figure 10–25.   Correction of a plunging tip.

A, Dislocation of the tip structures of the septal angle.

B, After resection of part of the lateral crus, the arrow shows an excess of upper lateral cartilage which will require resection in order to suspend the tip.

C, Lateral view, showing the prolapsed nasal tip.

D, Correction of the dorsal and caudal borders of the septal cartilage.

E, The dropped tip replaced in position. The remnant of lateral crus overlaps the upper lateral cartilage.

F, The medial crura of the medial cartilage are sutured in a tongue-and-groove fashion to the caudal border of the septum.

G, The suture placed through the medial crura and caudal border.

See illustration on the opposite page.

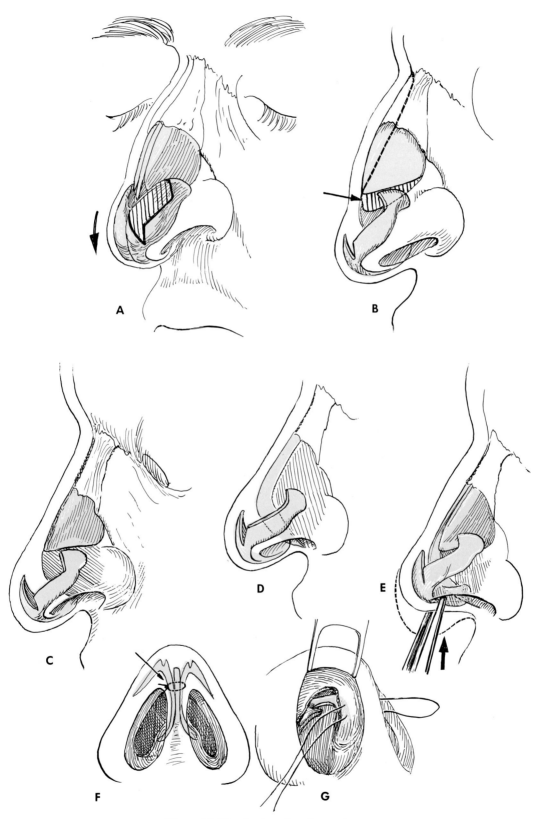

Figure 10–25. *See legend on the opposite page.*

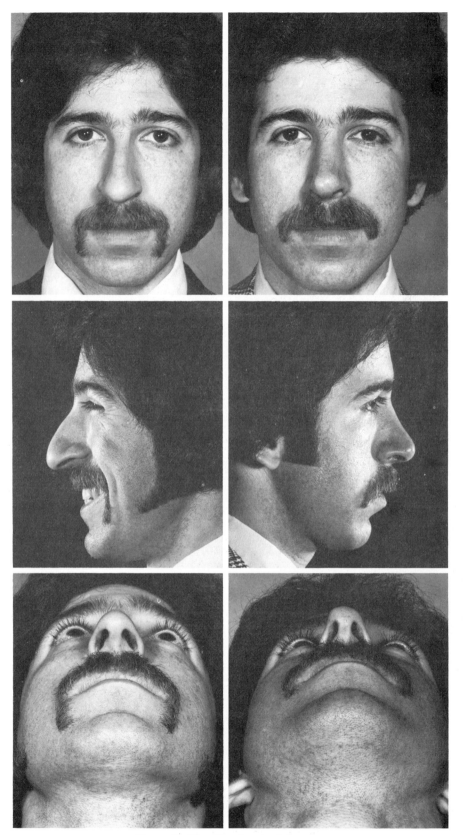

Figure 10–26. Plunging tip deformity.

Figure 10–27. *A* and *B*, The effect of animation on the nose.

C, The resected areas of cartilage and minimal bone of the hump are outlined as well as the portions of the alar cartilages and septum to be resected to allow upward rotation of the tip. Transection of the depressor muscles is also indicated by the arrow.

D, The effects of the resections on the tip are indicated by the arrows. With relaxation of the strong dorsum, the tip can relax and rotate.

E, The cephalic portion of the alar cartilages and a complete transection with a removal of the domes was required not only to reduce the forward tip projection, but to permit cephalic rotation of the lateral crural remnants.

F, Arrow indicates cephalic mobility of the tip cartilages achieved by the planned resection.

G, Resection of alar domes viewed from below.

H, Resection of alar domes completed. The remnants of the lateral crura are now more freely movable and can be rotated without the tethering effect of the domes, which were angulated caudally, making tip rotation difficult.

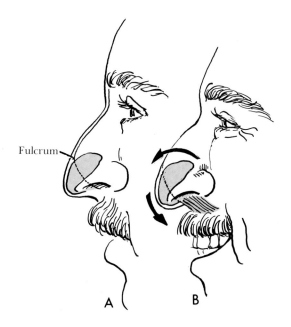

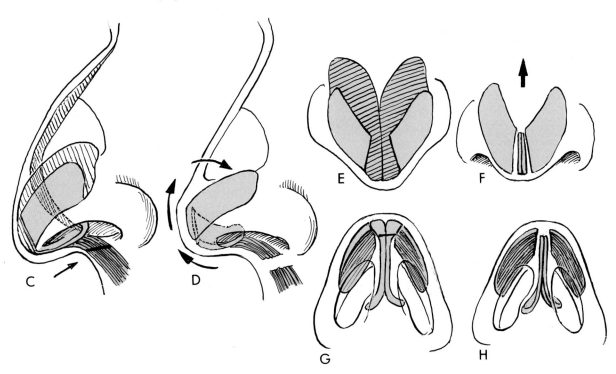

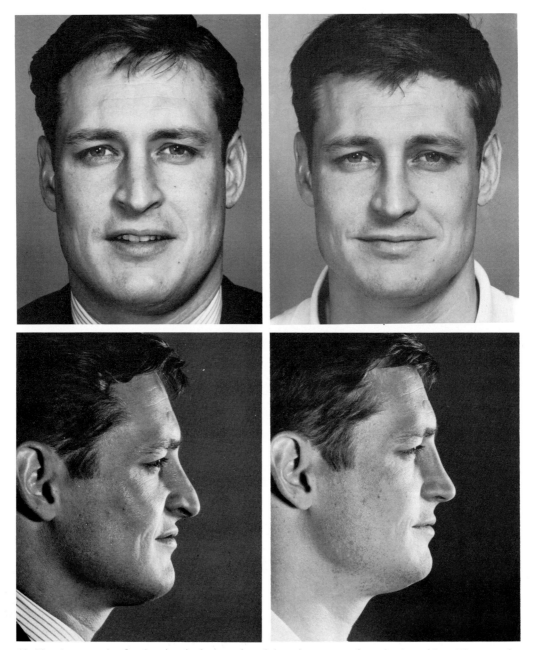

Figure 10–28.   An example of a plunging tip that constituted the primary part of a patient's problem. The operative procedure combined alar cartilage revision, reduction of the nasal dorsum, and tongue-and-groove insertion of the caudal septal border between the medial crura. A small alar base resection completed the correction. The result was somewhat limited by the short columella.

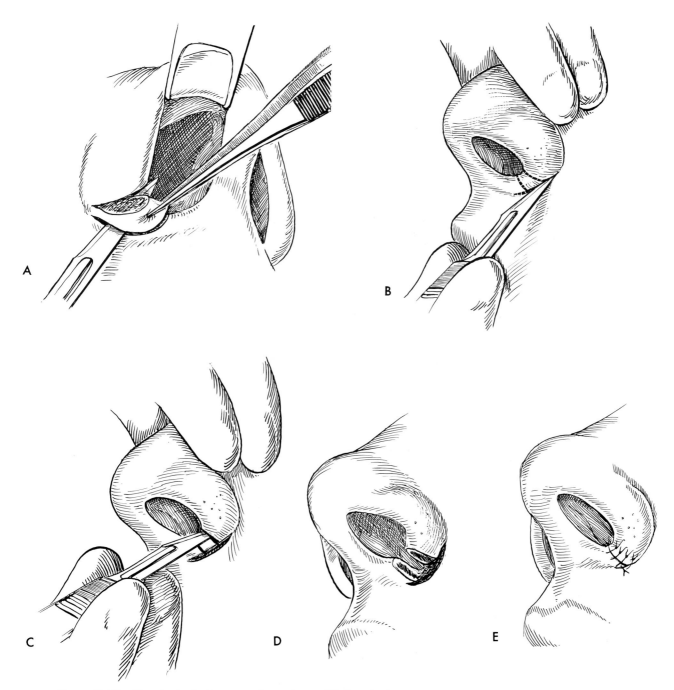

Figure 10–29. The classic alar base resection and a modified method.

A, Removal of an elliptical segment of the alar base gives the most natural result.

B, Removal of a square segment and closure by advancement of the nostril floor and the alar base.

C, Completion of the excision.

D, Freed medial and lateral flaps.

E, Closure by interrupted 5–0 nylon sutures. While it is possible to conceal the horizontal lines of the incision, these will always be more prominent than the lines of the classic elliptical resection.

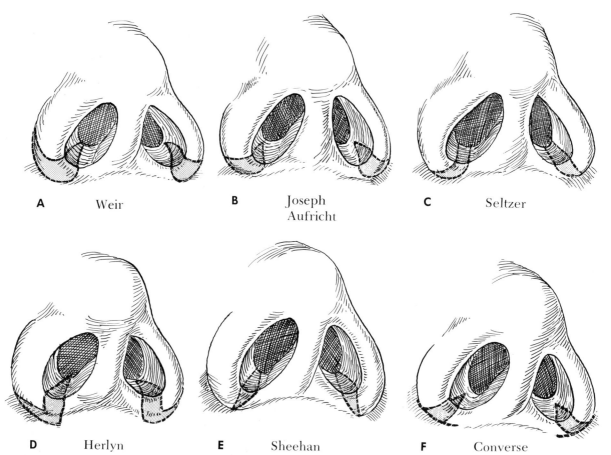

Figure 10–30.   The Nostrils and the Alae. The different types of alar base resection shown in the drawings are used to achieve different goals:

A, Reduction in flare.

B, Reduction in both width and flare.

C, Reduction in width.

D, Reduction in width with a V-shaped staggering of the excision for a less pronounced scar.

E, Resection of a portion of the nasal floor to lessen flare.

F, Closure of the defect by advancement flaps of nasal floor and nasal cartilage; this has the disadvantage of creating more scars in this region.

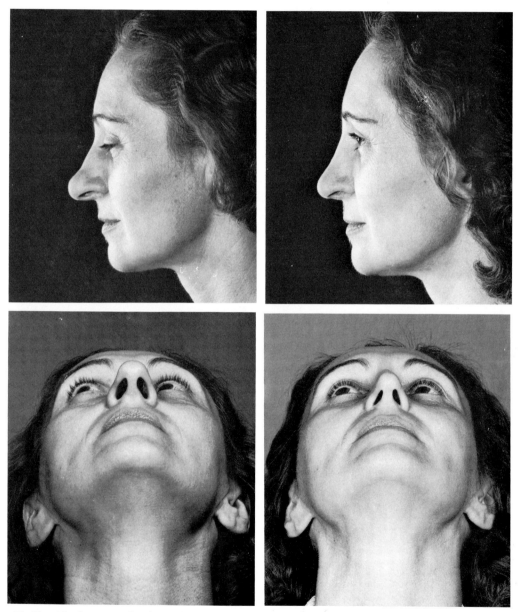

Figure 10–31.   Alar base resection in combination with Lipsett approach to the tip to correct the prominent nasal tip.

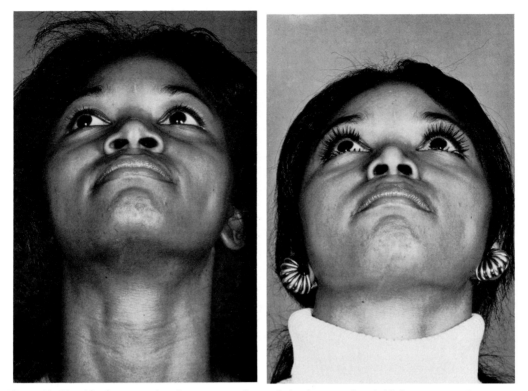

Figure 10–32. Alar base resection done as part of a nasal tip plasty produced this improvement in contour.

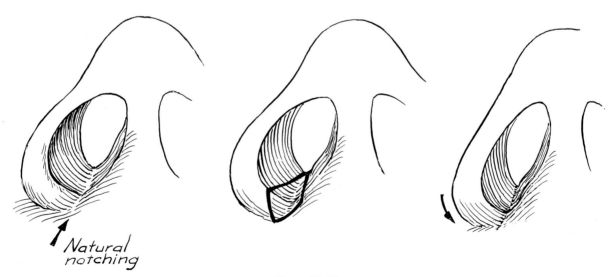

Natural notching

Figure 10–33.

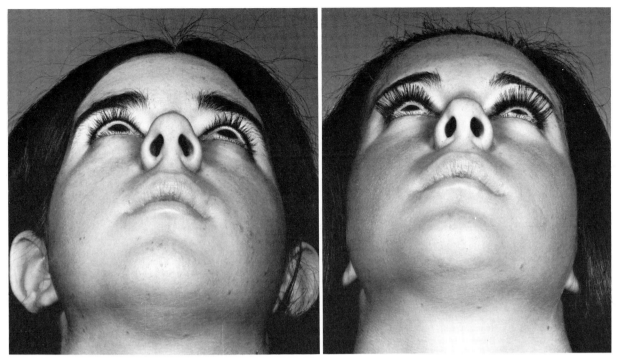

Figure 10–34.   This patient had a natural crease at the base of the alar roll. In such patients, this groove is used to place the incision. The final scar is unobtrusive.

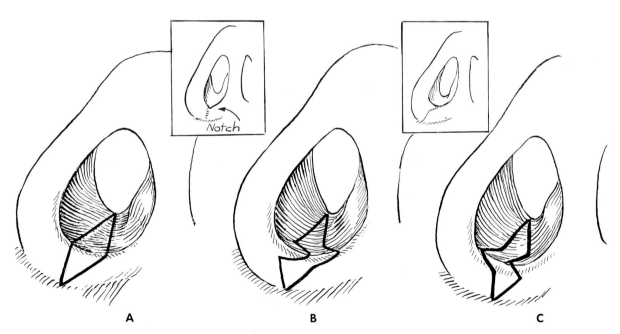

Figure 10–35.   Staggered incision to avoid postoperative notching.

A, When a natural notching or grooving exists in the floor of the nostril sill, the incision is best placed in the notch.

B, To avoid a postoperative notching, a staggered incision can be designed with a small wedge-shaped flap which retains the natural curve of the nostril sill.

C, The small flaps can be designed in the reverse.

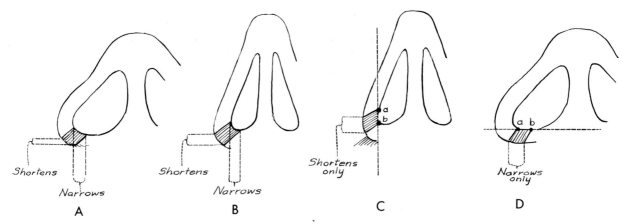

Figure 10–36. *A,* In the wide-angled nostril, reduction of height is minimal, but varies with the shape of the inner arc.

B, In the narrow-angled nostril, undesirable narrowing may occur when excision is done at the angle.

C, No narrowing will occur if points *a* and *b* are on the same vertical line.

D, No reduction in height will occur if points *a* and *b* are on the same horizontal line.

Figure 10–37. Reshaping a prominent nasal tip by resection at the alar base.

A and *B,* Resection of the alar base segment, numbered 1, will almost always result in a somewhat unnatural appearance of the remaining alar base.

C and *D,* Excision of a triangular segment of the alar base and associated nostril floor, numbered 2, gives a moderate reduction in width.

E and *F,* A combination of these techniques can result in a significant reduction of projection and alar base width. But there will still be some degree of unnaturalness.

The novice surgeon must be cautioned that the use of alar base resection should be infreqent, for this is a major factor in the production of the "operated nose" look. Alar base resection ought to be a last resort, rather than a method of first choice.

See illustration on the opposite page.

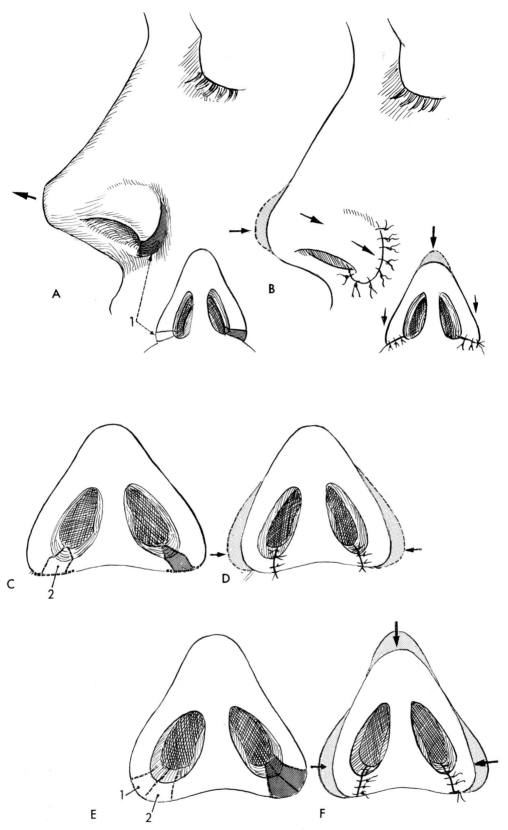

Figure 10–37.   *See legend on the opposite page.*

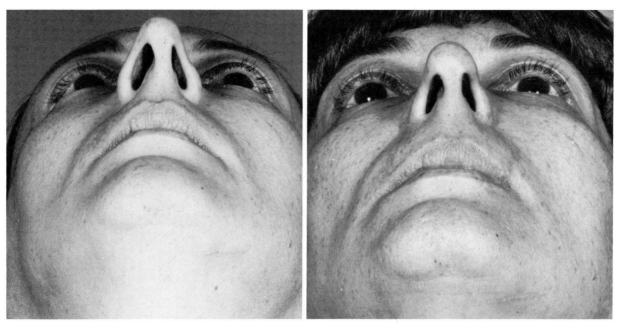

Figure 10–38.   The technique of alar base resection when applied to the forward projecting tip is demonstrated in this patient. The alar base resection is performed to reset the tip in a more normal position. Care must be taken not to crowd the airspace when the nostrils are long and thin, as in this patient.

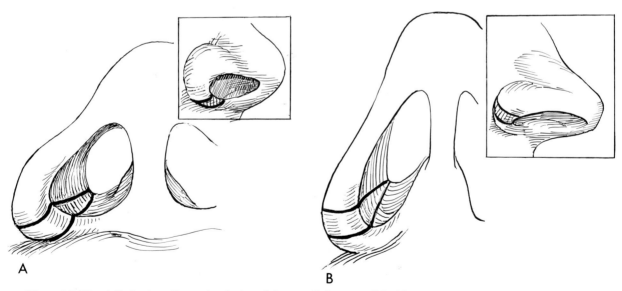

A

B

Figure 10–39.   *A*, Reduction of excessive flaring of the nostrils is accomplished by appropriate wedge excisions at the base of the nostril in the floor of the sill.

B, To reduce the tip projection, the wedge shape is designed more anteriorly (toward the tip). The resulting scar is usually acceptable if the repair is exact. This technique not only reduces the tip projection, but also reduces flaring of the ala.

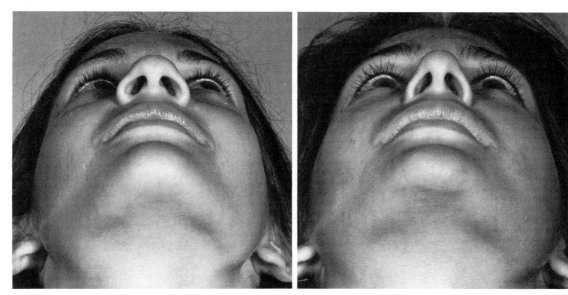

Figure 10–40.

pleasing profile. It must always be kept in mind during nasal reduction surgery that the nose must be considered as a three-dimensional whole. The surgeon should view individual techniques upon the nose only insofar as they affect the composite whole. Figure 10–32 shows a patient in whom a resection was performed as part of a tip plasty.

When in doubt as to whether or not an alar base resection should be done, it is generally wiser to postpone this procedure. A secondary reevaluation of the results of the original surgery can often dictate the advisability of this simple maneuver, which can be carried out as an office procedure several weeks following primary rhinoplasty.

The Natural Crease

Many patients have a natural groove or crease at the base of the nostril sill that facilitates placement of the incision so that the resulting scar will be less conspicuous. Figure 10–33 demonstrates such a natural groove. The incision is placed in the notch and the desired amount is excised to reduce

flaring of the ala, which is often accentuated during rhinoplasty when the dorsal profile is reduced and the nasal soft tissues relaxed. (Relaxation of the soft tissues promotes flaring of the nostrils.) The final scar lies in this natural notch and is difficult to see after healing is complete (Figure 10–34). Staggered incisions may also be made to avoid postoperative notching (Figure 10–35).

Variations in Design

The alar base resection can be varied in each patient, depending on what is to be accomplished (Figure 10–36). Figure 10–37 and 10–38 show the reshaping of a prominent nasal tip by resection at the alar base.

Flaring. Figures 10–39 and 10–40 show reduction of inordinate flaring of the nostrils. This can be a primary problem or one that is accentuated during rhinoplasty in which reduction of the dorsum with relaxation of the tip results in "settling" with increased flaring.

(For references, see pages 450 to 453.)

Chapter 11

Correction of the Deviated Nose

THOMAS D. REES, M.D., F.A.C.S.

THE SEPTUM AND NASAL OBSTRUCTION

Obstruction to the flow of air through the nose can be caused by several different mechanisms either individually or collectively. Obstruction can occur at the vestibule, at the point of air intake, at the internal valve, or anywhere within the nasal passages depending on the architectural derangement involved. Obstruction at the vestibule at the point of juncture of the alar cartilages, the lateral cartilages, and the septum has been discussed in the sections on anatomy and throughout the text at pertinent points. The physiology of nasal obstruction is covered thoroughly in the section on physiology by Dr. Baker. It is the aim of this section to examine the role of the septum in respiratory nasal obstruction.

The Deviated Septum

It has been commonly accepted that respiratory obstruction is most often caused by a deviation of the nasal septum to one side or the other in one or more planes (Figure 11–1). This theory has proved to be simplistic. It is now generally recognized that the septum probably is less often the culprit than formerly thought. In fact, the septum is rarely straight throughout its length. Of more critical importance in ascertaining the role of the septum in nasal obstruction is the determination of the exact location and plane of the deviation; that is, whether it is in the critical area for the perception of airflow or whether the mechanical obstruction is of such a magnitude that interference of the airflow of one side or the other is clearly caused by mechanical impingement. Corrective surgery on the septum should be undertaken only when a significant deviation and crowding of the air space

is obviously the problem, since septal surgery unquestionably increases morbidity in the postoperative course. The risk of epistaxis is increased by radical septal surgery, as is the danger of collapse of the osteocartilaginous vault from multiple osteotomies in conjunction with hump removal (Figure 11–2). A saddle-nose deformity can also result.

The experienced rhinoplastic surgeon must realize that many patients demonstrate severe distortions of the nasal septum with angulation in every conceivable plane and direction and yet have little or minimal difficulty in breathing. An example is the boxer with multiple deviations of the septum and unobstructed breathing. Similarly, the complaint of severe nasal obstruction is frequently seen in patients who have only slight to moderate degrees of septal deviation. Deviations or spur formation along the floor of the nose rarely cause significant symptoms, but minor degrees of deviation high along the dorsum, particularly where the septum meets the upper lateral cartilages, can result in severe complaints that are sometimes difficult to evaluate in view of the apparent patency of the remainder of the nares. The surgeon should make every attempt to analyse these anatomic deviations prior to surgery in order to make an intelligent assessment of the technical maneuvers required in the operative procedure (Figure 11–3).

History

An exact history of the nature of nasal obstruction is important. Persistent, chronic, unremitting obstruction of one nasal passage or the other is strongly indicative of a permanent mechanical obstruction of that side, most likely the result of crowding of the air space from deviation of the septum. On the other hand, intermittent obstruction that tends to shift from side to side —

284

Text continued on page 292.

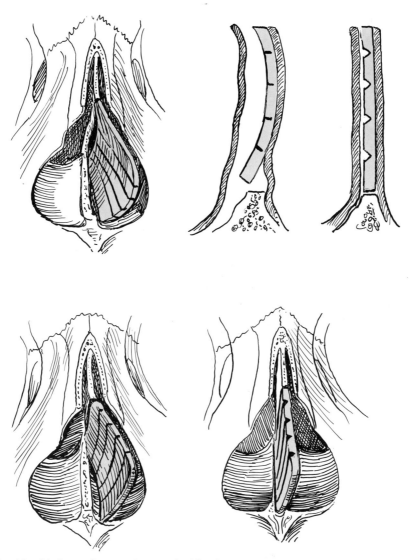

Figure 11–1. Considerable ingenuity must be exercised by the surgeon to design the technique in a given septal deformity that will offer the best chance of success. The deformity may be in one plane only, or several planes concomitantly. This illustration shows various techniques available for weakening the septal cartilage in every plane. These techniques are real and useful. They are not teleological. It is important to maintain the integrity of the mucoperichondrium on one side or the other since it provides the necessary vascular supply to the cartilage.

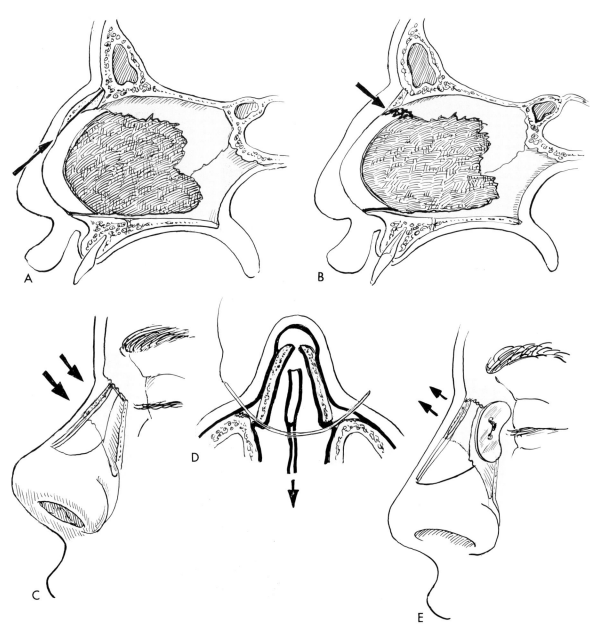

Figure 11–2. A radical submucous resection following hump removal and lateral osteotomy can be hazardous.

A, Following removal of the bony hump (arrow) and a classical submucous resection of the radical type, the nose is suspended only by a very thin perpendicular plate of the ethmoid.

B, During manipulation of the nose necessary during the operative procedure, this thin plate can easily be fractured (arrow).

C, With completion of the lateral osteotomies, fracture of the thin remaining ethmoid plate can result in collapse of the osteo-cartilaginous vault of the nose into the pyriform aperture in the direction indicated by the arrows.

D and *E,* Treatment for such a collapse is similar to that for severe mid-face trauma. A through-and-through wire is passed beneath the entire unstable complex. The nasal bones and cartilaginous structures are elevated with a blunt elevator, as in a traumatic case, and fixed into position by tying the through-and-through mattress wire over acrylic buttons or lead plates. Such sutures should be maintained in place for a minimum of two weeks and preferably for three weeks.

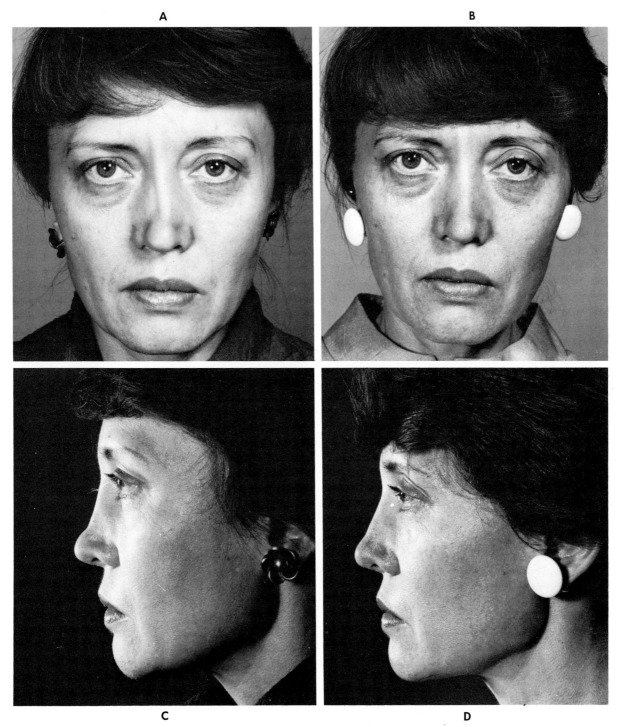

Figure 11–3. *A* and *C*, The severe nasal deformity with external deviation to the left in this patient was the result of a primary rhinoplasty. The surgeon failed to identify the marked septal deviation preoperatively and, therefore, failed to correct it. An infracture was also not accomplished, probably because of the septal deviation.

B and *D*, Correction was achieved by freeing the septum and replacing it in the midline, infracture, and placement of an autogenous, tiered, cartilage graft from the septum on the dorsum. (Courtesy of Dr. C. Guy.)

Figure 11–4.   *The Classical Radical Submucous Resection.*

A, The deviated nasal tip held in its deflected position by the septal angle.

B, The deflected dorsal border of the septum, with dislocation of the nasal tip into a central position.

C, Infiltration of the subperichondrial space by local anesthetic solution.

D, Mucoperichondrial flaps are raised with the anesthetic solution, a maneuver that will immeasurably aid the operator in dissection.

E, A transfixion incision is made along the lower border of the septum. It is frequently easier for the operator to begin the dissection by sharply removing the depressor muscles from the caudal border of the cartilaginous septum. After progressing superiorly for a distance of 4 or 5 mm, the operator will usually find a space appearing between the mucoperichondrium and the underlying cartilage.

F, Mucoperichondrial flaps are raised and the septal framework is exposed.

Submucous resection or septal plasty is best carried out after reduction of the hump, adjustment of the caudal septum and columella, and tip plasty, but before lateral osteotomy and infracture. Whenever possible, septal plasty (or readjustment of the position of the septum) is preferred over formal submucous resection (Killian).

See illustration on the opposite page.

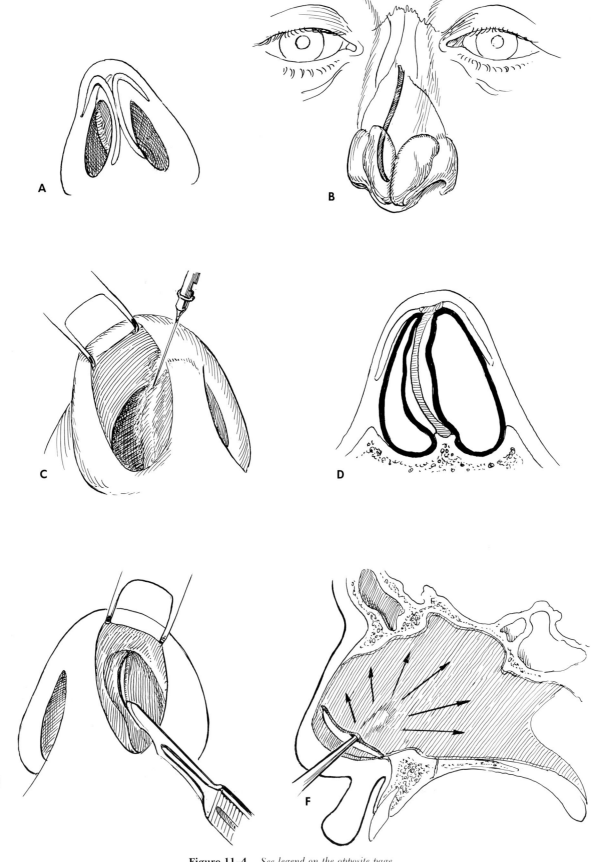

Figure 11–4.   *See legend on the opposite page.*

Illustration continued on the following page.

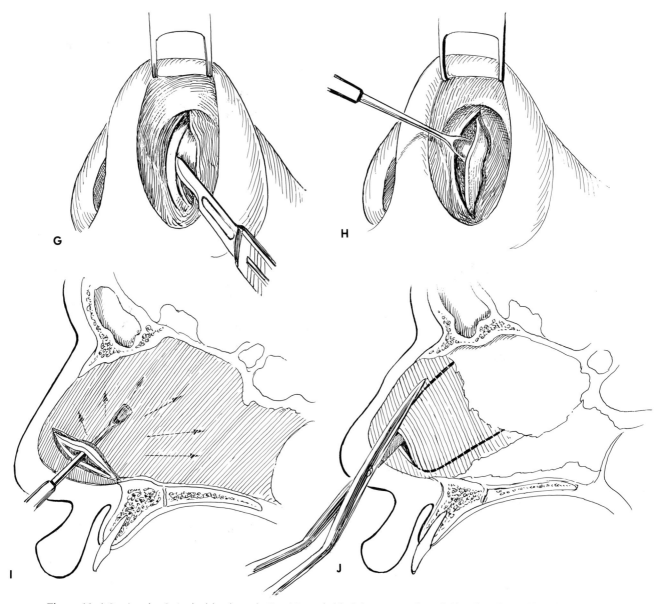

Figure 11–4 *Continued. G,* An incision is made 5 to 10 mm behind the corrected caudal border. Sharp dissection is required to separate the mucoperichondrium from the underlying cartilage, which is quite adherent in this region owing to the insertion of the depressor muscles.

H, Mucoperichondrial flaps are easily raised once the right plane is entered.

I, Similar flaps are raised on the opposing side after an incision is made through the cartilage. It is important to stagger this incision in relation to the first transmucosal incision so that the two do not overlie one another.

J, Resection of the deviated cartilage with Knight nasal scissors.

Illustration continued on the opposite page.

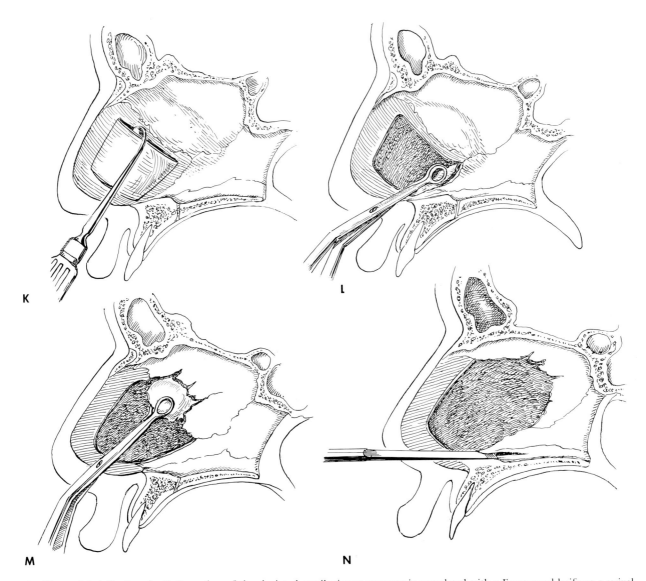

Figure 11–4 *Continued.* *K*, Resection of the deviated cartilaginous segment is completed with a Freer nasal knife or a swivel knife.

L, Deviated portions of bone and cartilage lying along the nasal floor are removed with Bruening forceps.

M, Where the submucous resection is more extensive than nasal plastic, the deviated bony septum is removed with Bruening forceps.

N, Further correction of the extensive osseous deformity may be achieved by passing an osteotome along the nasal floor.

particularly with the patient in a recumbent position at night or related to emotional stress or the menstrual cycle in females — is strong evidence of vasomotor rhinitis or allergic disease. Under these conditions, a mild to moderate deviation of the septum can contribute significantly to the problem but can usually be pinpointed to the involved passageway.

In chronic unilateral obstruction, a classic radical submucous resection at the time of rhinoplasty will often be helpful except in the case of high deviation along the dorsum (Figure 11–4). However, nasal congestion that results from vasomotor rhinitis will be slightly or not at all improved by radical submucous resection and rhinoplasty but is sometimes alleviated without submucous resection in the young patient. Another overriding factor is related to emotional stress, which can, under certain circumstances, be relieved by nasal plasty.

Severe deformities of the nasal septum may or may not be accompanied by the typical allergic or vasomotor nose with pale, swollen mucous membranes and hypertrophied turbinates. The inferior turbinate is frequently hypertrophied on the opposite side of septal deviation and often exhibits vasomotor changes. The typical appearance of vasomotor rhinitis or allergy is that of swollen baggy mucous membranes that may or may not be accompanied by a deviation of the septum. Edematous mucous membranes can be shrunk with topical nasal constrictors, and prompt relief of obstructive symptoms ensues. In addition, vasomotor rhinitis may be seasonal in occurrence. In the young female patient, it may be related to the menses with more severe obstruction during the immediate premenstrual period and the first few days of the menses.

Sensitive receptors in the lining of the nose indicate when there is interference with the eddies of the airstream. These are abundant in the anterior nose — in the region of the internal valve where the upper lateral cartilages meet with the septum — so that even minor obstructions of this critical angle can result in the sensation of obstruction although the passages beneath this point are wide open.

Collapse of the nostrils on inspiration occurs normally in some individuals or can be the result of loss of strength in the architecture of the alar cartilages following surgery or trauma. This cause of nasal obstruction is usually obvious on examination of the patient during inspiration.

Cartilaginous support of the critical triangle formed by the junction of the upper lateral cartilages with the septum must be maintained during surgery to allow for the eddying currents of in-

spired air to register on the receptors. Postoperative cicatrix or collapse secondary to overly ambitious resection of the upper lateral cartilages also destroys the apex of the triangle and results in the sensation of obstruction. Severe deviation of the septum above the internal valve to one side or the other with impingement on the lower and middle turbinates clearly causes mechanical obstruction to respiration and is more likely to be alleviated with radical submucous resection or various procedures designed to shrink the volume of the turbinates. It is well to remember that the mucous membrane lining of the turbinate is rich in a vascular venous plexis and is erectile in nature. It is this erectile property that accounts for the intermittent obstruction that is under direct vasomotor control and is influenced by many factors such as allergens, hormones, and emotional stress.

In the face of a severe mechanical deviation of the septum, it is sometimes preferable to perform a limited or radical submucous resection prior to, during, or subsequent to rhinoplasty (Figure 11–5). No more tissue should be resected than is necessary to produce a straight septum, and in particular only a minimal portion of the perpendicular plate of the ethmoid is to be removed, since a considerable risk is run of dropping the dorsum in completing this procedure.

The submucous resection is preferably performed through an L-shaped incision, the horizontal arm passing along the floor of the septum. Mucoperichondrial flaps are raised on the side of the septal deflection, taking care to place the incision sufficiently posterior to the transfixion incision to allow a healthy band of mucoperichondrium to remain. If there is a complicated deflection in the region of the transfixion incision itself, so that direct surgery on the caudal portion of the septum is necessary, it will of course be mandatory to do the resection through the transfixion incision (Figure 11–6).

Obstructive vomer spurs can be removed selectively when necessary without interfering with the remaining cartilaginous and bony structure of the septum (Figure 11–7). However, such spurs are usually found along the floor of the nose and are rarely the cause of significant nasal obstruction. The caudal septum is modified in most operations so that the surgery can technically qualify as an anterior submucous resection (Figure 11–8). In very severe deviations of the nasal septum, it is not always possible or wise to undertake radical submucous resection at the same time as nasal plasty. Accordingly, such severely obstructed septums can be resected either before or after rhinoplasty according to the choice of the surgeon. When almost

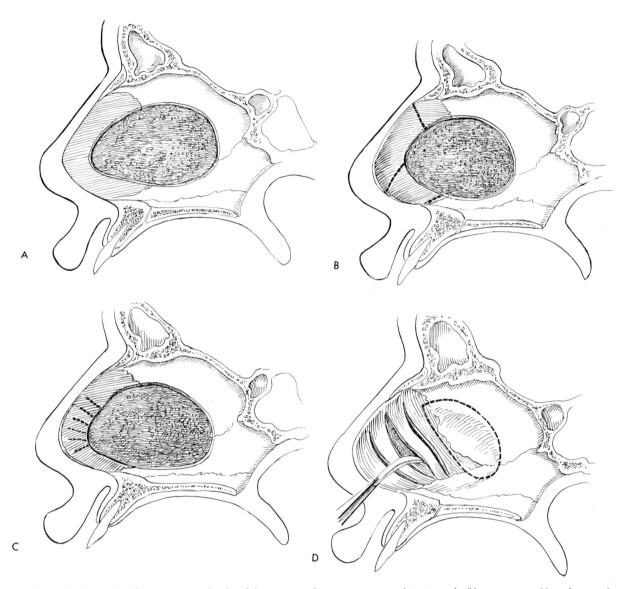

Figure 11-5. *A,* A submucous resection involving a somewhat more conservative removal of bony septum. Note the remaining wide, strong dorsal and caudal borders of the cartilaginous septum.

B, Septal angle deflection can frequently be corrected by multiple vertical cuts that do not touch the dorsal or caudal borders of the septum. Overlapping cartilage must be resected.

C, On occasion the operator may be forced to allow one or two cuts to touch the dorsal or caudal borders. It is important that on one side the mucosa is not raised from the septal cartilage in this region, so that support of the cartilage is maintained and no break in the profile line results.

D, Multiple oblique cuts are sometimes made to straighten a badly deflected septum. Some of the most seriously deviated segments may be resected.

(After Converse, 1964.)

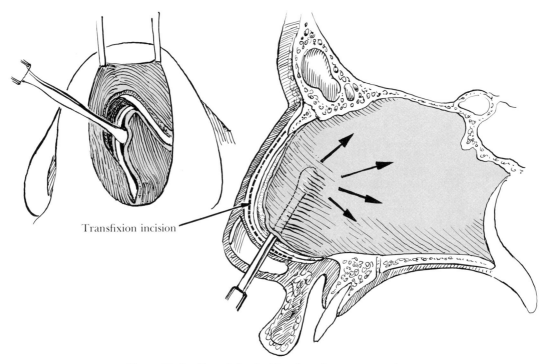

Transfixion incision

Figure 11–6. Transfixion incision for submucous resection.

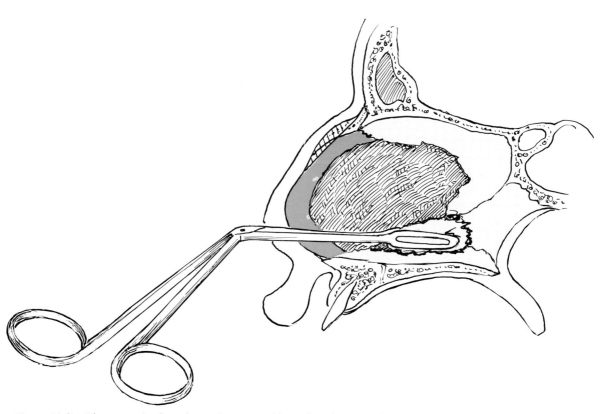

Figure 11–7. The vomer is often obstructive to one side or the other. It is also the keystone of the septal components. It is best removed with ring forceps after freeing it along the floor with a sharp osteotome. The vomer is quite thick and can be used as an implant to fill in contour deformities of the nose, or shaped to aid in tip support, as advocated by Sheen.

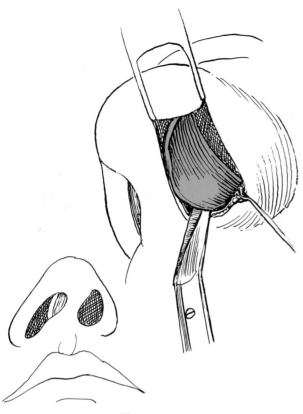

Figure 11–8.

total obstruction of one airway exists owing to deviation of the septum, the order of priorities perceived by the patient weigh heavily in the choice of which procedure comes first. It is the author's preference in such instances to perform a submucous resection first, maintaining an adequate dorsal and caudal strut of cartilage (at least 1 cm) to prevent nasal collapse. On the other hand, in some patients, when the role of the septum in a given obstruction problem is in doubt or unclear and it is apparent that a straight nose can be obtained cosmetically by rhinoplasty, the nasal plastic part of the procedure can be done first followed several weeks later by submucous resection if obstructive symptoms persist. It is astonishing in the author's experience how seldom the second procedure — i.e., radical submucous resection — is required in such patients, even in the face of what appears to be a significant septal deformity.

Many surgeons have traditionally believed that the standard radical submucous resection is required to permit more room inside the nose for breathing in almost every patient. They reason that reduction of the nasal hump along with infracture of the nasal bones encroached on the available breathing space. A study of coronal sections of the nose both before and after infracture reveals the

fallacy in this type of reasoning. The space encroached upon by infracture of the nasal bones occurs in the most dorsal (anterior) part of the nose and represents an insignificant reduction of the available airspace. It can be argued that this reduction occurs in a critical area from a standpoint of airflow; however, it is doubtful that even this reduction in space is significant. The cartilaginous septum is rarely more than 2 to 3 mm thick at most, and it is unlikely that resection of 2 or 3 mm of cartilaginous septum and even less bone from the perpendicular plate of the ethmoid represents a significant reduction in bulk unless, of course, the septum is severely deviated. Postponing a radical septectomy until after nasal plasty means that the surgeon is not limited in the amount of septal dorsum or inferior or caudal margin that can be removed during attempts at cosmetic improvement of the nose. Also, deviations of the dorsum that are uncorrectable by standard nasal plasty can often be camouflaged by various techniques such as septal overlap, upper lateral cartilage overlap, or camouflaging grafts of nasal septum (Figures 11–9 through 11–12).

Under certain circumstances, nasal plasty alone can do much to improve the flow of air. One such example is with the dropped or plunging tip, which in itself can represent an obstruction to airflow. Simple elevation of the tip opens the vestibule and provides a much clearer entrance passageway to inspired air. Insurance companies frequently demand that the surgeon assign percentage values to improvement achieved by the procedures as though they were completely separate operations. This attempt to define exact percentages is absurd.

Surgical manipulation of the septum by septal reconstruction, septal plasty, or repositioning of the septal elements are to be preferred whenever feasible over a radical submucous resection. These techniques, collectively known as septal plasty, obviate the necessity of elevating mucoperichondrial flaps from both sides of the septum — a step that frequently results in tears, perforations, and unstable scars prone to postoperative bleeding. The displaced or curved nasal septum can often be repositioned without elevating the mucoperichondrial flaps at all. In more severe problems, the mucoperichondrial flaps can be elevated from one side only and the septal elements can be repositioned by various methods of selective excisions, cross cutting, or weakening incisions. Such incisions can be multiple and extend in all directions, provided the basic integrity of the cartilaginous dorsum and caudal margins is maintained intact to provide support to this structure (Figure 11–13).

Text continued on page 304.

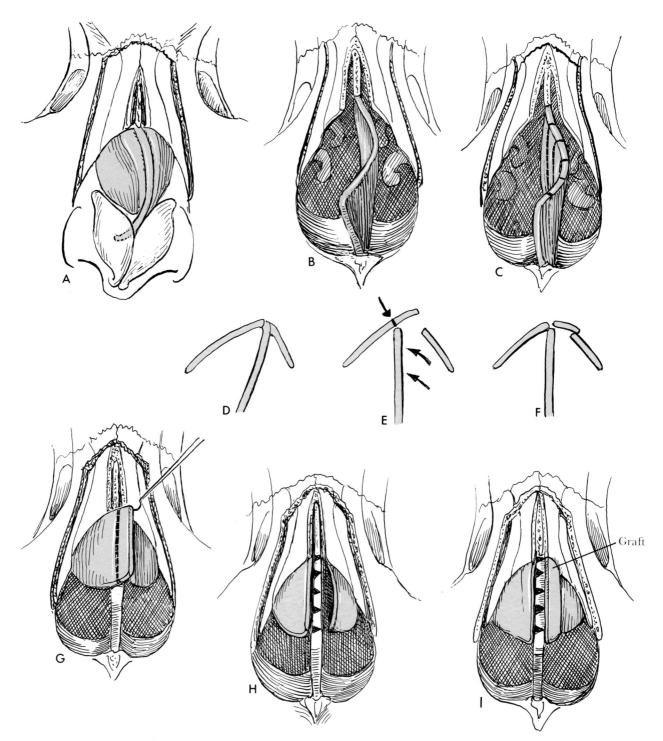

Figure 11–9. Some of the practical techniques available to straighten the crooked nose, or to at least camouflage the deviation in the final result. Unfortunately, it is not always possible to obtain a completely straight nose, mostly because of the vagrancies of the cartilage.

A, B, and *C,* The crooked nose is skeletonized, the septum is freed from the upper lateral cartilages, the bony hump is removed, and the septum is weakened in appropriate directions by cross cuts.

D, E, and *F,* Coronal representation of the deviation. The plan is to utilize the redundant upper lateral cartilage on the long side in a graft to fill the deficiency on the deviated side after repositioning the septum.

G, H, and *I,* The steps are shown from above.

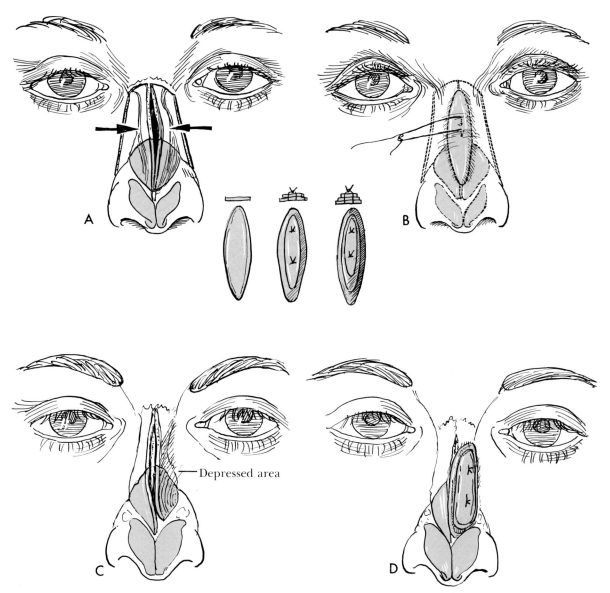

Figure 11-10. Another very useful method of camouflaging an imperfectly straightened nose is by implantation of autografts of cartilage or bone that are removed during nasal and septal surgery. For this reason, it is imperative that no piece of bone or cartilage be discarded during surgery. It is another good reason for conservatism in septal surgery during any primary operation, since the septum is an excellent source of autograft material, as is the concha of the ear.

A and *B*, Complete infracture of the deviated bone can be prevented by a high deviation of the septum. A single or multi-layered graft of septal cartilage can be used to fill in the midline after hump removal. The illusion of a straight nose is enhanced. Such grafts are well secured by a mattress suture brought through the dorsal skin (*B*).

C, Sometimes a significant depression on one side is unavoidable because of high septal deviation or severe comminution during the osteotomies.

D, An autograft of septal cartilage can be inserted off center to improve the contour.

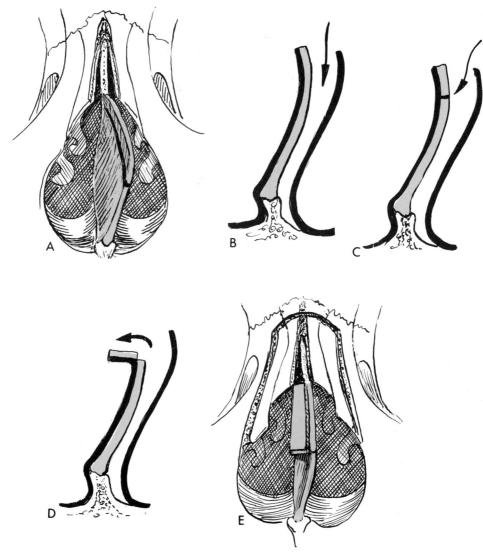

Figure 11–11. A useful technique for creating the illusion of a straight septum when it may not be possible by any technique of septal plasty to actually achieve straightness was described to the author by Shulman (1976). It has proven to be effective in several difficult problems.

A, The dorsal edge of the deviated cartilaginous septum is purposely left high during the rhinoplasty procedure. The solid line indicates the proposed real elevation line of the dorsum.

B, The mucoperichondrium is stripped from the deviated side.

C, The redundant dorsal strip of cartilage is incised through its length beginning at the junction of the nasal bones (arrow).

D, The dorsal strip is angulated toward the side opposite the deviation, hinged upon its intact lining.

E, While the septum beneath the dorsum remains deviated, the dorsal hinged strip camouflages the midline. The nose appears straight.

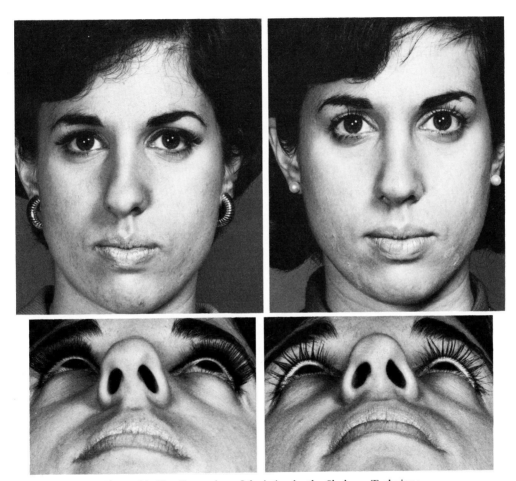

Figure 11–12.   Correction of deviation by the Shulman Technique.

Figure 11–13. A number of surgical options available for straightening the deviated cartilaginous septum are shown in coronal section. The technique to be utilized depends on the circumstances in each case. It is again emphasized that it is wiser to strip the mucoperichondrium from one side only to preserve the vascular supply to the cartilage and to prevent postoperative perforation, ulcers, bleeding, and unstable areas of mucosa.

A, Partial dislocation of the cartilaginous septum from the vomer groove.

B, Elevation of the mucoperichondrial and mucoperiosteal flap from the concave side. The perichondrium and periosteum are not confluent, so that separating at their juncture can be difficult.

C, The deflected vomer is cut with an osteotome, and the redundant inferior margin of the septum removed if necessary to provide room for movement.

D, The septum is fixed in its new position by suture, if necessary.

E, Correction of a buckling septal cartilage by wedge excision.

F, Septum straightened in midline after wedge removal.

G and *H*, Another undesirable feature of elevation of both mucoperichondrial flaps is the unequal tensions that can then act upon the transected cartilage. Overlapping can occur, with subsequent shortening of the vertical height of the septum and postoperative increased width of the septum where the fragments overlap.

I, J, and *K*, The Fry theory of the behavior of cartilage may be useful in achieving septal straightening. Stripping of the mucoperichondrium from the concave (deviated) side and cross-cutting of the septum partially or completely through allow the natural forces of the attached perichondrium to straighten the septum. Some opponents of this concept point out that the contracture that might occur during healing of the stripped side would tend to bend the septum into its original position.

See illustration on the opposite page.

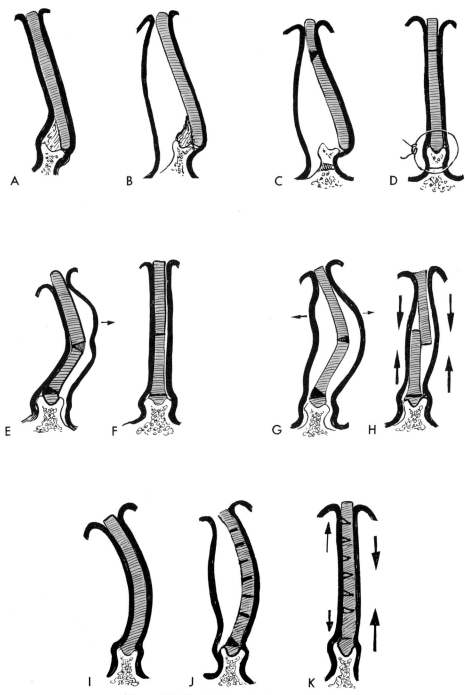

Figure 11-13.   *See legend on the opposite page.*

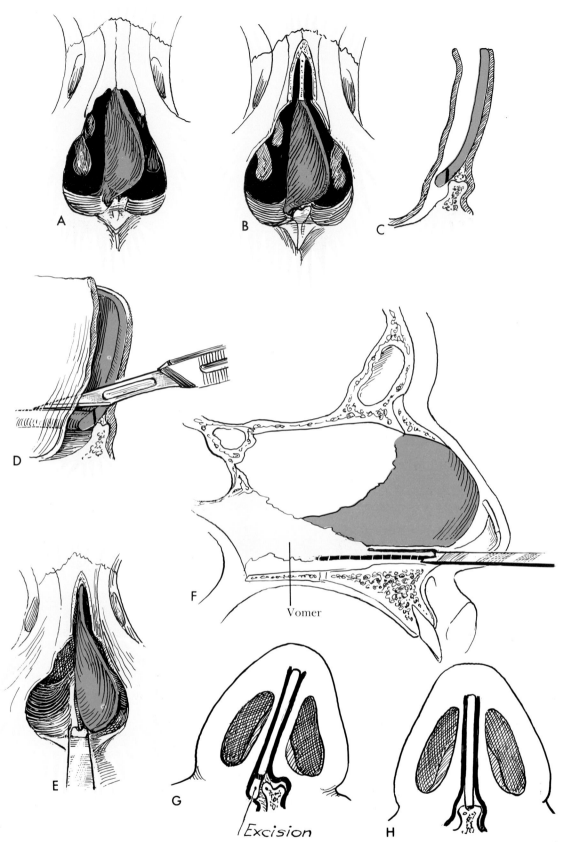

Figure 11–14. *A*, *B*, and *C*, The deviated cartilaginous septum is frequently displaced from its bony groove in the floor of the nose. Correction in such patients requires not only standard septal plasty techniques, but also replacement of the base of the septum in the midline.

D, The displaced spur of cartilage can be resected after freeing of the mucoperichondrium.

E and *F*, Resection of the palatine process and offending vomer may also be required to allow repositioning of the septum. A sharp osteotome is most useful for this purpose. As long as the mucoperchondrium is not disturbed on one surface of the septum, there is little danger of perforation or instability.

G and *H*, Replacement of the septum in the bony groove after resection of cartilage spur.

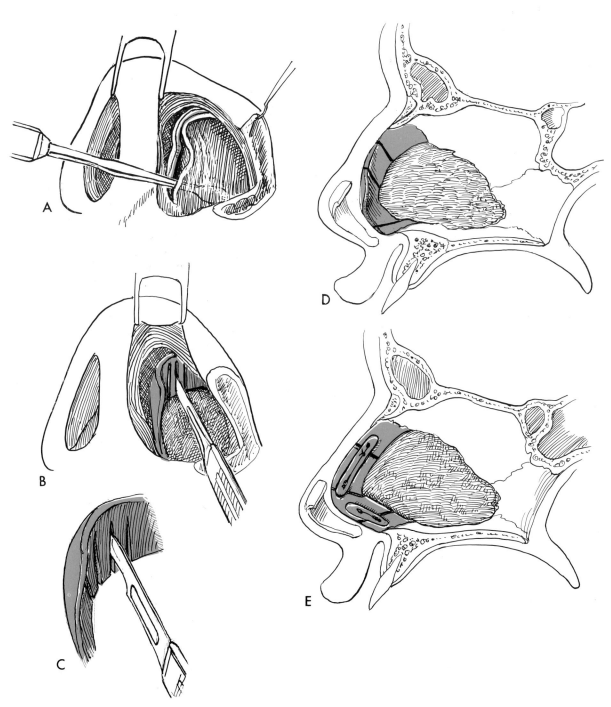

Figure 11–15.   It is often difficult to obtain and maintain a straight nose even after extensive mobilization and cross-cutting of the cartilaginous septum. Because of the innate elasticity of the cartilage and its relation to the perichondrium, a septum that has been straightened during surgery is apt to curl in the postoperative period and resume its original curve. Planas (1977) recommends an interesting trick to bolster the repositioned cartilage, which he attributed to Dupont et al (1966). *A–D,* The deviated dorsal strut of cartilage is scored after a partial submucous resection according to standard technique. *E,* The weakened cartilage strut is reinforced along its caudal and dorsal margins with carved plates of the thin bone of the resected perpendicular plate of the ethmoid. These are fixed in place with fine sutures passed through drill holes in the bone.

Selective resection of vomer spurs can be accomplished with minimal disturbance of the remainder of the septum, as already pointed out. Also, localized septal deviations can be shaved or partially removed where necessary. When the entire base of the septum is dislocated from the vomer groove along the floor, it is often possible to chisel the septum free and reposition it with a minimal disturbance to the mucoperichondrium and periosteum (Figure 11–14). It is always advantageous to maintain the integrity of as much of the septal anatomy as possible and avoid resecting large segments. Extensive resection of the cartilage and bone of the septum can result in unstable mucoperichondrial and mucoperiosteal flaps that may act as a valve-like structure that can occlude one side or the other by virtue of its excessive mobility. A number of useful techniques of septal reconstruction have been reported by Converse (1950, 1964), Dingman (1956), Becker (1951), Denecke and Meyer (1967), Planas (1977) (Figure 11–15), and others. The physiologic aspects of nasal obstruction were described in an excellent review by Baker and Strauss (1977) and are further amplified in the chapter on physiology by Baker.

After *in vitro* studies of the behavior of cartilage based upon its inherent system of response to stress, Fry (1967) proposed an intriguing theory that may prove helpful in septal reconstruction but

is as yet not totally confirmed in clinical practice. This interest was stimulated by the work of Gibson and Davis (1958) on the biomechanics of cartilage. These investigators established the principle that cartilage tends to bend or warp in the direction of its attached perichondrium when the perichondrium has been denuded from its opposite surface (Figure 11–16). Fry proposed that multiple cross cuts or "dicing" of cartilage disrupts the normal elastic forces on the side that is stripped of mucoperichondrium. He believed that the attached perichondrium on the opposite side would allow the innate elastic forces of the cartilage to bend toward that side. Accordingly, in a deviated septum, elevation of the mucoperichondrial flaps on the concave side of the septum with multiple cross cuts of the cartilage on that side would cause it to bend toward the opposite or undissected side with the mucoperichondrial flaps intact. He demonstrated that cartilage thus cut would bend toward the uncut side. This technique seems to work well in his hands in ear reconstruction and presumably would apply to septal reconstruction. Although such a technique has not found widespread clinical support, it bears continued investigation. A similar result can be expected from the crushing or morcellizing technique favored by some surgeons, in which once again the mucoperichondrial flaps are left attached on one side only, thus minimizing the

Text continued on page 319.

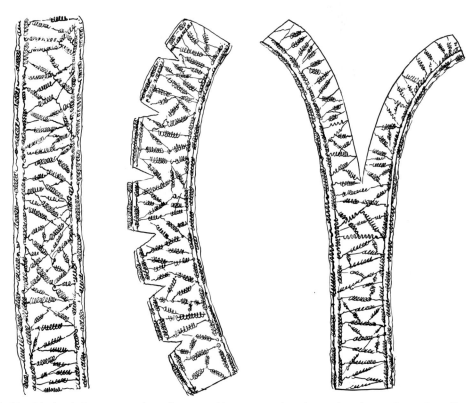

Figure 11–16. Mechanical representation of stresses (shown as springs in tension) in nasal septal cartilage with predicted effect of interruption of one surface. (After Fry, 1967.)

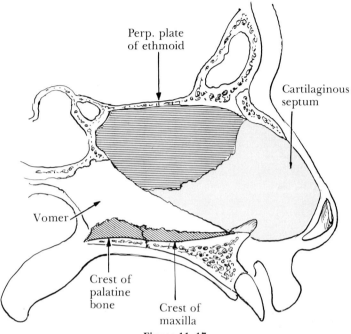

Figure 11–17.

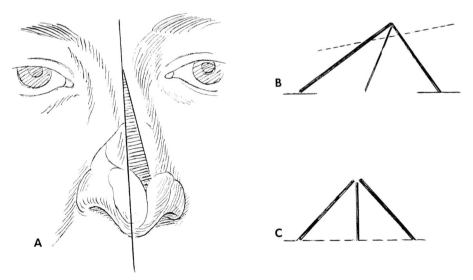

Figure 11–18. The externally deviated or twisted nose with unequal walls (*A*) can be likened to an off-center pyramid (*B*). The nature and extent of the deviation dictates the steps required to straighten the nose. In high deviations, simple removal of the hump (lowering the profile) sometimes suffices. Asymmetrical removal of the hump (*C*), allowing for the discrepancy between the nasal walls, is also very helpful.

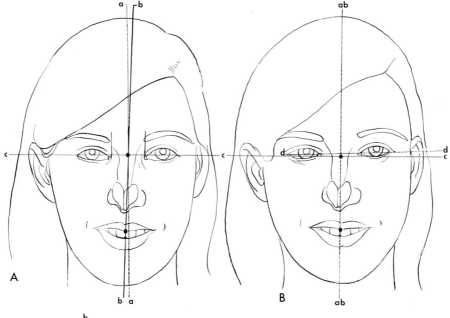

A

B

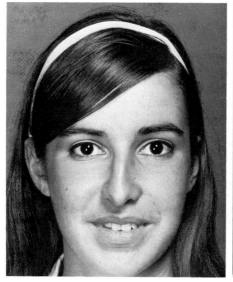

C

Figure 11–19. *A* and *B*, The aim of surgery in the deviated nose is to close the angle a-b in the final result.

Ideally, the triangle formed by the outer canthus (d) on either side with the midline (b) is an isosceles triangle, however, this is rarely the case in nature, since most faces are asymmetrical to some degree.

Note in the pre- and postoperative photographs of this patient that the postoperative nose is still deviated slightly to the right. Such a deviation may remain because the surgeon was unable to get the nose straight, or it may be that the patient's face was asymmetrical in the first place and thus the midline of the face is not straight. In this patient the midface plane is slightly crooked.

C, The center line "b" through face and line "d" through outer canthi are drawn. The triangle shows the acceptable position of the nose postoperatively. A slight depression is still visible in the area of left upper lateral cartilage.

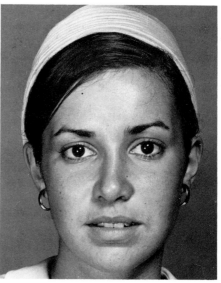

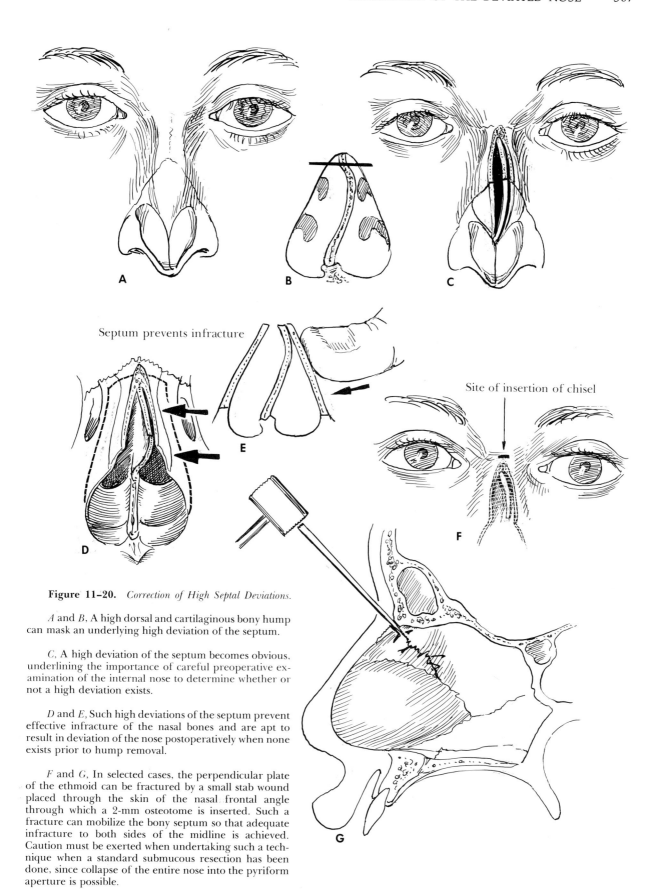

Figure 11–20. *Correction of High Septal Deviations.*

A and *B*, A high dorsal and cartilaginous bony hump can mask an underlying high deviation of the septum.

C, A high deviation of the septum becomes obvious, underlining the importance of careful preoperative examination of the internal nose to determine whether or not a high deviation exists.

D and *E*, Such high deviations of the septum prevent effective infracture of the nasal bones and are apt to result in deviation of the nose postoperatively when none exists prior to hump removal.

F and *G*, In selected cases, the perpendicular plate of the ethmoid can be fractured by a small stab wound placed through the skin of the nasal frontal angle through which a 2-mm osteotome is inserted. Such a fracture can mobilize the bony septum so that adequate infracture to both sides of the midline is achieved. Caution must be exerted when undertaking such a technique when a standard submucous resection has been done, since collapse of the entire nose into the pyriform aperture is possible.

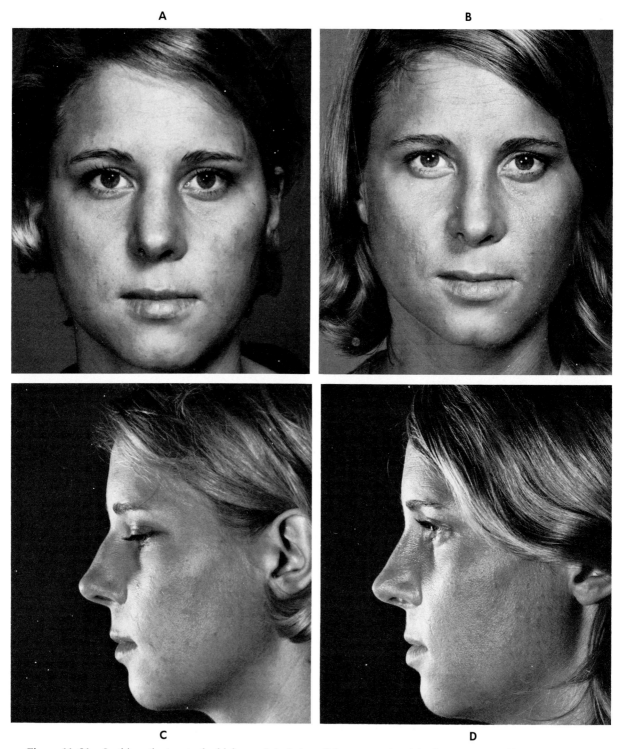

Figure 11–21. In this patient, note the high septal deviation of the nose to the right. It was corrected by the technique illustrated in Figure 11–20.

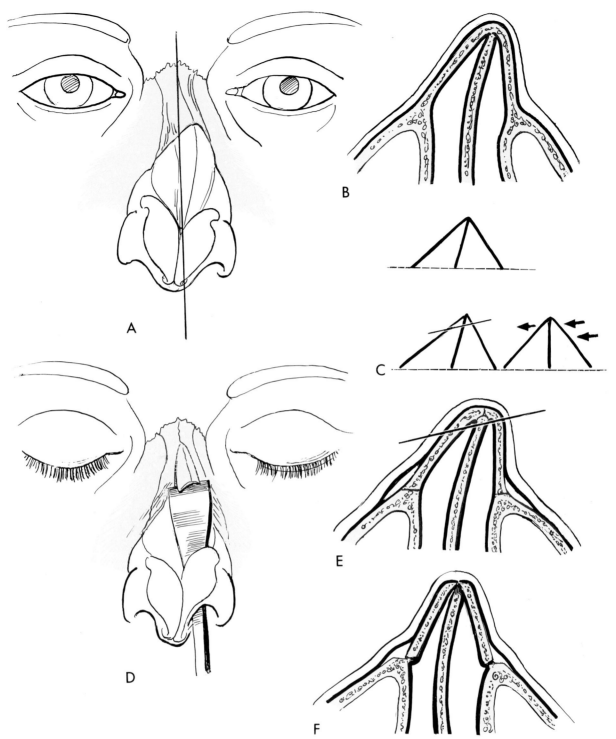

Figure 11–22. Often, an apparently marked deviation of the external nose can be corrected visually by an asymmetrical shaping of the dorsal hump.

A, The external deviation of the nasal dorsum in relation to the midline, which is represented by the vertical solid line, is shown.

B, A coronal section shows the nasal deviation along with warping of the septum to the affected side. *C,* The artist's illustration by triangles of the deviated nose. The arrows indicate the direction required in correction of the deformity.

D, The chisel or osteotome is manipulated on the bias, so that the majority of bony hump is resected from the side opposite the external deviation.

E, The obliquity of the cut is shown by the solid line.

F, After asymmetrical hump resection and infracture, the nose often assumes a midline position, provided there is not a significant degree of high deviation of the septum that buttresses against the nasal bone on the involved side, preventing a stabilized infracture.

Illustration continued on the following page.

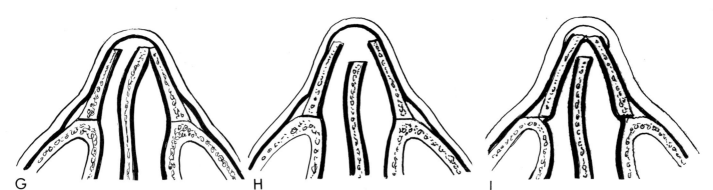

Figure 11–22 *Continued.*   *G*, In this instance, a high deviation of the nasal septum along the dorsum to the left prevents medial movement of the left nasal bone.

H and *I*, The bony portion of the septum as well as that part of the cartilaginous septum that is associated with the upper lateral cartilages can be trimmed at a level lower than that of the dorsal margins of the infractured nasal bone, as shown here, so that upon infracture, the dorsal border of the nose lies in a midline position.

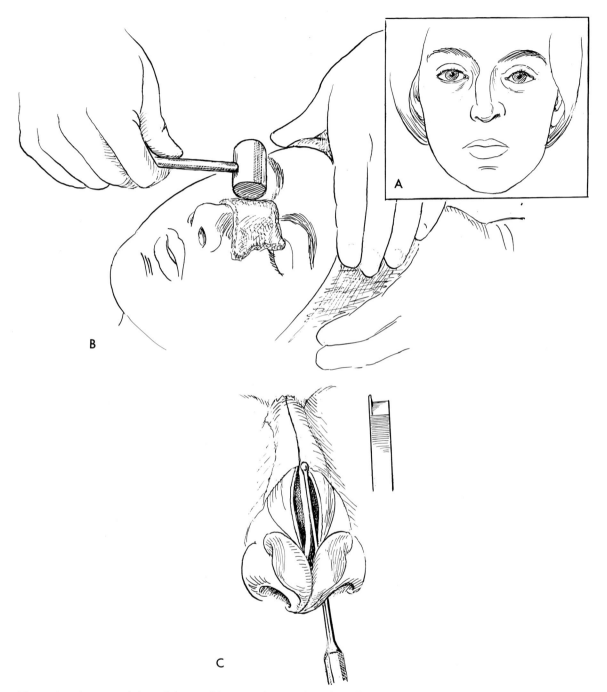

Figure 11–23. *A*, Deviation of the nasal bones and upper lateral cartilages of such a degree that repositioning the bones in the midline would not result in contour correction.

B, The Kazanjian maneuver: padding is applied over the nose and a sharp blow with a mallet comminutes the nasal bones. Care must be taken to protect the globe of the eye during this maneuver.

C, The guarded osteotome is passed along the nasal dorsum to separate the nasal bones and septum. The bones may then be straightened by manipulation and maintained in position by an external splint.

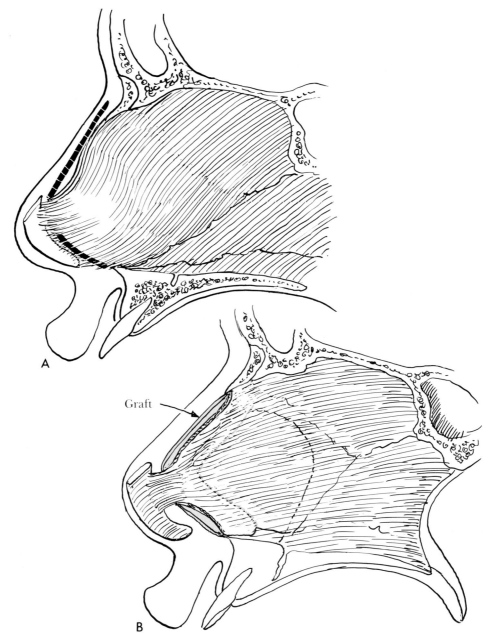

Figure 11–24.   When marked serpentine curvature of the dorsal border of the septal cartilage cannot be corrected by conservative methods, it may be necessary to resect the entire twisted septal cartilage and replace it with a straightened portion of the cartilage to provide support for the nasal dorsum. This procedure is rarely indicated and should be resorted to only if the surgeon believes that all other techniques would fail. Many procedures have been described which aim at minimizing the risk of collapse following such extensive surgery, and principal among these is the interrupted transfixion incision, with the mucoperichondrial flaps of the septum acting as a sling for the nasal dorsum (Converse, 1959).

A, Interruption of the transfixion incision. *B*, The mucosa in the region of the interruption acting as a hammock-like support for the nasal dorsum.

The septal transplant may be fixed in any of a variety of ways to the lateral cartilage, and many ingenious techniques of suturing have been described, such as transcutaneous ligation or drawing of the transcutaneously placed sutures into the nasal cavity with a hook (Kazanjian and Converse, 1959).

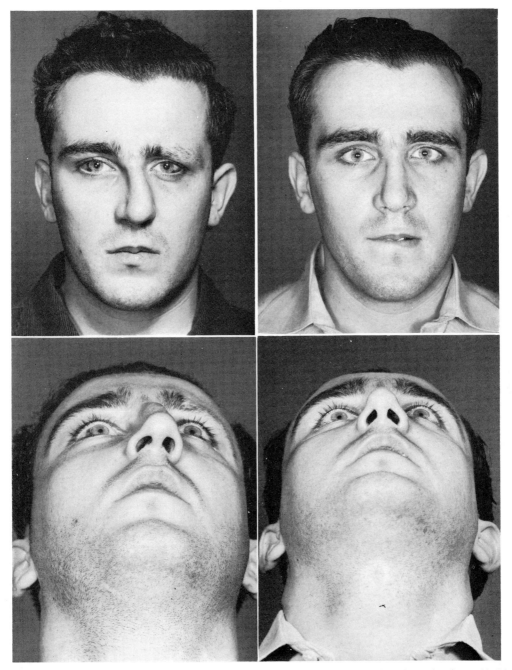

Figure 11–25. A badly deflected nose with a severely traumatized septum, corrected as shown in Figure 11–24, (Kazanjian and Converse, 1959).

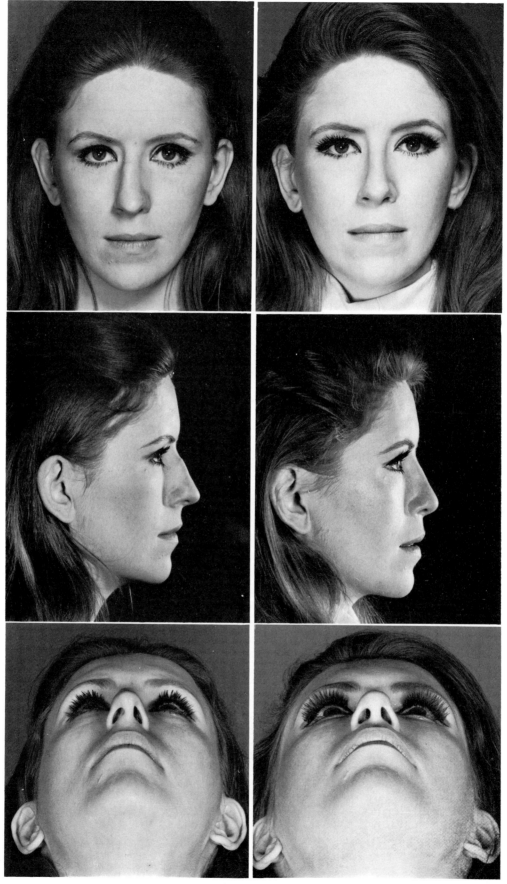

Figure 11–26.

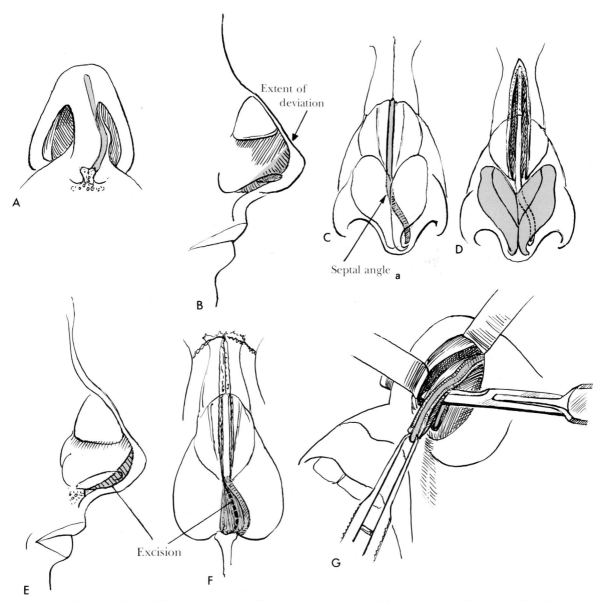

Figure 11–27. Deviations of the caudal margin of the septum, which are often where it has skipped out of the bony groove, can be corrected by a partial resection and replacement of the lower fragment after it is mobilized as a "swinging door."

A–D, Illustration of deflection of the caudal margin of the septum is demonstrated, as in the patient shown in Figure 11–26. The deviation occurs only in the lower septum and extends from just above the septal angle caudally.

E, F, and *G,* Such an obvious deformity is often easily correctable by simple, expedient trimming of the excess cartilage where it is redundant. Small "a" represents the line of deflection at which point it is sometimes necessary to effect the transection of the cartilage on the side opposite the deviation without elevation of both mucoperichondrial membranes to effect a "swinging door" correction. The patient in Figure 11–26 demonstrates the results of this technique. She also had a high deviation of the nose to the right, corrected by asymmetrical osteotomy.

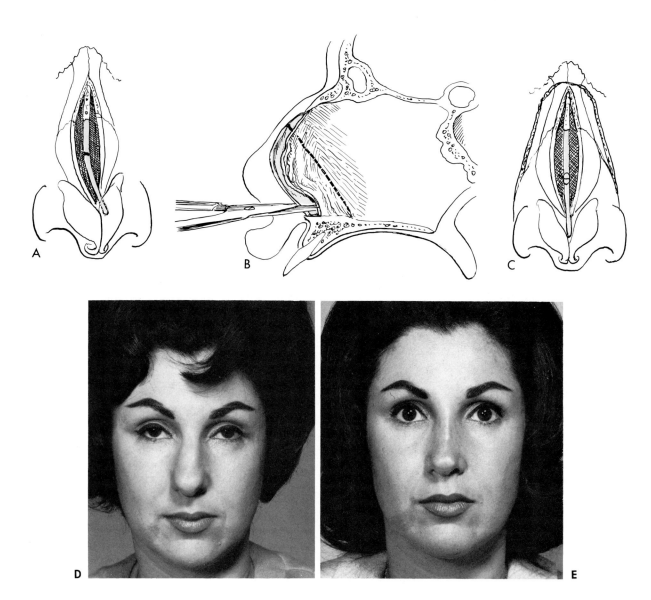

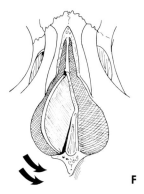

Figure 11–28. The "swinging door" technique is useful to correct deviations of the lower cartilaginous septum when the superior (bony) septum is more or less straight. In the illustration, the cartilaginous septum is sectioned completely through at the point of maximum deviation (*A*). In this instance it is below the junction of the bone and cartilage. *B*, Access is gained by developing a mucoperichondrial flap through the transfixion incision *on one side only*. The side elevated is on the side of the deviation whenever possible. The line of transection of the cartilage is shown by the dotted line, but it varies according to the deformity. The septum is then freed along the floor and swung to the midline, with the opposite lining intact. *C*, With the septum in a midline position, a fixation suture through the septal break is often useful.

D, E, and *F,* In this patient, a lower septal deflection to the right, mostly cartilaginous in nature, was corrected by the "swinging door" technique in which the cartilage was transected at the osteocartilaginous junction.

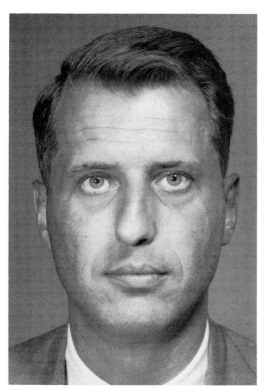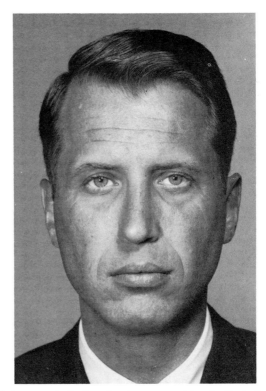

Figure 11–29. A deflection of the cartilaginous portion of the nose, including the tip, corrected by the "swinging door" procedure and nasal tip plasty.

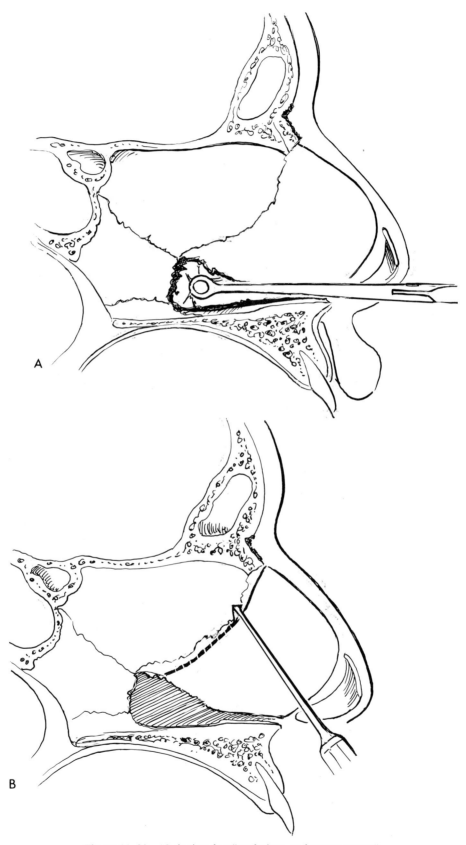

Figure 11–30. "Swinging door" technique and "spurectomy."

possibility of postoperative complications such as perforation, tears, and unstable ulcerations.

In summary, one should not hesitate to perform a conservative submucous resection, spurectomy, or septal reconstruction when necessary. When a formal submucous resection is undertaken, it is important to maintain a 1 to 2 cm dorsal and caudal strut when it appears obvious that radical submucous resection is necessary to provide breathing space. Great care must be taken not to perform extensive submucous resection in combination with extensive osteotomies of the bones, where the risk of dorsal collapse is great from inadvertent fracture of the remaining fragile attachment of the thin perpendicular plate of the ethmoid (Figure 11–2).

Figure 11–17 shows the normal anatomic landmarks and distribution of bone and cartilage of the nasal septum. Note that the vomer provides the keystone of support to the perpendicular plate of the ethmoid, which forms the greater bulk of the septum superiorly, and the quadrangular septal cartilage, which provides the majority of the remaining bulk of the septum anterocaudally. The septum nestles snugly in the groove formed by the crest of the palatine bone. More often than not, it is a mistake to consider the nasal septum as an anatomic entity to be dealt with separately in nasal deformities. The septum should be thought of as a component of the osteocartilaginous nose that plays an intimate role not only in dividing the nose into two separate chambers but also in providing support to the dorsum, particularly after an operation. Septal deformities are certainly the most difficult and often vexing problems facing the surgeon in nasal reconstruction, since the cartilage of the septum often has a "mind of its own" and can resist even the most dedicated and intricate corrective maneuvers that the surgeon can devise.

The problem of the twisted nose that is externally obvious can sorely try the ingenuity of the surgeon (Figure 11–18). The aim of reconstruction of the twisted nose is not only to obtain cosmetically a nose that is as straight as possible but one that functions well in the all-important process of respiration. Accordingly, a careful preoperative analysis of the anatomic factors in each individual case is important to provide guidelines and a surgical blueprint for the surgeon. Unfortunately, it is frequently necessary for the surgeon to alter any preconceived surgical plans he may have during the operative procedure to accommodate for unperceived exigencies that arise during each step of the operative procedure, since the pieces may not fall exactly into place as planned. The twisted nose must be considered as a unit in which all components play their part and in which various techniques must be available to obtain the desired result. (See Figures 11–19 through 11–30.)

(For references, see pages 450 to 453.)

Chapter 12

Postoperative Considerations and Complications

Thomas D. Rees, M.D., F.A.C.S.

THE FINAL STEPS IN THE OPERATION

After the transfixion incision is sutured, the final step in the procedure is removal of the redundant parts of the upper lateral cartilages. Mattress sutures of 4–0 silk or interrupted sutures of plain or chromic catgut can be used for suturing the transfixion incision.

It is usually necessary to overcorrect the tip slightly in an upward position, because the effects of gravity and scar relaxation will cause it to drop somewhat. Most patients prefer a nose that is slightly tilted rather than one that is too long, and they often return to express disappointment as the tip relaxes from its immediate postoperative position. In patients with plunging tips, the tip must be markedly overcorrected and the caudal portion of the septum must be sutured between the medial crura in a tongue-and-groove fashion.

A separate incision in the mucoperichondrium to elevate a flap for submucous resection of the septum is sutured with fine catgut.

The suturing of the alar base incisions varies somewhat, depending on the design of the resection. A 4–0 chromic catgut suture with the knot tied inside the nose and incorporating a substantial bite of muscle and alar base is used to relieve tension from the skin sutures, which are removed on the third or fourth postoperative day at the latest. Interrupted nylon sutures of 5–0 or 6–0 size are used for the skin.

The Upper Lateral Cartilages

The amount of upper lateral cartilage to be removed varies considerably from patient to patient and depends on how much of the lateral crus
320

of the alar cartilages was removed and on the need to shorten the side walls to correct a plunging tip (Figure 12–1). It must be appreciated that the upper lateral cartilages are a vital part of the respiratory anatomy, and that the junction formed by the upper lateral cartilages and the septum is critical in nasal ventilation and should be maintained. Extra caution must be used when resection of the lateral wing of the alar cartilage has been generous and when some nasal lining skin has been resected in the eversion technique. Excess cartilage that projects after the tip is set at the desired angle and the transfixion incision is sutured is the only cartilage that is resected. It is not necessary to suture the upper laterals to the septum.

Final Checking of the Nose

This is probably the most important single step in nasal plasty. The operator checks the nasal dorsum for spicules of bone or cartilage and for irregularities of contour. It may be necessary to smooth the nasal bones with a rasp or scissors, and care must be taken not to dislocate them. Finally, with a small curette the skin pockets are carefully swept for any bony, cartilaginous or soft tissue debris that may contribute to infection or contour deficiencies (Figure 12–2). This checking may be aided by gentle pressure to remove edema (Figure 12–3).

Suturing

It is always better to suture an incision, including nasal incisions, particularly those in the vestibular skin used to deliver the alar cartilages (Figure 12–4). Such incisions, left unsutured, may be

Text continued on page 325.

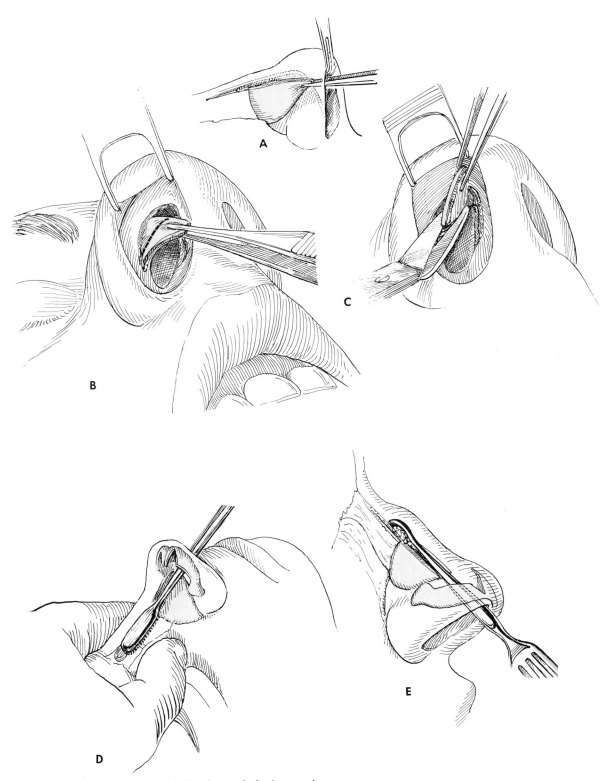

Figure 12–1. Finishing touches for the nasal plastic procedure.

A, Excess length of the upper lateral cartilages is estimated by visual inspection during gentle traction on their distal ends.

B, The excess amount of cartilage.

C, The excess is amputated conservatively.

D, Final smoothing of irregular nasal bones is completed when necessary with the rasp.

E, Bone and soft tissue debris is swept out by a small curette, and the entire region is carefully inspected with the aid of the Aufricht retractor to insure that all surfaces are smooth and that no small remnants of cartilage or bone remain. This measure is a most important step.

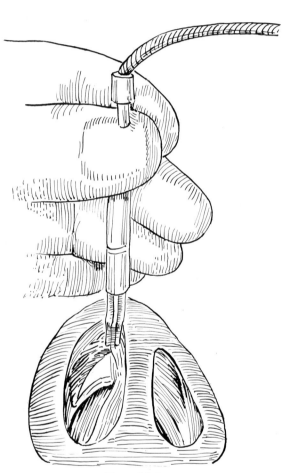

Figure 12–2.

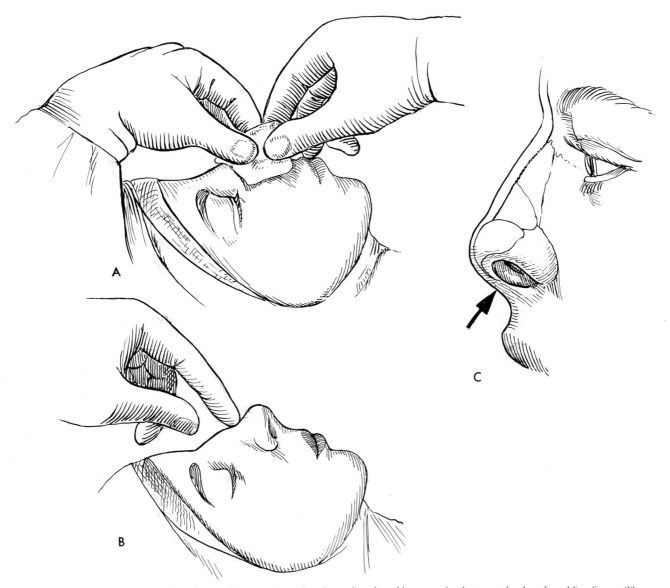

Figure 12–3. *A*, Operative edema of the nasal covering tissues is reduced by squeezing between the thumb and forefinger. The soft tissues are reapplied to the underlying nasal framework.

B, The finger is run along the new nasal dorsum and the soft tissues applied to it in order to determine the degree of correction achieved in the nasal tip and the dorsum. At this point it is important to palpate for any irregularities that will require secondary correction if left.

C, Pressure is carefully applied to reapproximate the margins of the membranous and cartilaginous septum, and the adequacy of the resection in this region is checked.

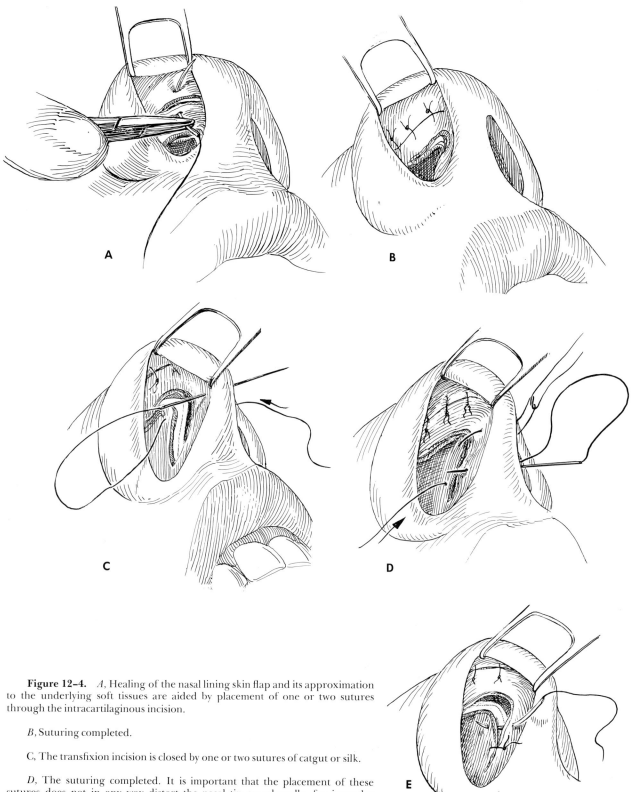

Figure 12–4.   *A*, Healing of the nasal lining skin flap and its approximation to the underlying soft tissues are aided by placement of one or two sutures through the intracartilaginous incision.

B, Suturing completed.

C, The transfixion incision is closed by one or two sutures of catgut or silk.

D, The suturing completed. It is important that the placement of these sutures does not in any way distort the nasal tip or columella, for irregular contour may result from carelessness in observing this point.

E, Closure of the transfixion incision by reapproximation of lining skin to mucosa on either side of the incision. This method results in a minimum of tip distortion and is applicable when repositioning of the tip angle is not required.

distorted by the tape supports or by the splint, with healing delayed across a gaping wound and scarring with distortion. Interrupted 5–0 catgut sutures are used in these incisions; one or two sutures suffice.

PACKINGS, DRESSINGS, AND SPLINTS

Tight intranasal packs are not necessary except on the rare occasion when a wide submucous resection requiring bilateral elevation of mucoperichondrial flaps is done. The usual technique of accordion packing with strip gauze of a nonadherent type can then be used to approximate the flaps. A simple folded piece of Telfa gauze is used to separate the incisions in the vestibule and the columella (Figure 12–5).

This procedure has proved to be all that is necessary. It is comfortable for the patient and suffices to separate raw surfaces. It also obviates outward pressure upon the nasal bones that can occur with tight intranasal packs. There has been no increase in postoperative bleeding with this technique.

It is not necessary to apply external taping to all noses. It is difficult to assume that such taping does have a splinting effect on the underlying skeletal or cartilaginous structures. The exception to this statement may be when there has been ambitious remodeling of the alar cartilages, altering the "spring" effect. Under these circumstances, traditional tape strapping probably has a salutary effect as a fixation dressing to splint the cut ends of the cartilage in the desired position until fibrous union begins. Sterile paper tape has greatly reduced skin reactions.

A malleable splint is placed over the taping or on the skin to approximate the skin flaps to the bone and to help to prevent hematoma formation beneath the skin flaps. It is fallacious to assume that casts or splints will maintain inadequately fractured bones in place. Fractures must be complete, and the bones must be placed where desired *during* the operative procedure. A splint cannot do a job that the surgeon failed to accomplish.

Molded plaster of Paris applied directly to the skin is an excellent splint (Figure 12–6). It can also be applied over paper taping, when used; plaster rarely causes skin irritation. It can be accurately molded to apply to the skin over the nasal skeleton and conforms at crucial points such as the glabella and nasofrontal angle where small hematomas are apt to occur. It is difficult to apply too much pressure with plaster, so that focal skin necrosis is avoided. After the plaster has been molded and allowed to dry, it is affixed to the skin of the fore-

head and cheeks with 1-inch paper tape applied in such a way that some pressure is exerted on the splint to keep it firmly seated. Aeroplast, or a similar sticky substance, is helpful in achieving adherence of the tape to the cast. A dental compound splint may be used alternatively; it also provides satisfactory support (Figure 12–7).

Some surgeons remove the nasal splints soon after surgery — three or four days postoperatively. The author prefers to leave all splints in place for seven to ten days because of the protection afforded the freshly operated nose. Edema is also controlled, and the patient has a sense of security knowing the new nose is being protected. Premature removal of the splint can accidentally elevate the skin flaps, so that accumulation of serum or blood can occur beneath. Healing is then prolonged.

All packs are removed on the second postoperative day, except when extensive septal reconstruction has been done in correcting the "crooked" nose. In such cases, the packing is left in place three or four days. It is not to be assumed, however, that this packing in any significant way prevents recurrence of warping of the cartilage or bending of the nose. Recurrence of the distortion is a risk throughout the healing period, including the prolonged period of scar contraction. It is inconceivable that packing for an extra day or two can influence the eventual outcome.

After extensive septal reconstruction, some surgeons employ prolonged intranasal splinting with thin plates of polyethylene, silicone, Teflon, or another similar material. These sheet splints are placed on either side of the reconstructed septum and are sutured into position. They are left in place for several weeks (if the patient can tolerate their presence). Such splinting seems a reasonable technique in selected cases. Surgical reconstruction of the twisted nose must at times, of course, be extensive, but postoperative splinting of parts cannot be accepted as a substitute for surgical correction.

Despite complete fracture lines, and what seemed entirely adequate infractures at the time of surgery, the nasal bones (one or both) sometimes seem to creep laterally soon after the splint is removed. This results in a widening of the upper nose, which can be unilateral or bilateral. When this lateral displacement of the bone occurs, it can sometimes be corrected by manual pressure applied by the surgeon at weekly or biweekly intervals. This is slightly painful for the patient but quite effective, unless the bone is being held outward by a high septal deviation. Some surgeons prefer the use of a nose clamp, which Aufricht

Text continued on page 332.

Figure 12–5.   *A*, Nasal packs of a single, folded piece of Telfa dressing placed in the nostril.

B, The packs in position, with a minimal amount protruding from the external nares.

C, Adhesive to support the soft tissues and to reduce dead space is applied to the exterior of the nose. The first tape to be applied is across the supratip region to appose the soft tissues to the dorsal portion of the septum.

D, The tip is supported by a sling of adhesive in the manner shown. This should be applied loosely about the tip and then tightened as shown in *E* to bring about accurate support of this area without skin wrinkling.

See illustration on the opposite page.

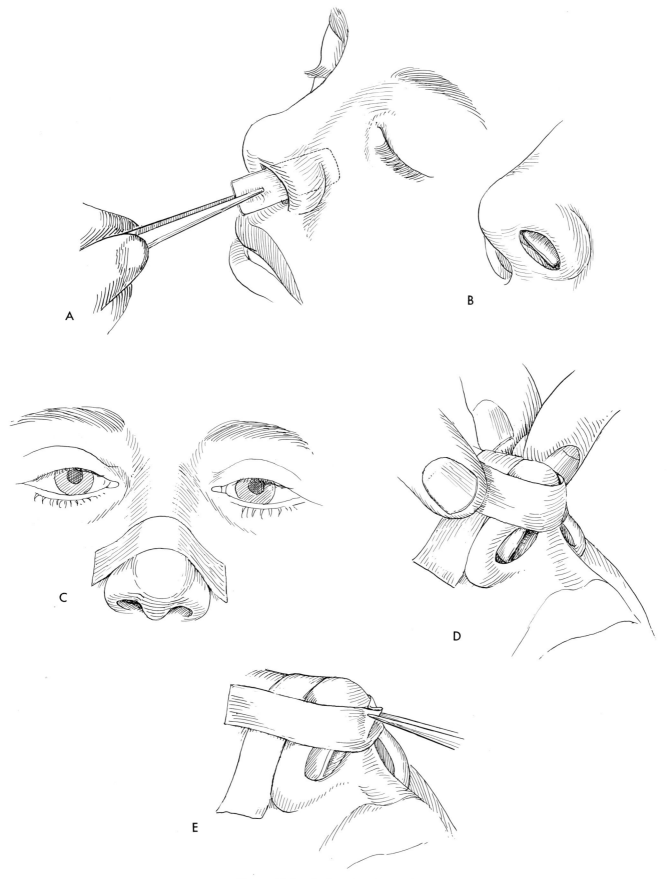

Figure 12–5. *See legend on the opposite page.*

Figure 12–6. *A*, The adhesive support completed.

B, Seven or eight layers of plaster of Paris cut to the pattern shown.

C, In the patient with a deep nasofrontal angle, it is often necessary to cut into the precanthal area of the plaster splint to facilitate accurate approximation in this region. A piece of flannelette or Telfa dressing is placed over the nose and the forehead in the manner shown to keep the plaster from adhering to the underlying adhesive tape.

D, The plaster of Paris is placed in tepid water to speed hardening, and the splint is molded into position. Aeroplast is applied after the plaster hardens to facilitate the adhesion of paper tape to the plaster.

E, The splint is held in place with additional adhesive strips. Prior to application of these strips, the skin should be protected with one of the many varieties of skin varnishes.

See illustration on the opposite page.

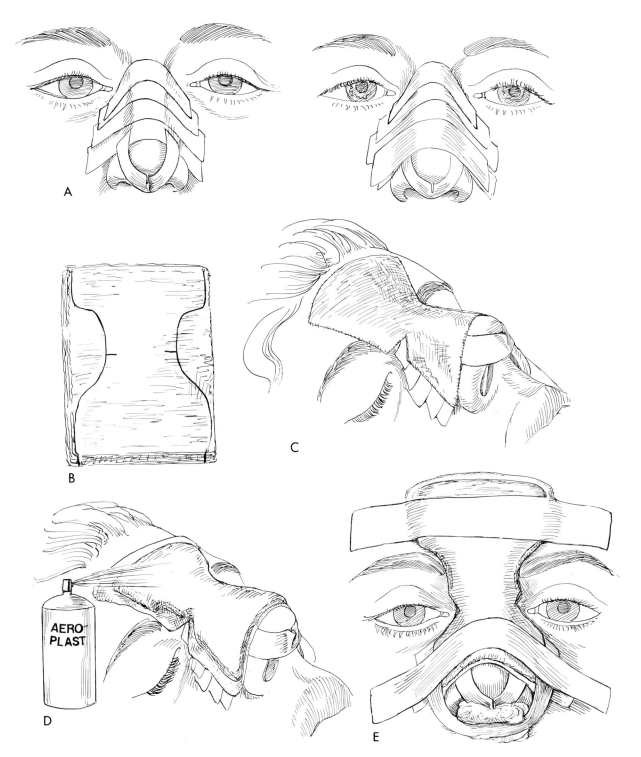

Figure 12–6. *See legend on the opposite page.*

Figure 12–7.   An alternate method of splinting the nose with dental compound.

A, A pattern is cut in Asche's soft metal to an approximate size, as shown.

B, A completed splint, showing the Asche's soft metal acting as a carrier for the dental compound.

C, The heat-softened (black) dental compound carried by the Asche's soft metal is placed over the nose and molded into position. Hardening is speeded by applying ice compresses. The soft metal carrier facilitates the handling of the dental compound and prevents transfer of excessive finger pressure to the nasal structure.

D, Transparent skin varnish is applied to the forehead and cheeks.

E, Adhesive applied to support the splint.

F, A 2 × 2 inch gauze is used to catch any nasal leakage.

See illustration on the opposite page.

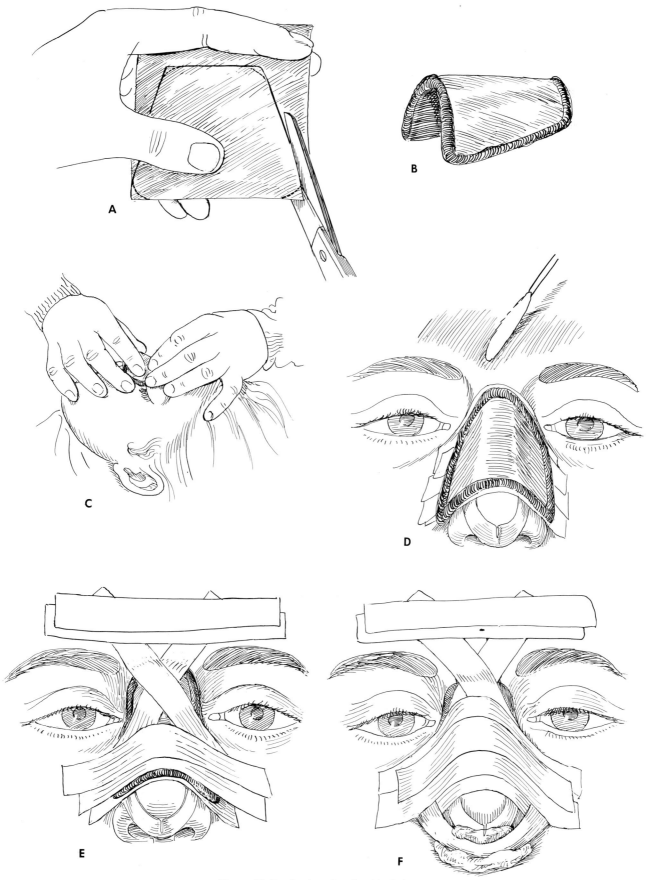

Figure 12–7. *See legend on the opposite page.*

(1971) has attached to a pair of glasses. Nose clamps, if use is left to the discretion of the patient, can be dangerous if they exert too much pressure. It is my feeling that they are generally not very effective and are certainly no substitute for thorough fracture lines and proper infracture.

On the tenth postoperative day, when all sutures and the splint are removed, patients are advised to cleanse the nose gently with half strength peroxide solution and cotton-tipped applicators, after which the vestibule is coated with a fine layer of sterile petrolatum or oil.

The patient is instructed not to blow the nose until the second postoperative week. The use of nose drops is discouraged. Often the nose is stuffy, simulating a head cold, but this is caused by congestion and vasomotor changes in the mucous membranes as a result of surgical trauma. This problem usually clears within the first four weeks. If it persists, however, other causes such as allergic rhinitis or mechanical obstruction aggravated by surgery should be sought.

In patients with severe preexisting allergic rhinitis aggravated by surgery, a course of antihistamines is maintained throughout the healing period. In very severe problems, the inferior turbinates are injected with a steroid solution. Postoperative nasal obstruction symptoms are common. When they persist for many months, however, the surgeon is apt to blame a septal spur or an apparent minor deviation of the septum. He may therefore suggest a submucous resection. This procedure may be very helpful if a true obstruction exists, but it has been disappointing in many cases. Its worth has generally been overemphasized. It is not advisable to take the attitude, "when in doubt, do a submucous resection."

Many postoperative nasal obstruction problems are not structural but rather are physiologic and can be treated with patience and medical care. Allergic problems often respond to only one or two of the many and varied antihistamines available. It may be necessary to try several different compounds before the effective one is discovered.

There is often a good deal of emotional overlay involved in nasal obstruction secondary to congestion of the mucous membranes. Such problems are highly challenging and sometimes obstinate to treat. The help of a psychiatrist can sometimes be obtained if the patient and family can be coaxed into accepting such help.

When artificial heating is used in homes, the nasal mucous membranes often dry out during the night, causing small encrustations to form. These become separated, and often, punctuated raw areas are produced that cause bleeding. Patients are advised to humidify their rooms. Placing a pan of water under the bed or a chair or on a radiator often helps. Use of a cold steam humidifier is most helpful.

POSTOPERATIVE CARE

PHYSICAL ACTIVITY

Moderation in physical activities is advised after surgery. This does not mean that the patient should be limited to a totally sedentary life for many weeks, as some surgeons recommend. Most strenuous physical activities are limited for three weeks. Beyond this point, reasonable activities are begun. The exceptions, of course, are body contact sports such as soccer, volley ball, and football. These sports are limited for from four to six months.

The nose knits slowly at the fracture lines and can quite easily be disturbed during this period. However, sports that rarely cause injury to the nose such as horseback riding, swimming (not diving), and tennis are permitted after the third week. Patients are advised that if the nose is injured, it can be reduced promptly (even more effectively than before rhinoplasty), so that they should not be overly concerned. Figure 12–8 shows a standard form given to patients explaining postoperative care.

COMPLICATIONS OF RHINOPLASTY

General Considerations

Unquestionably, rhinoplasty is technically the most difficult of all operations in plastic surgery — partly because the operation must be conceptualized as a three-dimensional technique requiring what is essentially a blind approach. This is further compounded by the difficulty in predicting the final result; many factors combine to produce this result including the surgeon's skill; anatomic variations in the skin, subcutaneous tissues, and cartilages of the nose; healing idiosyncrasies of the patient; and complications. The final result of rhinoplasty is evident only after months or years, during which time the nose changes continuously. This long-term gradual metamorphosis is extremely important for the surgeon to recognize, since a common cause of failure — the overoperated nose — is due to steadfast determination at the operating table to achieve a result that fits a preconceived vision, without real appreciation of the long-term effects of the healing process.

Thomas D. Rees, M.D., F.A.C.S.
176 East 72nd Street
New York, N. Y. 10021

Le 5-1611

PLASTIC AND RECONSTRUCTIVE SURGERY

INSTRUCTIONS FOR PATIENTS HAVING

AESTHETIC SURGERY ON THE NOSE

I.   Do not take aspirin or any medications containing aspirin for two weeks prior to surgery. Aspirin interferes with normal blood clotting. Aspirin containing drugs include: Alka Seltzer, Anacin, Bufferin, Darvon Compound, Empirin, Excedrin, Midol and numerous others. If you are in doubt about a drug, please check with your pharmacist. Tylenol is a good substitute for aspirin.

II. Notify us of any signs of infection such as a cold, boil, etc. or fever during the week prior to surgery.

III. THE FIRST 48 HOURS AFTER YOUR OPERATION:

What to expect:
Swelling and black and blue discoloration around the eyes are likely and may be worse the second morning after surgery. The white of your eyes may appear red.

A certain amount of bleeding from the nose occurs which will gradually stop. The "nasal diaper" gauze can be changed as needed.

You may be uncomfortable, but you should have minimal pain. Medication will be prescribed for discomfort.

What to do:
Stay in bed with your head at about the level of two pillows.

You may go to the bathroom at this time with assistance if needed.

Take only liquids during the first twenty-four hours after surgery and then begin soft foods if you wish.

IV. THE FIRST TWO WEEKS AFTER SURGERY:

Brush teeth gently. (A Water Pik is excellent.)

Do not blow your nose.

Sleep with your head elevated on two pillows.

-2-

IV. THE FIRST TWO WEEKS AFTER SURGERY - CONT'D

After the first two days almost anything can be eaten. However, soft foods require less chewing and will seem easier to manage.

Do not clean your nose with Q-tips, etc. until the splint is removed.

Sneezing may occur, try to sneeze through your mouth.

Glasses may rest on the splint or be taped to your forehead after the splint is removed. Do not allow glasses to rest directly on your nose for six weeks following surgery. Contact lenses can usually be inserted after a few days.

After the splint has been removed you may clean just inside each nostril once a day with Q-tips soaked in a solution of ½ hydrogen peroxide and ½ water.

You may gently wash your face around the splint with a cloth and plain water. Following removal of the splint, wash the nose gently twice daily with any mild soap. You may resume your normal facial care at this time. You may shower as soon as the splint is off, but avoid putting your face in the full force of the shower spray for three weeks.

Hair may be shampooed on the day the splint is removed, but put your head back not forward. Shampooing is easiest in the shower.

Facial and eye make-up may be used as soon as the nasal splint is removed.

You may cook, shop, and care for your personal needs as desired when the nasal splint is off, but avoid strenuous exercise and activities for four weeks. At that time swimming, tennis, golf, running, horse-back riding and other sports are permitted that do not require direct body contact. Body contact sports such as volley-ball, football, wrestling, etc. are prohibited for six months.

Hemorrhaging from the nose is very rare and usually not serious. Should it occur, try to remain calm, keep your head elevated and apply iced compresses to the side of bleeding. Place gauze or towel under the nostril to absorb the blood.

You may sunbathe following surgery but avoid sunburn. Use a sun screen (Pre-Sun, U-Val) until the swelling has subsided.

Figure 12–8.

In no other cosmetic operation are the preoperative evaluation and patient selection more crucial to minimizing complications than in rhinoplasty. Much has been written about the neuroses and psychoses of the rhinoplasty patient, and a careful evaluation of the patient's motivations and self-image is essential. The surgeon must determine whether the patient is emotionally suited to the operation and to what degree the nose can be improved in contour. A poor decision at this time can result in the ultimate failure of the operation, although a technically successful contour has been achieved. Age is an important consideration, for the patient of 40 years or older presents an entirely different set of problems than does the teenager. Bones are more brittle, skin is inelastic, cartilage is calcified, and vessels are fragile in advancing age, increasing the possibility of complications.

Anatomic factors that may influence the result of rhinoplasty are the thickness of the nasal bones, the presence or absence of the nasion depression, and the thickness and position of the septum. Deviations of the cartilaginous septum pose the most difficult and challenging problem. Despite all surgical maneuvers, attainment of a completely straight dorsum may not be possible, and some curvature or external deviation of the nose may still be present immediately postoperatively or become apparent only after several weeks or months. Evaluating the tip preoperatively and predicting with any degree of accuracy the postoperative result requires considerable experience. The most difficult tips to correct are in those patients with thick, oily skin and a marked excess of subcutaneous fatty tissue; extremely inelastic skin with large pores does not conform well to the new, smaller cartilaginous and bony framework. Blemishes, scars, pigmentation, and irreparable asymmetries should be pointed out to the patient preoperatively; otherwise, these faults might be wrongly attributed to the surgery.

A thorough physical examination including anterior and posterior rhinoscopy is important in order to evaluate septal abnormalities and nasal obstruction. If a structural abnormality such as a deviated septum warrants correction, and the patient also has allergic or vasomotor rhinitis, he should be told that the operation will improve but not cure his nasal obstruction. The attitude, "when in doubt, do a submucous resection" is fraught with error, for many preoperative and postoperative nasal obstruction problems are physiologic rather than structural and can be treated with patience and medical care.

It is simply not possible to perform a standard operative procedure on every patient and obtain satisfactory results. The surgeon must appreciate individual anatomic limitations and problems, and he should command at least three or four basic surgical approaches in order to treat each nasal plastic problem adequately. Even the most experienced and expert surgeons must accept the necessity of secondary operation in a certain percentage of rhinoplasty patients. The most common deformities requiring secondary surgery are minor irregularities of the dorsum such as depressions or elevation of the septal dorsum or upper lateral cartilages, asymmetry of the nostrils or tip, and malposition of the bones. Secondary surgery should not be performed before six to twelve months, since low-grade edema can persist for long periods. Secondary surgery before edema is resolved only aggravates the vicious circle of edema → resolution → scar tissue.

Early Postoperative Complications

Hemorrhage. The most common troublesome complication of rhinoplasty is hemorrhage or epistaxis, which can occur any time from immediately after surgery to several weeks later. As in face lifting, prophylaxis is the best treatment. It is very important to advise rhinoplasty candidates to discontinue ingestion of any drug or medication containing salicylates for 10 to 14 days prior to surgery. These medications include aspirin, Bufferin, Alka Seltzer, Excedrin, and others listed in the letter to patients. Usually, bleeding occurs during the first 48 hours or at 10 to 14 days postoperatively. Excluding blood dyscrasias, bleeding that occurs during the first 48 hours is particularly apt to come from the raw edge of the anterior septal mucosal incision. If septoplasty or submucous resection has been performed in conjunction with rhinoplasty, the chances of bleeding are increased considerably. Blood dyscrasias, particularly occult diseases such as von Willebrand's disease, can cause troublesome, even serious bleeding during or shortly after surgery. A history of excessive or prolonged bruising either spontaneously or following minimal trauma, or a positive family history of bleeding, indicates the need for a thorough preoperative hematologic workup.

The second period in which epistaxis is most common is from the 10th to the 14th postoperative days, when the eschars along the incisions separate. When vigorous bleeding occurs, the nasal cavity is suctioned free of clots, and an attempt is made to locate the exact bleeding point, using a nasal speculum under good lighting. The nose may be gently repacked with epinephrine-soaked cotton pledgets, which usually control the bleeding. It is then wise to insert a pack of Oxycel or some similar material, which forms a natural clot. This may be teased out several days after the bleeding ceases. If hemorrhage is severe and the bleeding site cannot be located, the nose must be packed with a non-adherent or greased gauze extending as far posteriorly as possible and exerting pressure against the splint or cast. Posterior bleeding must be controlled with nasopharyngeal posterior packs as well as anterior packing. For persistent bleeding, the patient may require hospitalization and sedation. Uncontrolled epistaxis from the posterior septum can occur as the result of radical septal surgery, particularly in the older patient prone to hypertension. Transsinus ligation of the internal maxillary artery may rarely become necessary in such patients. Postoperatively, patients must be admonished not to blow, pick, touch, or insert applicators into the nose.

Hematoma. Uncontrolled hemorrhage may result in hematoma, which could cause displacement of the alar cartilages or distortion of the nasal tip with the eventual thickening of excessive scar tissue. Septal hematomas, if not properly evacuated, may later cause nasal obstruction and lead to septal perforation. Prompt treatment of hemorrhage and careful inspection of the septum following submucous resection will minimize these complications.

Hematomas under the dorsal skin flaps can occur immediately if the dorsal splint is not accurately applied, or even several days following surgery if the skin flap is elevated from the underlying framework during removal of the cast or taping.

Infection. Infection following rhinoplasty is surprisingly rare, although one of the most potentially contaminated areas in the body is transgressed. Klabunde and Falces (1964) reported 5 infections in 300 cases (1.6 percent), although this seems high. Flowers and Anderson (1968), in reviewing 1000 rhinoplasties, found eight (0.8 percent) instances of localized infection somewhere along the course of the lateral osteotomy. Even before the advent of antibiotics, infections following rhinoplasty were infrequent. When an infection does occur, it is usually found in a hematoma site or in areas surrounding retained bone dust or loose bony fragments. To prevent this, bone dust, spicules, and clots should be removed from the osteotomy site and nasal dorsum with a curette, frequently called a "nasal sweeper."

Fortunately, the majority of potentially invasive organisms of the nose are controlled by appropriate antibiotics. It is best to postpone surgery on patients with active pustules or infection around the nose. Localized abscesses can occur at the

transfixion incision in the columella, the tip (between the undermined domes of the alar cartilages), and the base of the prefrontal process of the maxilla along the lateral osteotomy. These should be treated with incision and drainage, local heat applications, and broad-spectrum antibiotics — pending culture results when the appropriate specific antibiotic should be given. The offending organism is most often *Staphylococcus aureus*. A most dreaded but rare complication is septic cavernous sinus thrombosis, which, if undiagnosed, can lead to brain abscess and death. It must be treated vigorously with massive doses of broad spectrum antibiotics.

Periostitis. Along fracture lines in the nasal bones, periostitis can begin as a low-grade infection and smolder for weeks or months. This is most apt to occur when the saw osteotomy technique is used, and sawdust or debris is left behind. The presenting symptoms are swelling, pain, and later, erythema. When periostitis is recognized, vigorous broad spectrum antibiotics should be given. Inadvertent or purposeful comminution of the nasal bones can very rarely result in a sequestrum that becomes the site of a localized osteomyelitis. Intensive antibiotic therapy may control the infection; however, removal of the sequestrum may be required if conservative therapy fails.

Edema and Ecchymosis. This is a universal occurrence following rhinoplasty, although there is a tremendous variation among individuals as to the extent and the amount of time required for swelling, edema, and ecchymosis to subside. Swelling of the tip in a patient with thick, sebaceous skin may take many months to resolve. For most patients, it takes six to twelve months before all swelling has cleared and the final result can be seen. However, it is not unusual for patients to have residual swelling for up to two years postoperatively. Gentle support and reassurance by the surgeon are necessary to support the patient. Ecchymosis usually subsides promptly in two to four weeks after surgery. However, there are some patients in whom dark circles remain beneath the eyes — presumably from blood breakdown products — for many months, even up to a year or more. The cause is unknown, but it usually occurs in patients of Mediterranean heritage, especially Italians. Except in those patients with a family predisposition to darkly pigmented eyelid skin, this condition is rarely permanent. A tendency toward increased pigmentation of the lower eyelid skin should be recognized before surgery, and the patient should be advised of the possibility of prolonged "black eyes." There is no effective treatment to hasten the absorption of blood pigments.

Skin Problems. Minor skin complications include tape reaction, skin pustules, and the formation of telangiectases. Tape reactions have been minimized by the use of paper tape, but they may still occur in highly sensitive individuals. Allergic reactions are treated with topical steroid creams and systemic antihistamines. Pustules should be expressed as they occur, and a drying desquamating soap is prescribed. Patients with a diathesis toward capillary telangiectasis will sometimes develop these small spider lesions after rhinoplasty. They may be treated by electrodesiccation using an epilating needle, which is passed under magnification into the lumen of the vessel. Several treatments may be required.

Skin necrosis over the dorsum resulting from excessive pressure from the splint or tape or from circulatory problems can occur but is very rare. The best treatment is a conservative "watch and wait" attitude. An eschar will form that eventually separates as healing progresses beneath. The final scar may require excision or even full thickness skin grafting. If a full thickness slough of dorsal skin is evident with danger that the nasal bones and cartilage will become exposed, the slough can be excised and the defect can be covered with a local or island flap.

Necrosis of the tip skin can result from excessive dissection of the tip and undue surgical trauma. This represents a surgical disaster, and little can be done either at the time of the slough or subsequently to obtain an acceptable result. Such patients become nasal cripples and often begin an odyssey from surgeon to surgeon seeking help.

Injury to Lacrimal Apparatus. Because of the proximity of the lacrimal apparatus to the lateral osteotomy site during rhinoplasty, lacrimal sac injury is not uncommon, according to Flowers and Anderson (1968). They demonstrated anatomically in cadavers and then clinically in patients undergoing rhinoplasty that significant disruption of the lacrimal sac occurred during osteotomy; 21 of 27 patients showed lacrimal obstruction on one or both sides on the second postoperative day. However, at two weeks postoperatively only one patient had an obstruction, which cleared at three months. They concluded that postoperative obstruction of the lacrimal apparatus was functional, of short duration, and without sequelae. Although there is no report in the literature of permanent damage to the lacrimal apparatus, it could conceivably happen with a careless osteotomy or technical error. A study of the skull confirms the improbability of injuring the nasolacrimal duct during the operation because of its well protected location below the maxillary rim.

Septal Perforations. Septal perforations are less common today than they were several decades ago because of the infrequency of radical septal resection for septal deviation. Also, the use of antibiotics for adequate early treatment of nasal infection has reduced the complication of septal perforation. The main causes are improperly executed submucous resections and unrecognized septal hematomas. Small anterior septal perforations may cause a disturbing whistling noise with respiration. Treatment includes use of local or buccal mucosal flaps if the patient is symptomatic.

Late Postoperative Complications

Nasal Obstruction. With rhinoplasty, nasal obstructive symptoms are common in the early postoperative period. Almost all patients experience partial nasal obstruction from transient edema of the mucosa, coagulated blood, or crusting along the incision lines. This problem usually resolves spontaneously in several weeks without treatment.

Patients with allergic disorders or vasomotor rhinitis may have an exacerbation of nasal obstruction postoperatively. In a review of 1000 consecutive rhinoplasties, Beekhuis (1976) found that approximately 10 percent of patients developed a persistent enlargement of the inferior turbinates postoperatively, causing an obstructive vasomotor type of rhinitis. The obstruction usually began at the time of surgery and persisted for several months if left untreated. The use of intranasal, intramucosal injections of long-acting corticosteroids as described by Baker and Strauss (1977) is the treatment of choice for these patients, and it will alleviate the majority of symptoms.

Altered Sense of Smell and Anosmia. The olfactory area is located high in each nasal cavity, far from the operative field of rhinoplasty, and interference with the sense of smell should thus be an unusual complication. However, Champion (1966) questioned 200 patients who underwent rhinoplasty and found that 10 percent had temporary anosmia lasting 6 to 18 months, and one patient had permanent anosmia. He did not perform olfaction tests on these patients. Goldwyn and Shore (1968), however, did further studies on this problem using olfactory testing in patients undergoing rhinoplasty and/or submucous resection. They found that at two weeks after surgery, 80 percent of patients had normal sense of smell, and at two months postoperatively, no patients complained of anosmia or demonstrated it upon testing. They concluded that submucous resection and/or rhinoplasty rarely produces permanent anosmia. Postoperative bleeding and edema can cause temporary anosmia lasting a few weeks. Nevertheless, a careful preoperative history questioning for anosmia could prevent a postoperative complaint.

Callus Formation. Occasionally, bony callus can form at the site of bony hump removal or along lateral osteotomy sites. This is usually the result of an exaggerated response to bone dust, periosteal tags, or blood clots that were not carefully removed at surgery. This can result in a residual bony dorsal hump or sometimes in irregularities along the lateral osteotomy site that appear several months after surgery. Treatment requires rasping of irregularities or repeat osteotomy.

SECONDARY RHINOPLASTY

The frequency with which secondary rhinoplasty is performed varies considerably. Few hard statistics are available as guidelines. The novice surgeon will certainly find it necessary to reoperate more often than the experienced surgeon; however, no one becomes experienced enough to eliminate secondary surgery altogether. Klabunde and Falces (1964) found that approximately 10 percent of the 300 patients they reviewed needed one or more secondary procedures. As skill and experience increase, the incidence of secondary surgery should decrease proportionately — ideally to a 5 to 10 percent level.

Secondary rhinoplasty is certainly one of the most difficult and unpredictable challenges in plastic surgery. There are no studies to indicate the level of patient satisfaction achieved following secondary surgery. It is probable that such patients are rarely *completely* satisfied, since there are inherent limitations of the result imposed by scar tissue, tissue loss, and so forth. A significant number of patients who have had multiple nasal plastic procedures by different surgeons are neurotic. Repeated procedures in such patients often can result from pressures exerted on the surgeon by the patient for more surgery and for not altogether "realistic" reasons. Such patients tend to be passively aggressive; they are surgery seekers. They pressure the surgeon to perform a secondary procedure early, often before the final results of the primary procedure can be fully evaluated and the wound reaction has subsided. Such ill-timed secondary surgery often results in further deformity compounding the original problem, and frequently leads to yet more surgery.

Revision rhinoplasty is unquestionably more difficult than primary surgery. The surgeon must face many technical factors that complicate the picture, some of which may be beyond his control. The effects of scar formation and distortion of the normal anatomy and tissue depletion are primary factors to be considered. It is helpful to know the technique employed at the first operation in order to help evaluate these factors; however, such information is infrequently available. Many surgeons are loath to undertake secondary surgery in patients other than their own because of the difficulty in achieving results that are rewarding to both surgeon and patient if the deformity is severe. If there is extensive scarring and distortion of the soft tissues, minimal improvement can be gained by a secondary procedure.

EVALUATION

Careful preoperative evaluation of the combination of problems is exceedingly important in secondary rhinoplasty in planning the technical approaches that might insure some measure of success. These problems should be assessed in an organized way. For this purpose, the author prefers to divide the nose into its component anatomic parts. These include the (1) osteocartilaginous framework, excluding the tip, (2) internal nose, including the septum, the turbinates, and the internal valve, (3) lobule, including the tip, the columella, the caudal septum, and the cartilages contained therein, and (4) lip and other associated structures. It is most important to determine how much normal tissue has been excised, the degree of scarring and distortion present, the physiologic status of the mucous membranes, the degree of respiratory obstruction from septal deviation and enlargement of the turbinates, and, most importantly, whether the nose will require augmentation or tissue replacement with grafts. Autogenous grafts should be used without hesitation to replace missing elements or to provide support. An excellent source of graft material is the nasal septum. Unfortunately, the septum is often subtotally absent in the secondary case, since radical submucous resection during the primary procedure is common. Thus, an argument against *routine* submucous resection is evident.

The "crucified" nose presents a highly complex technical and psychologic problem requiring innovative surgical planning to achieve results. The novice surgeon would be well advised to refer such severe problem patients to an experienced surgeon with special interests in this problem. Unfortunately, very few surgeons are intrigued with secondary nasal problems. Of course, every surgeon is obligated to use every means at his disposal to resolve problems arising in his own patients.

TIMING

Secondary rhinoplasty should be delayed as long as possible following the primary operation to permit the edema to subside and the wound scar to mature. Six months is considered a minimum by most surgeons; however, it is difficult to set hard and fast rules. Structural defects may be observed early in the postoperative course; however, subtle changes in contour that vary with the influence of recurrent edema may continue for many months. Minute changes can and do continue for years, and corrective surgery need not be postponed for such extended periods. It is nevertheless most unwise to reoperate during the peak of wound activity, because the vicious cycle of edema ↔ scar is exacerbated by surgical intervention. Some surgeons such as Pollet and Weikel (1976) advocate reoperating the nose for any obvious deformity as early as three weeks following primary rhinoplasty, reasoning that "at this time most of the edema has resolved from the nose, the period of maximum wound contraction has occurred, and only 15 percent of wound strength is present in the originally created wounds." Further, "Experience has shown that the nose is extremely easy to operate on at this time, using the previous planes of dissection." In making such a statement, they acknowledge that this preference for early surgery was made at the risk of inviting great controversy. Whereas such timing may be preferred by a surgeon with the extensive experience that Pollet had, the author feels strongly that for most surgeons, such early intervention is fraught with hazards.

Prior to undertaking secondary surgery, it should be emphasized that the principles of patient preparation that apply to primary rhinoplasty apply to secondary rhinoplasty as well. That is, the patient should be advised again that the results of surgery cannot be perfect and that no warranties or guarantees can be made regarding the outcome. The reasons for dissatisfaction following the primary operation may still be present after a secondary procedure, particularly if they are of emotional or psychologic origin. It is well to provide a more detailed informed consent for secondary procedures than for primary procedures. Likewise, the patient should be prepared for the possible use of autogenous grafts, which may be required from such donor sites as the ear and the iliac crest. The possible use of alloplastic materials must be understood.

Most surgeons do not charge another operative fee when reoperating on their own primary patients, a practice with which the author concurs. But when performing secondary surgery on patients of other surgeons, it is generally accepted practice to charge a fee commensurate with the difficulty of the surgery. The responsibilities in such cases rest heavily on the surgeon.

CLASSIFICATION

It is convenient to classify secondary nasal deformities according to anatomic compartments, but such a classification must allow for inclusion of specific structures in one or more categories, since it is based more on surgical convenience than along strict anatomic lines. Thus, the nasal septum is included not only as a component of the internal nose, but also as part of the osteocartilaginous vault insofar as it contributes to both internal respiratory function and structural support. Problem areas are classified as follows:

1. The soft tissues of the nose, including the skin, subcutaneous fat, connective tissues, and musculature

2. The osteocartilaginous vault, including the nasal bones, the upper lateral cartilages, the frontal process of the maxilla, the glabella, and that portion of the bony and cartilaginous septum that provides support for the external framework

3. The internal nose, including the lining mucous membrane, the turbinates, the septum, the internal valve, and so forth

4. The lobule and adjacent structures, including the tip, the columella, the nostrils, the alar cartilages, and the vestibulum, the membranous septum, and the caudal margin of the septum. The upper lip and associated musculature are intimately associated with problems of the lobule.

Any combination of the above can of course exist, as in the case of the septum.

THE SKIN AND SOFT TISSUE

The first step in primary or secondary rhinoplasty is elevation of the soft tissues from the underlying framework. Soft tissue coverage can be considered as a flap subject to the healing behavior of all flaps. In the young patient, this skin flap is elastic and tractile and it readily accommodates to the underlying cartilaginous framework sculptured during the procedure. In the older patient, there is less elasticity of the skin; accordingly, redundancy may result, requiring more extensive undermining to redistribute the excess or occasionally necessitating external incisions to excise it. The behavior of the skin flap in the postoperative course depends on its anatomic composition and how it is handled during surgery. If the skin and subcutaneous tissue are thick and/or contain large numbers of sebaceous glands and appendages, postoperative sequelae such as prolonged edema and fibrosis may result. Sheen (1975) pointed out that external bulges, such as supratip swelling, hanging columella, and dropped tip may mask the structural abnormalities. Under such conditions, further sculpting with reduction of the underlying bony or cartilaginous structure can only increase the problem of skin draping and accentuate the "bulge" deformity.

The thickness of the skin and subcutaneous tissue bears a direct relationship to the amount of postoperative swelling that may be expected, particularly in the supratip region. Probably the most common cause of supratip swelling ("Ram's" tip or "Polly" tip) is edema of the skin and subcutaneous tissue. Such a problem can be anticipated in patients with thickened skin and subcutaneous tissue. Treatment of supratip deformity will be discussed more fully subsequently.

THE OSTEOCARTILAGINOUS FRAMEWORK

The shape of the nasal pyramid is formed by junctions of the nasal bones and the septum, the maxilla and frontal bones, and further caudally by the junction of the upper lateral cartilages with the cartilaginous septum, which extends to the lobule. Deformities of the bony hump are closely related to the other components of the nasal framework and can be either "real" or "relative." For example, Berson (1943), Goldman (1950), Converse et al. (1954), Calzolari (1965), and others have pointed out that a depressed vault in the lower cartilaginous part of the nose can simulate a hump. The significance of the hump also depends to a great extent on the length of the nose. Lipsett noted that a lesser amount of hump can be removed if the septum is shortened first. Therefore, it is often desirable to correct the cartilaginous nose before removing a hump, especially a small one. This is the author's practice in most primary rhinoplasties. The degree of projection of the tip is also critical in determining the amount of hump removal; the nose with a recessed tip requires relatively more hump removal than one with a projecting tip, in which hump removal should be extremely cautious.

Deformities of the bony or cartilaginous support of the nose that may serve as indications for secondary surgery include malposition of components, contour deformities, insufficient primary resection, or excessive primary resection of either bone or cartilage. Insufficient resection of the bony or cartilaginous hump during rhinoplasty may leave a secondary hump requiring further removal, whereas removal of too much hump may result in a saddle-nose deformity or supratip defect that can be corrected only with bone or cartilage grafts or prosthetic implants.

Should the surgeon suspect during the course of primary surgery that too much bone or cartilage has been resected from the dorsum, he should replace it then and there. Skoog (1966, 1974) routinely replaced the hump after first removing it and trimming it. It survives as a free graft extraordinarily well. Another alternative is the immediate insertion of components from the septum, which can include either bone from the vomer or ethmoid plate or cartilage from the quadrangular plate or both. The use of bone or cartilage from the nose itself to replace deficiencies has long been advocated by experienced rhinoplastic surgeons. Autografts of bone or cartilage from the nose and particularly the septum seem to be privileged, since they apparently survive almost *in toto* and undergo minimal absorption in contrast to other types of autografts such as iliac bone or costal cartilage. Conchal cartilage from the ear is also an excellent graft source. Excessive hump removal often occurs in those patients who have minimal small humps to begin with, particularly if the saw technique is employed. There is much less likelihood of excessive removal if the hump is removed with sharp osteotomes or rasps rather than the saw (Figure 12–9). A "bird beak" nose resulting from gross overresection of a dorsal hump is shown in Figure 12–10. Such a result is much more apt to occur when the saw is used than a rasp or sharp osteotome. Such defects may require a substantial iliac bone graft, as there may not be enough material available in the septum to raise the dorsum high enough. Sometimes sufficient septal cartilage and bone can be obtained to achieve correction (Figure 12–11).

Secondary corrections of the dorsum may simply require uncovering the dorsal framework and rasping away a small point of bone or trimming a cartilaginous projection, or further hump removal, which certainly in secondary surgery is best accomplished with rasps. When excessive dorsum has been removed, the profile can be built with autogenous grafts from the septum, ilium, rib, or ear (the septum is preferred). If previous radical sep-

Text continued on page 345.

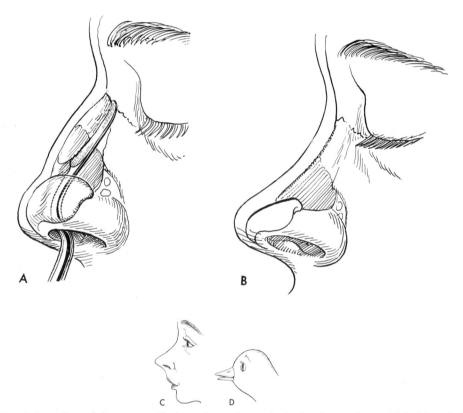

Figure 12-9. *A*, Resection of the osteocartilaginous hump in continuity by the nasal saw. With this technique the upper lateral cartilages are not detached from the nasal septum but are removed in continuity with the osseous hump.

B, Great care must be exercised in the use of the nasal saw, since it is easy for inexpert hands to remove too much of the nasal dorsum, as in this drawing.

C and *D*, Removal of excess nasal dorsum produces a so-called "birdlike" deformity.

Humps that are mostly cartilaginous and thus involve the lower third of the nose primarily are best removed after tip plasty and in a most conservative fashion. Conversely, humps that are mainly osseous and involve the upper portion of the nose can be removed before tip plasty, when it is much easier to judge how much dorsum to remove.

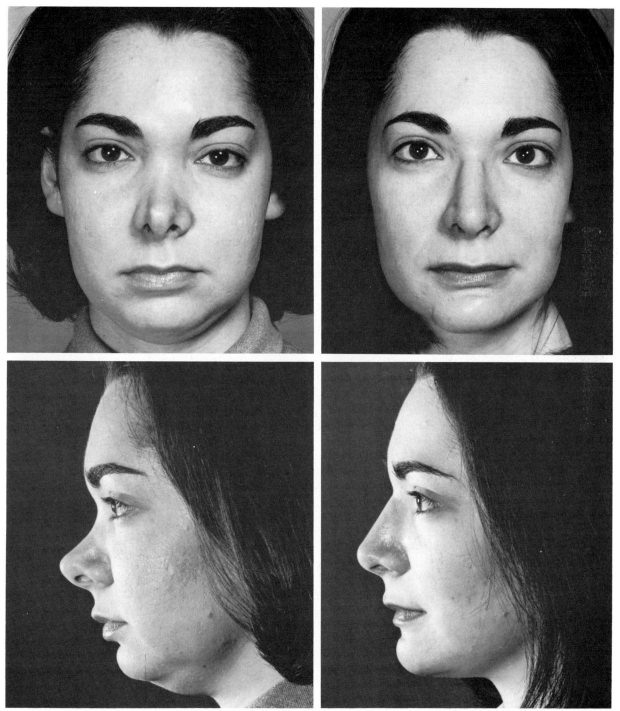

Figure 12–10. Overresection of a dorsal hump by the saw technique. Reconstruction required a generous iliac bone graft. (Courtesy of Dr. C. Guy.)

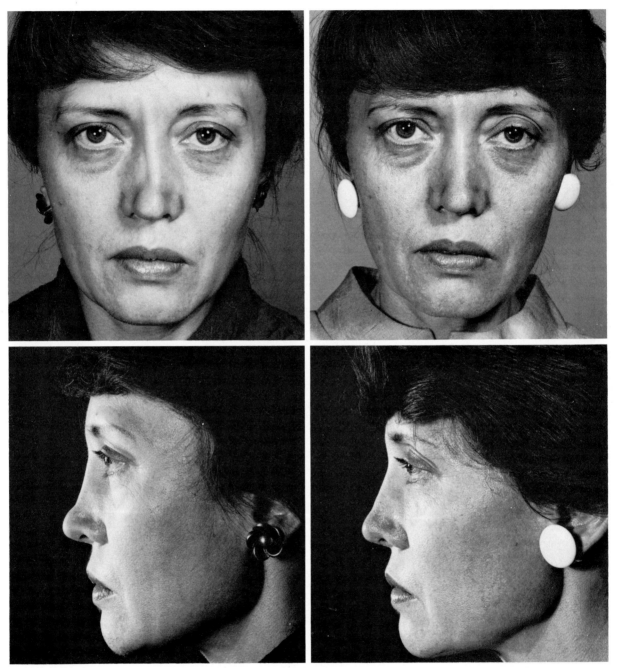

Figure 12–11.   The bony hump was overresected in this patient, leaving a marked underlying curvature of the septum clearly visible from the front view. A simple lateral osteotomy was not successful because of the septal deflection, which did not permit the nasal bones to come in.

Correction was achieved by infracture, septal plasty with a limited submucous resection, and use of the elements removed from the septum as an augmentation graft to the dorsum. Autogenous bone was also required. (Courtesy of Dr. C. Guy.)

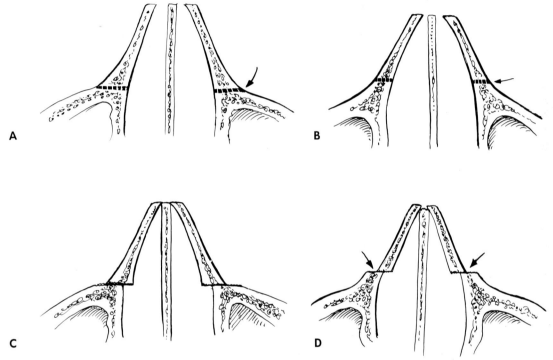

Figure 12-12. A common stigma of rhinoplasty is a visible ridge that can result from a lateral osteotomy at too high a level. The osteotomy must be made through the thick portion of the nasal process of the maxilla in order to prevent this "stair-step" deformity. Osteotomy at this level by a surgeon inexpert in the use of a saw will be both tedious and difficult, and an osteotome will be easier to use.

A, The desirable lines of osteotomy. *B*, An osteotomy made too high on the bony vault. *C*, Ideal lines of osteotomy following infracture. *D*, Lines of osteotomy that will result in a typical "stair-step" deformity.

(From Rees, T. D., Krupp, S., and Wood-Smith, D.: Plast. Reconstr. Surg. *46*:332, 1970. Reproduced with permission.)

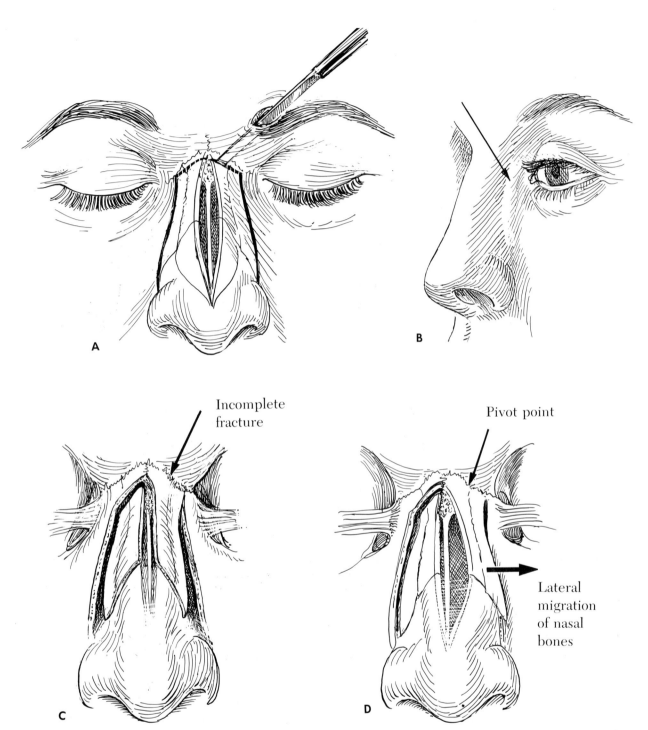

Figure 12–13.   Lateral drifting of the nasal bones after rhinoplasty may result from an incomplete superior fracture at the root of the nose, or from a "greenstick" fracture. *A*, Direct superior osteotomy with a 2-mm. osteotome passed through the medial aspect of the eyebrow insures a complete fracture and prevents postoperative drifting. *B*, Lateral osteotomy should be low on the prefrontal process of the maxilla in order to prevent a "stair-step" deformity. *C*, Postoperative widening of the bony vault may also result from incomplete fracture of the nasal bones or the nasal process of the frontal bone. This is particularly true if the bones are thick. *D*, Lateral migration may easily occur if a "greenstick" fracture is created, because the bone tends to pivot on the nasal process of the frontal bone.

tal surgery eliminates the septum as a graft source, iliac bone or auricular cartilage are excellent choices. The conchal cartilage has been championed by Brent (1978) as an excellent donor site for nasal deformities. Iliac bone is reserved for large saddle defects, but such grafts are subject to absorption of variable degrees. Alloplastic materials are a poor choice in secondary rhinoplasty with the relative hypovascularity of a scarred recipient bed. Extrusion is frequent under such circumstances.

Comminution of the nasal bones may result in palpable irregularities requiring rasping or further comminution by percutaneous insertion of fine 2 mm osteotomes.

Reduction of redundant dorsal border of septal cartilage is one of the more common indications for secondary rhinoplasty. This defect is discussed in the section on supratip deformity.

Stair-Step Deformity

Prominent ridges along the frontal process of the maxilla on the lateral side of the nose are commonly called stair-step deformities (Figure 12–12). These actually result from the lateral osteotomy having been placed too high (ventral) on the frontal process of the maxilla. The lateral osteotomy should be done as close as possible to the maxilla. The osteotome should be directed flush along the anterior face of the maxilla into the nasomax-

illary groove. If the lateral osteotomies are inadvertently made too far anteriorly during primary rhinoplasty and a stair-step ridge results, a small 2 or 3 mm osteotome is used to fracture the projecting lip of the frontal process of the maxilla by directing the osteotome at a deeper angle (Figure 12–13). Stair stepping can be corrected secondarily by comminuting the frontal process with a fine osteotome or by rasping the bony ridge with a fine rasp through a subperiosteal tunnel in the pyriform aperture.

Postoperative Widening. Postoperative widening of the bony framework is usually the result of a high deviation of the septum, which may have been unrecognized at the primary operation. Although it is difficult to correct, this problem can sometimes be solved by fracture and repositioning of the bony septum. Narrowing of the nasal bones, particularly at the nasofrontal angle, may have been prevented by incomplete osteotomy of the frontal process of the maxilla with a "greenstick" type of fracture. Marked thickness of the bone also may have prevented narrowing at the radix, and resection of a medial triangle or web of bone with osteotome or bone forceps may be necessary to allow room for medial displacement at infracture (Figure 12–14). These techniques have been reviewed by Levignac (1958) and Converse et al. (1964).

When the saw is used for the lateral osteoto-

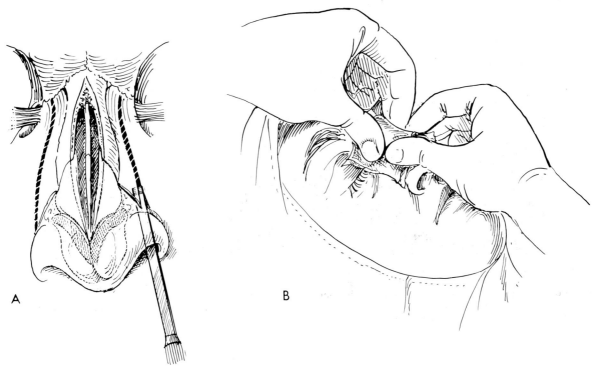

Figure 12–14. Narrowing of the nose after hump removal requires a complete lateral osteotomy to the level of the inner canthus. *A,* Lines of fracture of the lateral osteotomy. *B,* Complete infracturing by pressure concentrated on the upper halves of the nasal bones.

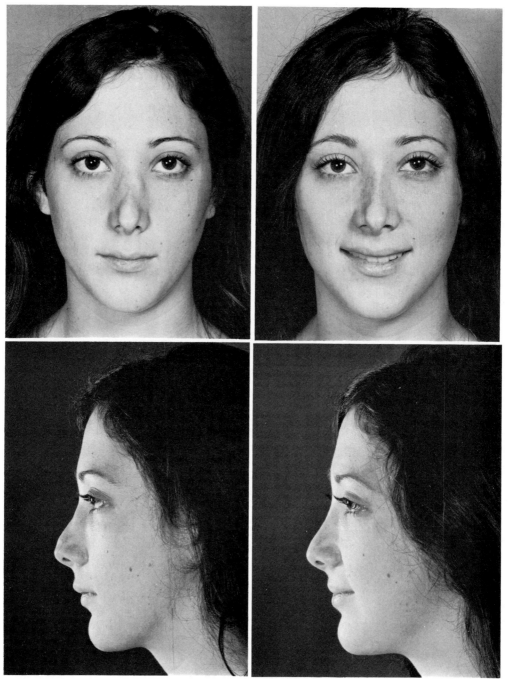

Figure 12–15.   A favorable case for secondary repair. The first surgeon removed too much of the bony hump and practically none of the cartilaginous dorsum. He left only a minimal dorsal strut after completing a submucous resection. The secondary operation consisted of lateral osteotomy with infracture, trimming of the alar cartilage, and a careful lowering of the dorsal border of the septum. The slight dorsal hump was left, for it was feared that further lowering of the dorsum could result in sufficient weakening of the dorsal septum to bring about collapse of the nose.

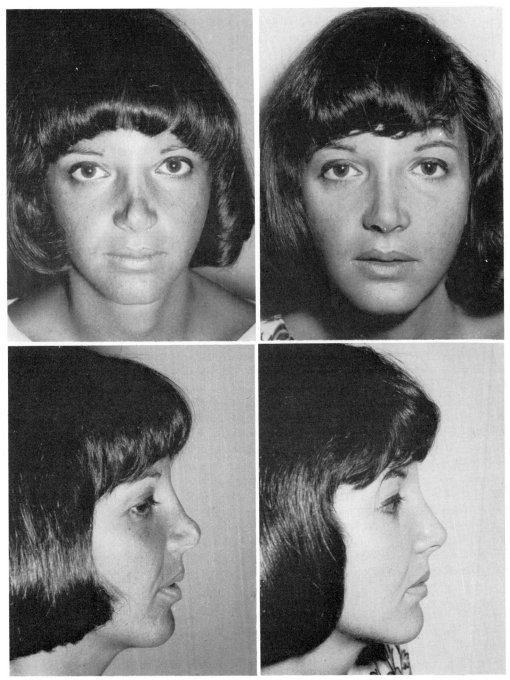

Figure 12–16. Another favorable case for secondary repair. The first surgeon apparently removed the hump unequally, so that a small dorsal bony hump remained, with a depression of the dorsal cartilaginous septal border. In addition, the alar cartilages were asymmetrically and insufficiently remodeled, and infracture was not done. The secondary procedure comprised lowering of the bony dorsum, nasal tip plasty, and lateral osteotomy with infracture.

(From Rees, T. D., Krupp, S., and Wood-Smith, D.: Plast. Reconstr. Surg. *46*:332, 1970. Reproduced with permission.)

my, thorough curettage and removal of all fragments and debris of bone and periosteum should be done. A low-grade inflammatory reaction can occur in the "sawdust." Such a periostitis can be stubborn to treat and may require intensive antibiotic therapy. It can also result in swelling along the frontal process of the maxilla on either side of the nose, simulating a stair-step deformity.

Saddle Nose

The saddle-nose deformity can be caused by either excessive lowering of the profile (hump removal) or by accidents (surgical or traumatic) that precipitate circumstances in which the fractured nasal bones can drop into the pyriform aperture. To achieve adequate infracture, it is sometimes necessary to comminute the nasal bones during primary or secondary surgery. Comminution may be inadvertent, and when combined with radical submucous resection with accidental fracture of the thin perpendicular plate of the ethmoid, the entire osteocartilaginous complex can behave similarly to a midface pyramidal fracture with depression of all elements into the pyriform aperture. To avoid this complication, it is important to preserve the periosteal attachment over the external surface of the nasal bones until a stabilized infracture has been achieved. In this way, the soft tissue will support even comminuted fractures of the bones (Lewis, 1954; O'Connor and McGregor, 1955).

Correction of saddle nose deformity is best accomplished with autogenous bone or cartilage grafts. The "flying wing" technique for correction of minor degrees of saddle deformity resulting from traumatic loss of septum or from excessive resection of cartilaginous septum during surgery has been popularized in textbooks. The procedure has a place and is effective, provided sufficient lateral crus of the alar cartilage remains to provide bulk. The technique illustrated in Figure 12–17 is to be limited to the most minor cases. Great care should be taken to adjust the cartilage flaps and to suture them into position so that they are symmetrical.

Saddle defects are best repaired by implants. When the deformity is great, a carefully carved block graft of autogenous iliac bone remains the best corrective material available (Figure 12–18). Smaller depressions can be improved with single or multilayered graft of cartilage obtained from the septum or the concha of the ear. Alloplastic materials are frequently extruded after insertion into the scarred, soft tissue of the nasal dorsum. The nasal septum is an excellent source for graft augmentation of the nasal dorsum to correct mod-

erate degrees of saddle deformity or the relative saddle deformity of supratip swelling where lowering of the septal cartilage or excision of scar tissue will not suffice (Figure 12–19). If the septum is not available because of primary rhinoplasty procedures, distant donor sites of bone and cartilage must be sought. These include the auricular cartilage, the iliac crest, and the anterior tibia. Rib bone is poor for nasal implant in adults, as it tends to absorb and to fracture. Costal cartilage can be used as "eye round" grafts to minimize curling and distortion (Figure 12–20). However, the disadvantage of a thoracic scar, particularly in women, is a significant drawback. Bone grafting of the dorsum of the nose is illustrated in Figure 12–21.

Other problems that occur with the bony framework of the external nose following primary rhinoplasty include incomplete lateral osteotomy, incomplete fracture at the junction of the nasal and frontal bones, and incomplete or unstable infracture of the nasal bone. These problems can best be overcome by reestablishing the fracture lines, insuring that the bones are in the desired position and stabilized there. (See Figures 12–22 and 12–23.)

THE CARTILAGINOUS FRAMEWORK

Irregularities of the dorsum of the nose may occur from sloppy trimming of the dorsal margins of the lateral cartilages or the dorsal lower septum. These are corrected simply by rasping or trimming the offending prominence with a scalpel or curved scissors.

Sometimes, an external deviation of the nose may be apparent after rhinoplasty where none was visible before. Deviations of the dorsal border of the septum forming a C- or S-shaped curvature are often exceedingly difficult to correct, as previously discussed. Complete freeing of the septum along the vomer groove combined with multiple incisions in the deviated cartilage may help to straighten it. It is preferable to remove cartilage only when necessary to open an airway. Techniques to correct such deviations have been reviewed by Converse (1950, 1964), Becker (1951), Dingman (1956), Planas, (1977), and others. The problem of the deviated septum has been well reviewed elsewhere in this book and will not be repeated here. Suffice it to reiterate that when radical septal resection appears indicated, it is best to plan it as a separate procedure. Septal plasty with repositioning of the fragments is preferred over radical extirpative operations on the septum.

The overshortened nose is one of the most

Text continued on page 360.

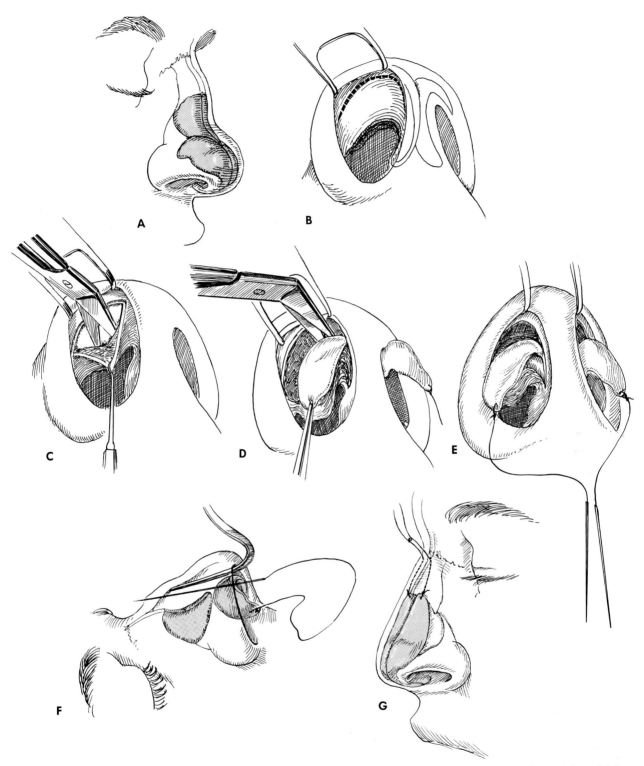

Figure 12–17.   The "flying wing" correction of minor degrees of saddle deformity. The lateral crus is dissected free of lining and converted into a single pedicle flap (*B* to *E*). These flaps are then rotated into a pocket surgically created between the dorsal skin covering and the septal border, where they are fixed by sutures (*F* and *G*). The sutures can be fashioned as pull-out sutures passing through the dorsal skin.

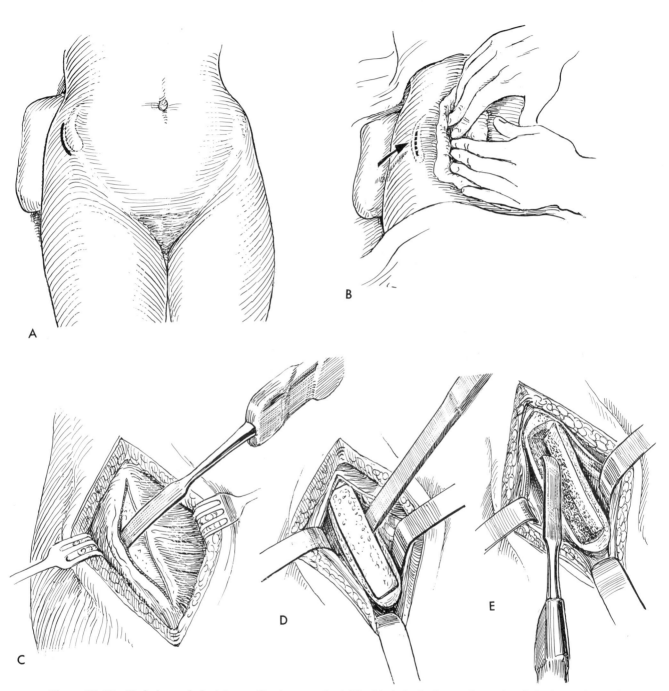

Figure 12–18.   Technique of obtaining an iliac bone graft. *A*, The ideal site is shown; the patient is in the supine position and the incision is placed just below the iliac crest so that it will not be irritated by the pressure of belts or undergarments. *B*, The skin is displaced medially by pressure on the iliac fossa, and an incision is made through skin and subcutaneous tissues to the iliac crest. *C*, The periosteum is raised from the iliac crest. *D*, A suitably sized segment of bone, with the underlying cancellous bone, is removed. *E*, Hemostasis is aided by heavy pressure with the osteotome, which helps to bring about closure of the underlying cancellous bony spaces. The wound is closed in layers, with or without drainage, depending upon the degree of hemostasis obtained.

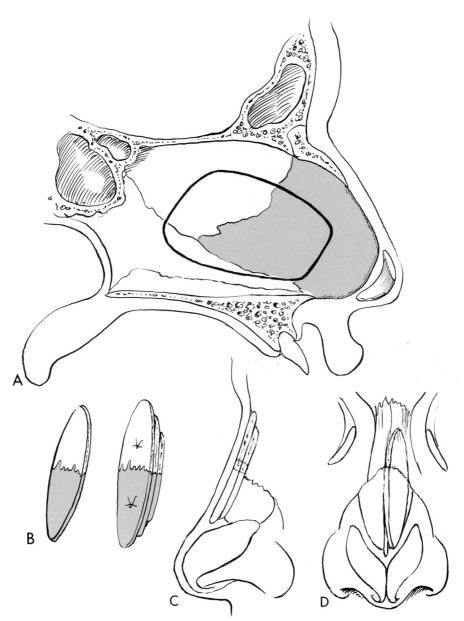

Figure 12–19. Graft augmentation for correction of saddle deformity. *A* The area available for graft material is indicated by the solid line. It includes a portion of quadrangular cartilage, vomer, and perpendicular plate of the ethmoid.

B, Single-tiered or multi-tiered grafts can be fashioned by suturing them together. Mixed grafts of bone and cartilage can be used as well as grafts of either substance (Sheen).

C, Lateral view showing graft in place along dorsum.

D, The graft can also be placed asymmetrically to correct deformities with deviation of the nose (see section on nasal deviation).

Figure 12–20. Saddle defect repair. Prosthetic materials are rarely used because of the pressure of scar tissue and loss of pliability of the skin. Autogenous grafts, either septal or costal cartilage, or bone, are the materials of choice. Layered strips of septal cartilage rarely warp but are scanty in amount and difficult to shape, while costal cartilage tends to warp unless "eye round" cartilage is used (Gibson). Iliac bone is unquestionably the best material; it can be shaped exactly to suit, it is hardy, and it withstands contamination admirably. Some absorption and even spontaneous fracture can be found to occur on long-term follow-up, but those disadvantages are outweighed by the biological advantages of this excellent graft material.

The upper drawings illustrate the technique of placing a costal cartilage graft. *A*, Depression of the nasal dorsum.

B, Elevation of the soft tissues and periosteum via an intercartilaginous incision.

C, Cartilage from the costochondral junction carved to the appropriate shape for the particular patient.

D, The implant in position.

The remaining drawings demonstrate the insertion of a septal cartilage implant.

E, Depression of the cartilaginous dorsum.

F, Built-up dorsal cartilage implants held together with 4-0 plain catgut sutures.

G, The implant in place.

See illustration on the opposite page.

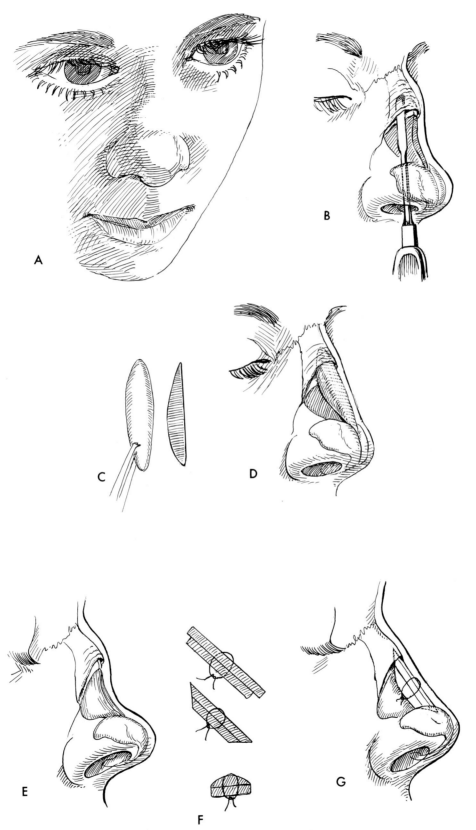

Figure 12–20. *See legend on the opposite page.*

Figure 12–21. Bone grafting of the dorsum of the nose.

A, A saddle nose deformity.

B, The interdome region is exposed through a rim incision.

C, Soft tissues in the interdome region are divided.

D, After the soft tissues are raised from the dorsal aspect of the cartilaginous framework, a periosteal elevator is used to sweep the periosteum laterally from the nasal bones and to expose bare bone.

E, The shaped iliac bone implant; its shape varies considerably from patient to patient.

F, It may be necessary to remove a portion of the nasal bone in order to allow a sufficiently thick strut of iliac bone graft to be placed over the dorsum without overcorrecting the profile. The transnasal wires are placed in position by two small percutaneous punctures on either side of the nose.

G, The iliac bone graft in place and maintained in position by circumferential wire. Wiring is not essential to the success of the procedure and should be employed only when excess tension is believed present over the caudal aspect of the bone graft, which would make it difficult to maintain osseous contact above.

See illustration on the opposite page.

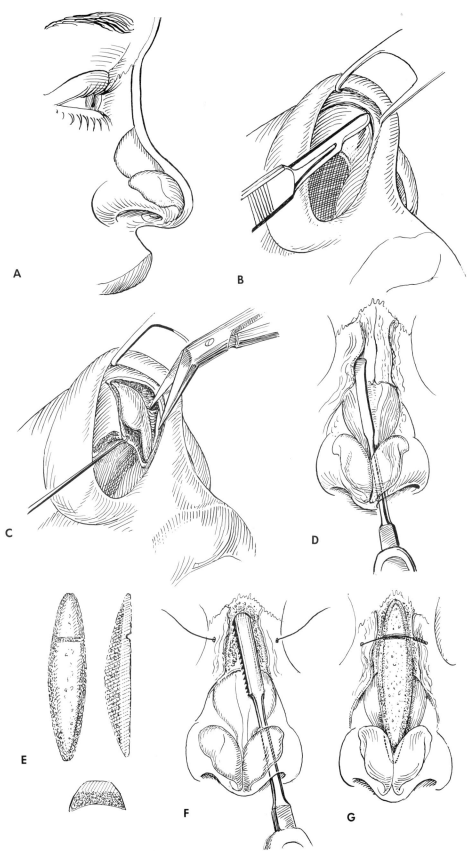

Figure 12–21. *See legend on the opposite page.*

Illustration continued on the following page.

Figure 12–21 *Continued.*

H, Another view of the bone graft secured in place by circumferential wire.

I, Projection of the tip is maintained by 4-0 plain catgut sutures passed over the cantilevered tip of the nasal bone.

J, The nasal tip prior to correction.

K, The nasal tip after correction, showing how it is suspended from the bony strut.

L, The operative procedure completed, showing the tip projection achieved.

M, Periosteum undermined and raised.

N, The carved bony implant.

O, The implant held in position by the pressure of soft tissues over its upper end. It must be noted that such an implant will not stay in place where much tension exists on its lower end.

P, Undermining soft tissues in the columella to expose the nasal spine.

Q, An iliac bone graft with a nasal spine extension to support the tip.

R, The procedure completed and the support of the tip aided by the passage of a catgut suture between the alar domes.

See illustration on the opposite page.

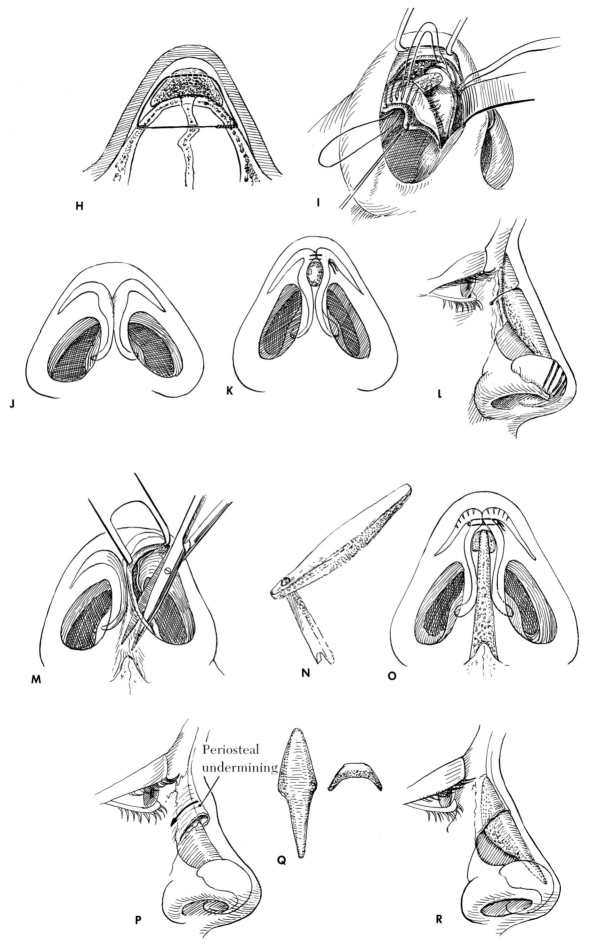

Figure 12–21 Continued. *See legend on the opposite page.*

357

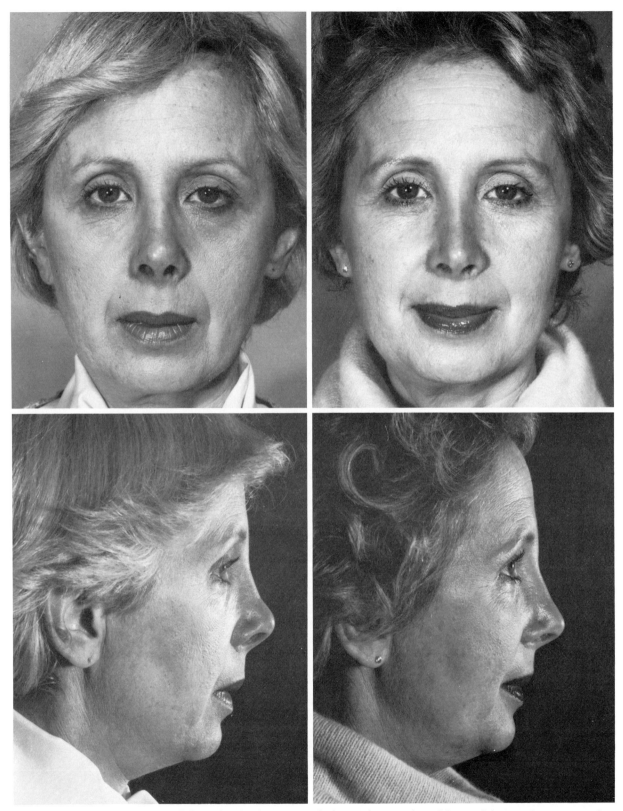

Figure 12–22.   This patient and the patient in Figure 12–23 had excessive resection of the nasal dorsum (hump removal), as well as overshortening. The dorsal profile can be built up with septal grafts (Fig. 12–19) and/or iliac bone grafts (Fig. 12–18). Unfortunately, it is very difficult to lengthen the nose once the caudal septum has been resected. (Courtesy of Dr. C. Guy.)

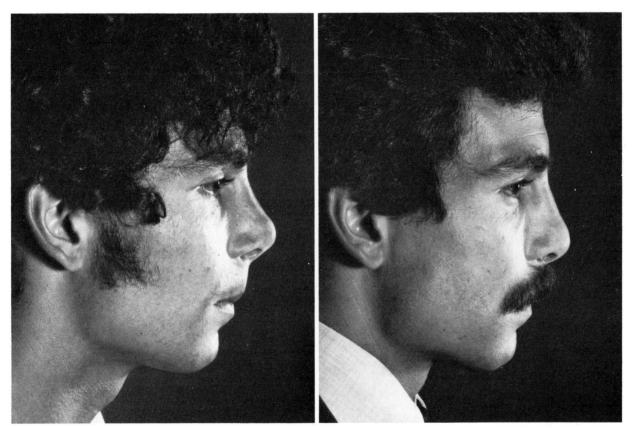

Figure 12–23.

difficult problems to correct in secondary surgery. Usually, too much caudal septum has been resected and the membranous septum has been destroyed. Various techniques have been described to provide the missing tissue such as composite grafts from the ear, the chondromucosal turnover flap of Millard, and others; however, often the surgeon must struggle to gain as much length as possible with what has been left. Often, augmentation of the dorsum even slightly with a small autogenous graft is required, and this helps the situation considerably. (See Figures 12–10 and 12–11). At best, the end results are only an improvement on what should not have occurred in the first place.

If sufficient lateral crus and lining are available, the Millard flaps are most helpful in such problems (Millard, 1972).

The Supratip Deformity

The most common cause of supratip swelling is normal postoperative edema. A significant number of rhinoplasties develop mild edema with swelling of the supratip region, which may persist for several weeks or months. Such edema is more prone to occur in the thick-skinned nose. Supratip swelling from edema is readily treated by intralesional steroid injections in very small doses (Figure

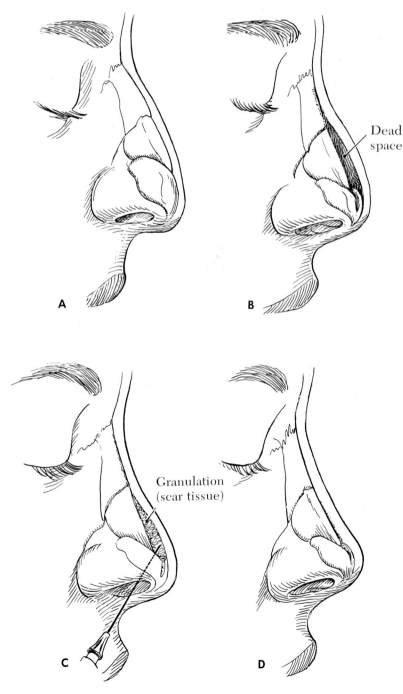

Figure 12–24. Intralesional injections of steroid compounds have proved helpful in hastening resolution of granulation tissue causing supratip swelling. *A*, The preoperative anatomy. *B*, Potential dead space between skin and cartilage created by the operation. Dressings help to eliminate this space. *C*, Granulation tissue in the dead space. Injection of triamcinolone directly into this tissue at weekly intervals for two or three weeks, usually in a dose of 5 mg per injection, will help to eliminate this tissue. *D*, The result after dissolution of the granulation tissue.

12–24). Subcutaneous granulation tissue and fibrosis — which develops in a surgical "dead space" between the septal border and the skin when the skin is not sufficiently resilient to drape over the new underlying cartilaginous framework — is also a common cause of supratip swelling. This type of problem is also amenable to steroid injection, particularly if the skin is thin and elastic.

Sheen believes that excessive hump removal is the commonest cause of supratip prominence. Certainly, overenthusiastic profile reduction of the skeletal framework creates a situation in which the soft tissues cannot drape well, and "bulges" of soft tissue or cartilage are exaggerated (Figure 12–25). His conviction may be related to the type of long-term problem most commonly seen in his practice. The author considers overreduction of the hump to be an important cause of supratip prominence, but not *the* most common cause. Other factors frequently include an elevated septal angle, a dropping columella, and the formation of supratip scar tissue, particularly in thick skinned individuals. These problems are shown in Figure 12–26.

Another common cause of supratip prominence following surgery is insufficient lowering of the dorsal margin of the cartilaginous septum (Figure 12–26). Surgical trimming to lower the profile of the cartilaginous septum alleviates the problem. The deformity is called a "parrot beak" or "polly tip," in reference to a Polly parrot. Other causes of this deformity include insufficient trimming of the dorsal borders of the upper lateral cartilages, excessive resection of the alar cartilages including the domes and transition areas between the medial and lateral crura, redundancy of the lining of the nose at the junction of the septum and lateral crus, and a short columella that results in a downward tethering of the tip aggravated by a complete transfixion incision that heals as a straight line scar with contracture.

Supratip (Ram's tip) deformity occurred in the patient in Figure 12–27 because of a high elevation of the cartilaginous septal border at and just above the septal angle. The skin was thin and the scar tissue was minimal. An infracture had not been accomplished. The caudal septum was deviated and the nose had been overshortened, probably fixed too high on the septum with a mattress suture.

Correction consisted of replacing the caudal septum in the vomer groove, trimming down the high dorsal cartilage, and performing an infracture. The alar cartilages were also readjusted; however, no cartilage was removed.

A common reason for the supratip deformity caused by many surgeons is that the dorsal septal border is left slightly too high. It is usually wise to lower the cartilaginous dorsum to where it seems best, then resect another millimeter or two. Of course, if too much bony dorsum has been removed, it must be augmented.

To avoid the "Polly tip" in patients with thick skin, Wright (1967) advised shaping the nasal tip before reduction of the nasal profile (dorsum), a practice followed by the author in most rhinoplasties. Pitanguy (1965) recommended excision of his "fibrous ligament" from the dorsum. If and when such a ligament is present, it unquestionably contributes to supratip swelling.

Correction of supratip elevation may be very difficult, involving lowering of the high septal dorsum, excision of scar tissue, and resection of the upper lateral cartilages. Increasing tip projection by rearrangement of the alar cartilages and lengthening the columella may be helpful. Implantation of alloplastic materials or autogenous grafts to increase tip projection is rarely advised, as extrusion or resorption is the usual end result. Some of the factors contributing to supratip deformities and their correction are shown in Figure 12–29.

Injection of small doses of steroid solution into the edematous subcutaneous area of the supratip region during the first few weeks following surgery has proven to be of considerable value in controlling the edematous component of this deformity. It should be emphasized that the doses utilized are very small and should not be repeated more than once or twice monthly so that the effect of the previous injection can be carefully assessed. The author prefers to use Triamicoline diluted with either saline or Wydase solution, which is injected using a fine 30 gauge needle with a tuberculin syringe directly through the skin of the supratip area and in doses not exceeding 2 to 2.5 mg. Larger doses or more frequent injections can result in troublesome subcutaneous tissue atrophy with depression, thinning, and atrophy of the skin. Such a deformity frequently reverses itself after several months without treatment.

THE INTERNAL NOSE

The nasal lining should be protected and preserved during secondary as well as primary surgery. Destruction of the lining is a surgical disaster.

Scarring of the Vestibule. When the vestibular lining is unduly sacrificed and has healed with scar deformities, correction may be exceedingly difficult. Such deformities include webbing across the apex of the triangle of the vestibule or from the

Text continued on page 367.

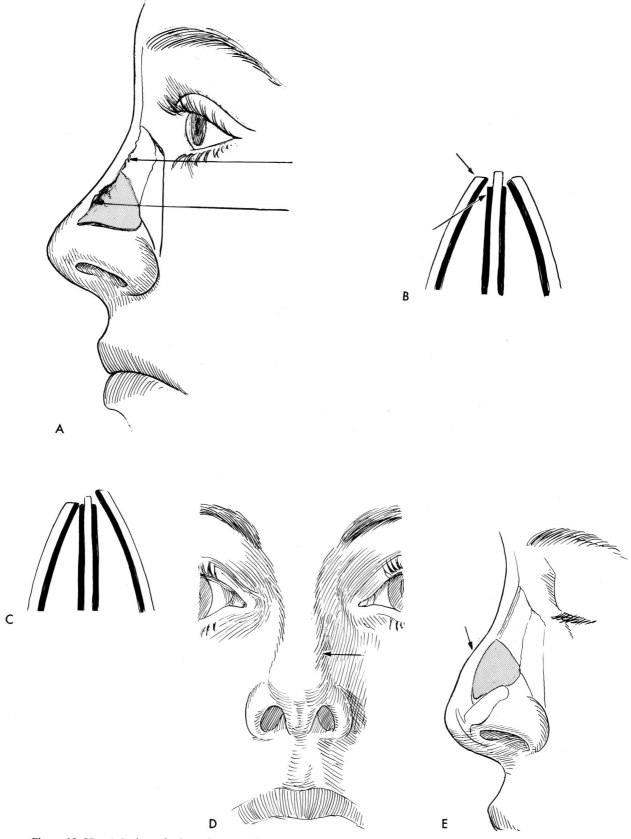

Figure 12–25. *A*, An irregular bony dorsum with excess protrusion of the upper lateral cartilages. No intervention is necessary in a patient whose irregularity is palpable but not visible. *B*, Ideal postoperative relations of cartilage and mucosa. *C*, An irregular upper lateral cartilage border. *D*, Fullness of the supratip area that may result from excessive upper lateral cartilage. *E*, In the thin-skinned patient, a supratip hump may be more noticeable.

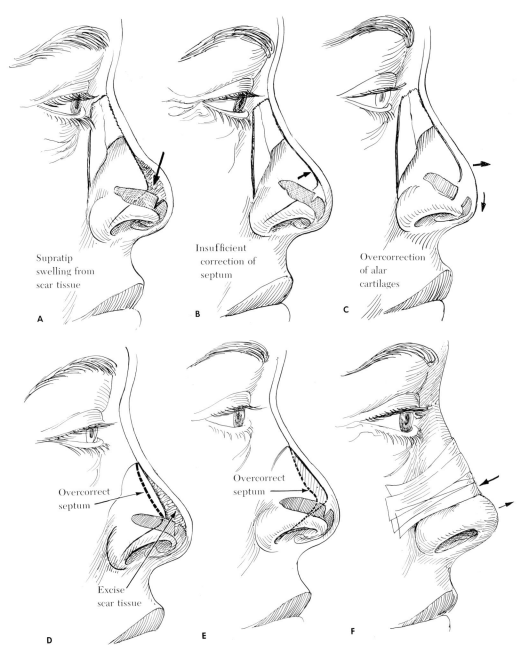

Figure 12–26. Supratip swelling, commonly called "polly tip" or "ram's tip," is perhaps the most common reason for a secondary nasal plastic operation. It is usually the result of scar tissue formation in the dorsal dead space secondary to granulation tissue (*A*), inadequate reduction of the dorsal septal border (*B*), or excessive resection of the alar domes (*C*). The first two problems are usually correctable by a secondary procedure (*D* and *E*) and fixation of the soft tissues to the nasal framework. However, when too much alar cartilage has been removed, correction is almost impossible.

(From Rees, T. D., Krupp, S., and Wood-Smith, D.: Plast. Reconstr. Surg. *46*:332, 1970. Reproduced with permission.)

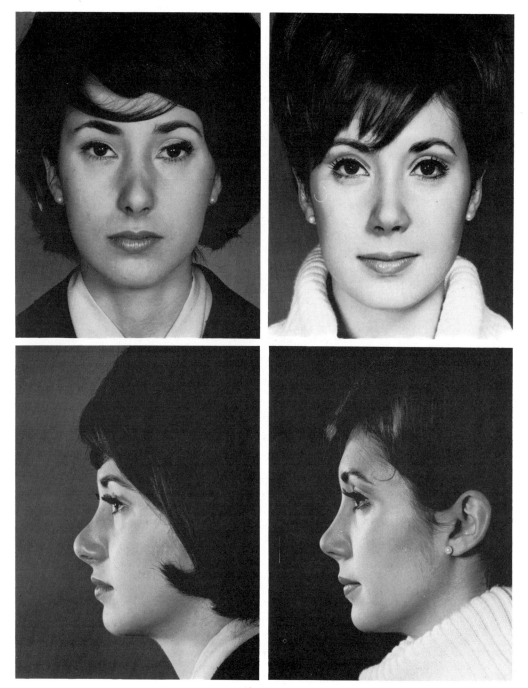

Figure 12-27. Removal of a bony hump with failure to perform infracture and lateral osteotomy; additionally there was insufficient lowering of the cartilaginous dorsal border of the septum. The secondary operation consisted of completion of lateral osteotomy, infracturing, and lowering of the dorsal border.

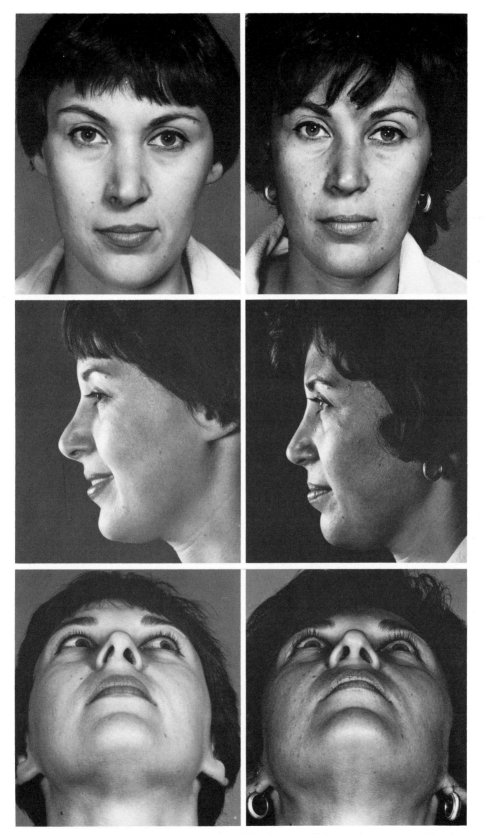

Figure 12–28. Supratip deformity caused by high elevation of the cartilaginous septal border.

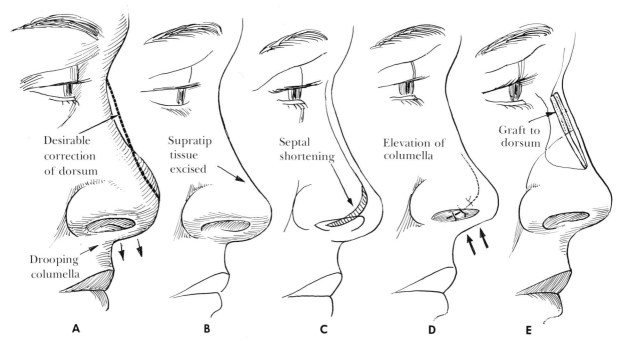

Figure 12–29. *A,* Supratip deformity from overresection of the nasal bridge, insufficient shortening of the lower nose, and bulging of the soft tissue above the alar cartilages from thick skin, scar, edema, or a high septum.

B, The supratip cartilage elevation and as much soft tissue or scar as is necessary to correct the defect is trimmed.

C, The caudal septum is shortened appropriately.

D, The columella is elevated to a more graceful position.

E, The dorsal profile is elevated with implants of bone or cartilage from the septum or auricular concha.

transfixion incision to the floor of the nose, or indeed any other location at which soft tissue has been lacking and raw areas have developed. Correction of this soft tissue loss requires either Z-plasty or transposition flaps, composite grafts, cartilage grafts, or full-thickness free skin grafts. The tissue defect is reestablished by resecting the unyielding scar. The raw defect is then reconstructed. Free composite or full-thickness skin grafts should be used whenever lining is deficient and cannot be repaired by local flaps (Figure 12–30). Such free grafts should be used without hesitation, as they "take" surprisingly well in the vestibule of the nose.

Repair of the "crucified tip" is unquestionably one of the most difficult tasks in secondary rhinoplasty and can tax the ingenuity of any surgeon. Once the lining is restored, adequate support to the soft tissue must also be provided by cartilage or bone grafts from the septum, the ear, or elsewhere

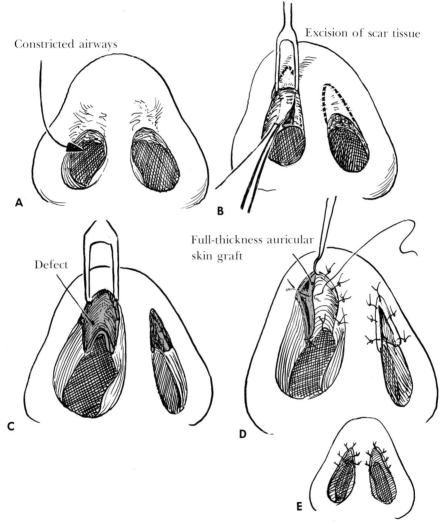

Figure 12–30. The repair of heavily scarred tip deformities in which there is considerable loss of lining and heavy scar infiltration requires a return to basic principles before implants can be utilized to improve the skeletal contour. Scar tissue and synechia must be replaced by healthy soft tissue lining. The simplest method is to use a free full-thickness skin graft, since flaps cannot be fashioned thin enough. The postauricular full-thickness skin graft takes readily after excision of scar. An acrylic or other plastic splint mold of the defect must be worn for several months until the graft has undergone full contraction and maturation. A model for such a graft is obtained at surgery with dental wax, which serves as a temporary splint.

A, Heavy scar tissue and synechia often restrict the airway.

B, The scarred vestibule is carved out.

C, The defect.

D, The free graft is sutured into position.

E, The immediate result. An immediate splint of dental wax is made with a duplicate from which a permanent splint can be crafted by a prosthodontist.

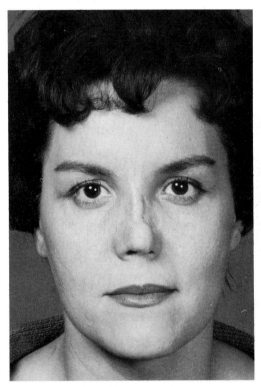 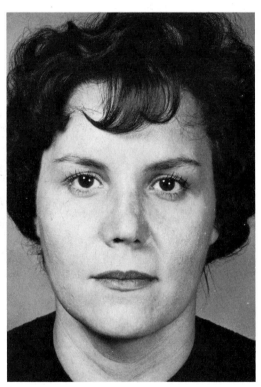

Figure 12–31. A series of inexpert surgical procedures resulted in scarring and actual skin slough in this patient. The situation was improved by full-thickness skin grafting and careful insertion of "matchstick" iliac bone grafts beneath the skin graft. (Courtesy of Dr. Ross Campbell.)

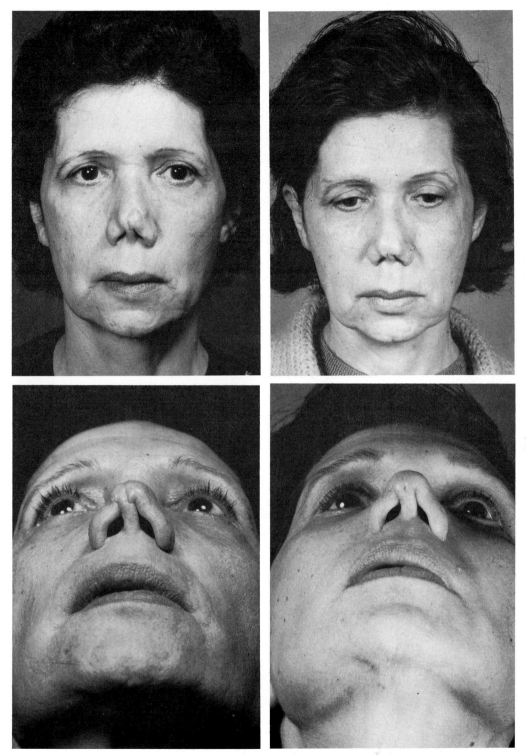

Figure 12–32. Severe nasal deformity following a number of inexpert operations on the nose. The postoperative views, taken after composite grafts from the concha were placed beneath the skin, illustrate the minimal success to be expected in such a difficult problem.

(Figure 12–31). The concha of the ear is an excellent source of graft material (Figure 12–32). Banked sclera has also been used to provide support to both the tip and the upper lateral cartilage area. Occasionally, vestibular collapse can be so severe and scar tissue can be so extensive that support can be provided only by a prosthetic vestibular splint after reconstitution of the soft tissue lining. Such an insert can be devised by a prostho-dontist. It provides an airway at the critical junction of the nasal cartilages and the septum.

Reconstruction of the Internal Valve. Destruction of the internal valve either by excessive resection of upper lateral cartilage, septum, or lining or formation of heavy scar tissue that interferes with the natural action of the valve is a major problem. Perception of respiration is obtunded because the natural air eddies of inspired air are deflected.

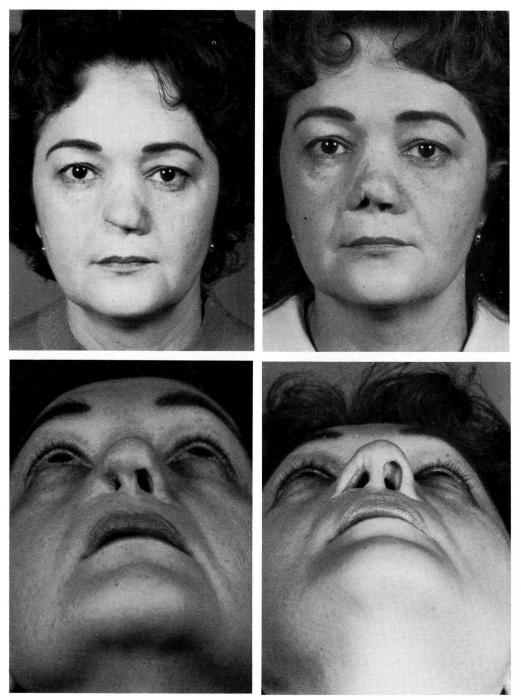

Figure 12–33. A mutilated nose, the result of many inexpert procedures done in rapid order. The right nostril was almost completely blocked, and loss of cartilage support on the left resulted in a flaplike action during inspiration. Postoperative views were taken after a chondrocutaneous composite graft to the right nostril; also illustrated is the use of a continuously worn acrylic shell prosthesis in the left nostril to prevent collapse.

Reconstruction of this important triangle formed by the upper lateral cartilages and septum is exceedingly difficult. Various methods have been devised to support and bolster the upper lateral cartilages in an effort to restore support or prevent collapse during inspiration. Tissues that are available include the thin perpendicular plate of the ethmoid, septal, and auricular cartilage. Correction of the cicatricial webbing of the internal valve may be required prior to insertion of such implants. Subperichondrial dissection of the nasal lining is extremely difficult in secondary as well as primary operations. Usually, when the internal valve is deficient, excessive mucosal lining has also been removed. In severe cases, the use of a small intranasal prosthesis sling as a permanent replacement may be the only final alternative if all other forms of reconstruction fail (Figure 12–33).

Septal Deviation. The management of nasal obstruction after rhinoplasty is discussed in the section on complications. Minor deflections of the septum may be impossible to correct. The success of secondary surgery on the nasal septum depends on the extent of the primary septal surgery. Elevation of mucoperichondrial flaps is much more difficult the second time around; tears and perforations are more common. If a sufficient dorsal and caudal strut remains, secondary attempts to correct obstructive deviations or external twists can be undertaken with great care. The fiberoptic light and magnifying loops are great aids, particularly in secondary surgery of the nose. All too often, however, curvature of the lower nose in the secondary case has recurred following or despite primary attempts to straighten the septum; therefore, further direct surgery to the septum is likely to fail. There is a significant number of patients in whom a straight septum simply cannot be obtained. In these patients, the illusion of a straight nose can often be achieved by various camouflaging techniques discussed in the section on nasal deviation and septal deformities. Such camouflage techniques can be put to excellent advantage in the secondary case, particularly with onlay grafts of single or multitiered layers of septal cartilage (see Figure 12–19).

THE NASAL TIP

Deformities of the nasal tip following primary rhinoplasty are second in frequency to those of the nasal dorsum already described. Deformities of the tip that may be seen after primary operation include pinching, asymmetry, prominent cartilage points, "knuckling," the square or box tip, and contour depression of the skin resulting from scar-

ring of the dermis — including pitting, depressions, and lumps. Such tip deformities are directly related to scar contracture from anatomic interruption of the alar cartilages or destruction of the lining of the vestibule or both. Knuckling may occur after complete transection of the alar cartilage width at one or more points.

Tip projection and shape can be lost as a result of excessive excision of alar cartilage, soft tissue, thick skin, or scar tissue. Implants to improve the contour of the amorphous tip have been advocated by many surgeons, most recently by Pollet (1972), Sheen (1975), Meyer (1977), and others. (Some frequently use such an implant in primary surgery if they feel that the shape of the tip warrants it.) Cartilage is most useful for these grafts, and different shapes and sizes have been suggested.

Deficient lining of the tip or vestibule can be replaced by full-thickness grafts. Sheen advised using elements of the nasal septum in a shaped vomer graft to restore symmetry to the amorphous tip that results from overdissection and resection of the nasal cartilages (1975, 1976). However, he subsequently found that the absorption rate of such bone was considerable, and that cartilage is probably superior as a permanent implant (Figure 12–34).

The Boxed Tip. A boxed tip deformity may result from primary rhinoplasty, but usually, the squared alar cartilages without clear definition of the angulation of the domes persists from failure of correction at the primary operation (Figure 12–35). It can be improved by various procedures designed to reshape the obtuse angle between the medial and lateral crura (Figures 12–36 through 12–39). The boxed tip may be corrected by resection or transection of the alar domes — a safer procedure in the secondary than in the primary operation since collapse of the soft tissue with pinching or impingement of the airway is less likely to occur in the secondary patient because of the added soft tissue support provided by a cicatricial matrix. Patients with thick skin or excess subcutaneous fat and connective tissue can afford loss of considerably more of the lateral crura of the alar cartilage without nostril collapse than can the thin-skinned individual. Excessive resection of the alar cartilage in the thin-skinned patient can be disastrous, since little support remains. Tip deformities as well as nostril collapse on inspiration easily result. Contour deformities of the remaining cartilage are easily seen through the thin skin. The Pollet (1977) technique as well as multiple cross hatching (weakening) of the cartilages can reshape the cartilage to form an acute angle in the boxed tip deformity. When complete transection of the

Text continued on page 380.

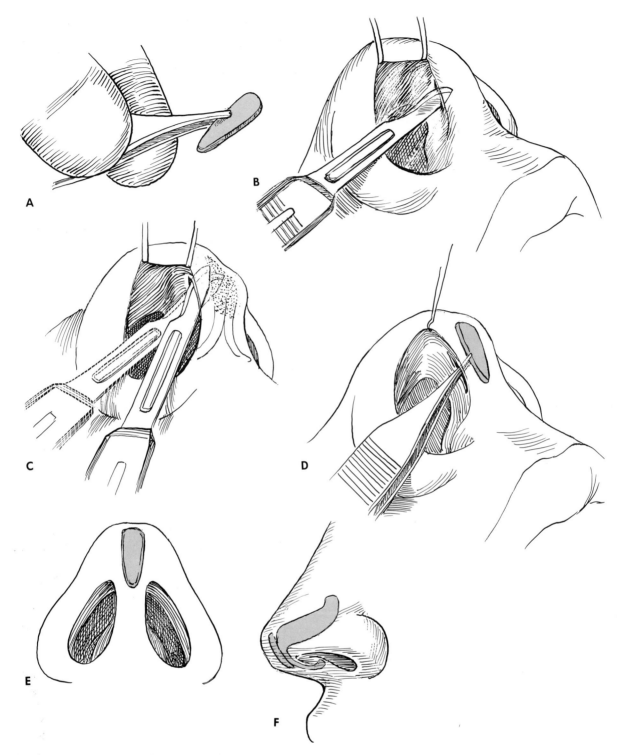

Figure 12–34.   *A,* A graft is fashioned from autogenous cartilage to provide tip projection. Septal cartilage is best. If septal cartilage is not available, the concha of the ear may do.

B, An incision is made in the columella along its caudal margin, just at the junction of the tip and columella.

C, A pocket is dissected.

D, The graft is inserted into the pocket through the columella incision. A slight cephalic tilt is achieved. Sheen cautions against expanding the pocket into the columella, which could allow the graft to shift inferiorly and thereby lose projection. If the pocket must be expanded, he recommends that the dissection be increased laterally. The goal of this maneuver is forward projection of the tip.

E and *F,* The graft is shown in place. Ideally, it is in the midline and anterior to the remnants of the alar cartilage. If desired, it can be fixed with a mattress suture of fine nylon or chromic catgut. (After Sheen.)

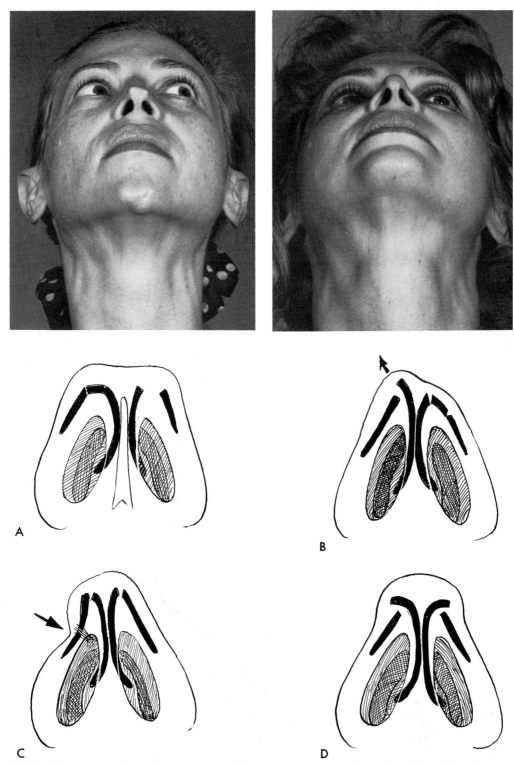

Figure 12–35. The asymmetric nasal tip and some of its common causes. *A*, Unequal excision of alar dome cartilage, with weakening of the dome support on the (patient's) left. *B*, Disruption of the continuity of the lateral crus of the alar cartilage, with projection of a portion of the cartilage expressing itself as a palpable skin irregularity. *C*, Damage to the skin overlying the lateral crus of the alar cartilage, resulting in dimpling. *D*, Breaking of the continuity of the lateral crura and failure to adequately resect their medial portions results in a so-called boxed tip.

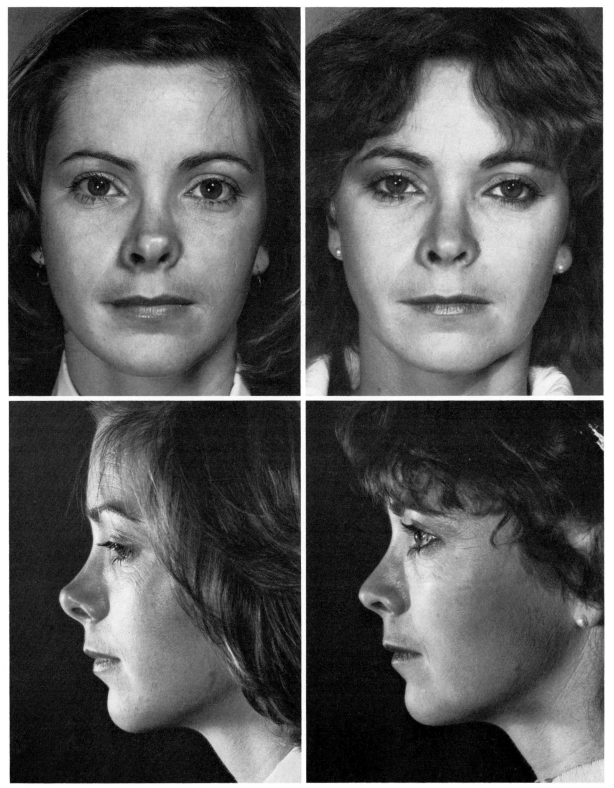

Figure 12–36.   This patient had overshortening of her nose at primary operation, as well as removal of too much dorsal bone and cartilage. The alar cartilages were resected, leaving only the domes present, which because of her thin skin were highly visible.

This excellent correction was achieved by Dr. Cary Guy who reshaped the tip by excising a portion of the most forward part of the alar domes and obtaining an exact reconstruction of the cartilaginous angle between the medial and lateral crus. He also gained length on the nose by thorough undermining, refixing the columella at a lower angle, and augmenting the dorsum with cartilage from the septum.

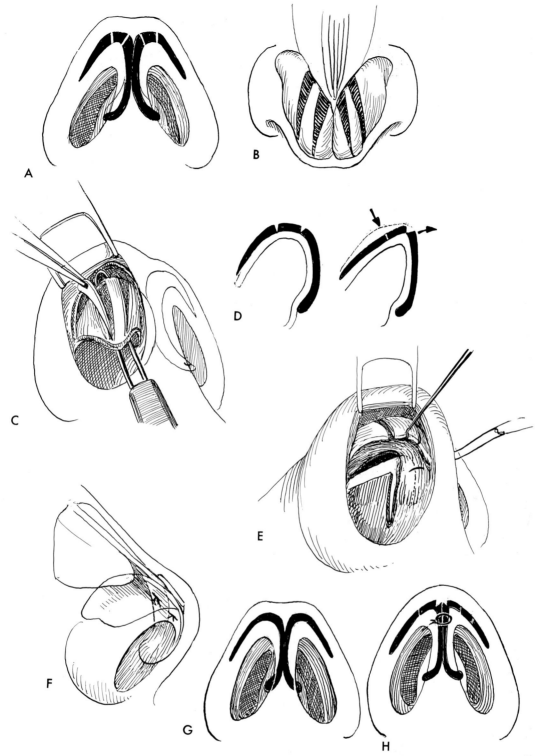

Figure 12–37. Modification of the squared and bifid tip.

A, Planned lines of incision through the lateral crura of the alar cartilages and the alar domes.

B, Excision of strips of alar cartilage to bring about an elevation of the rim and recession of the tip.

C, Strips of cartilage are removed, taking care to preserve the vestibular lining skin.

D, Medial motion of the medial crura brings about a flattening of the prominent alar dome region.

E, The two medial crura are sutured together by plain 4–0 catgut sutures.

F, Completed suturing of the medial crura, in this instance embracing the caudal border of the septum.

G and *H,* Preoperative and postoperative contours compared.

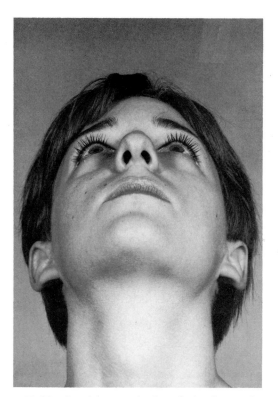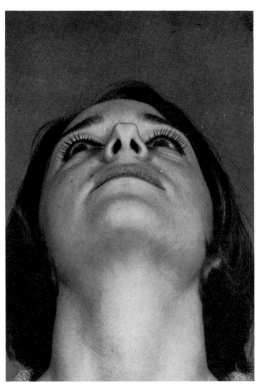

Figure 12–38. Development of a "boxed" tip after nasal tip plasty in which bifidity was not corrected and the alar "spring" was broken.

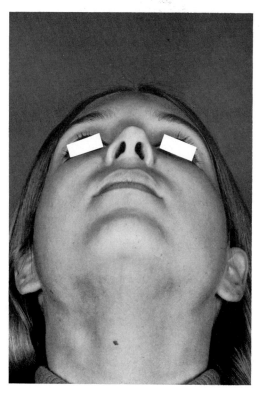

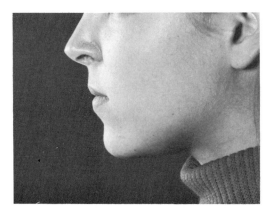

Figure 12–39. A complete breaking of the continuity of the alar cartilage may result in a small spicule of cartilage distorting the nasal tip skin, as in the postoperative view of this patient.

The rule in tip plasty is to be conservative, since there is nothing harder to repair than an overoperated nasal tip. If too much cartilage or lining has been sacrificed, little can be done to salvage the situation. Some surgeons have claimed that all the lateral crus can be resected without impairing the tip, either cosmetically or functionally. While this may be true in patients with thick, rigid skin and subcutaneous tissue, or in secondary operations in which considerable scar tissue is present, it is not true in the average patient with more delicate tip cartilage and skin. Alar collapse can and does occur, and it is always preferable to leave a small margin of the cartilage to act as a spring. It is also better not to break this spring, although in fact this is often necessary, particularly at the domes. Dicing or morseling the cartilage so that it can be shaped or molded is a reasonable alternative.

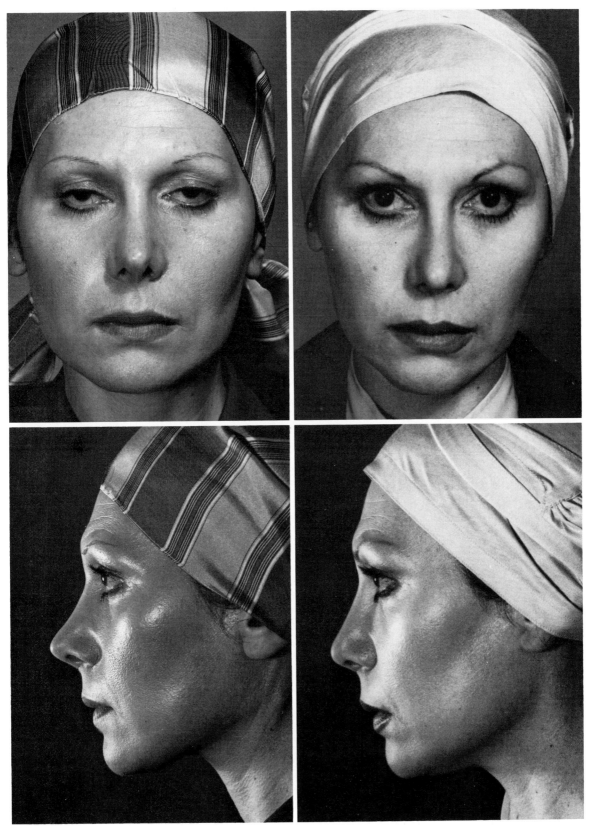

Figure 12–40. A sharp, pointed tip resulted in this patient after primary rhinoplasty because the septal angle was high and pointed and because a remnant of dome left on the left alar cartilage buckled owing to loss of support of the lateral crus and the forces of contracture.

Correction was achieved by simply excising the buckled dome, reconstituting an alar rim with the small remnants left, and lowering the septal angle. (Courtesy of Dr. C. Guy.)

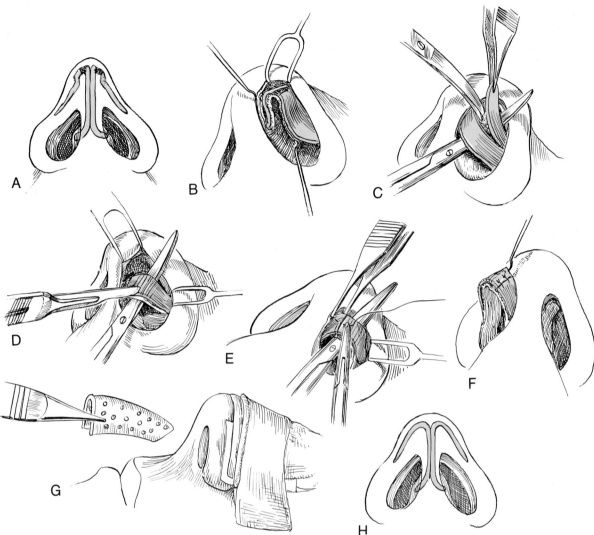

Figure 12–41.   The technique described by Williams (1977) is applicable for the correction of knuckling of the alar domes, when sufficient alar cartilage remains. When all of the alar cartilage has been sacrificed, implants must be used, such as the three-tiered implant described by Pollet (1972) or the nostril buttress grafts described in Figure 12–45. The Williams technique was devised to correct the pinched tip that is one of the drawbacks of an inexpertly performed alar flap technique (Lipsett); however, it is equally effective in correcting the pinching or knuckling that can occur as a primary deformity in a few patients, or after any tip procedure in which the cartilaginous remnants near the dome become trapped in scar contracture during the healing period and buckle as a result.

A, The deformity.

B, An alar flap, double-pedicle, is developed with a para-rim incision.

C, Should any redundancy of alar cartilage be present, it is removed from the cephalic portion of the lateral crus.

D, The cartilage is scored, as in the original Lipsett procedure, by cross-cutting it. This allows a new dome to be shaped.

E, The point of fracture where the cartilage has collapsed is repaired.

F, The repair creates a new dome.

G, A splint is inserted to maintain the shape.

H, The new alar cartilage.

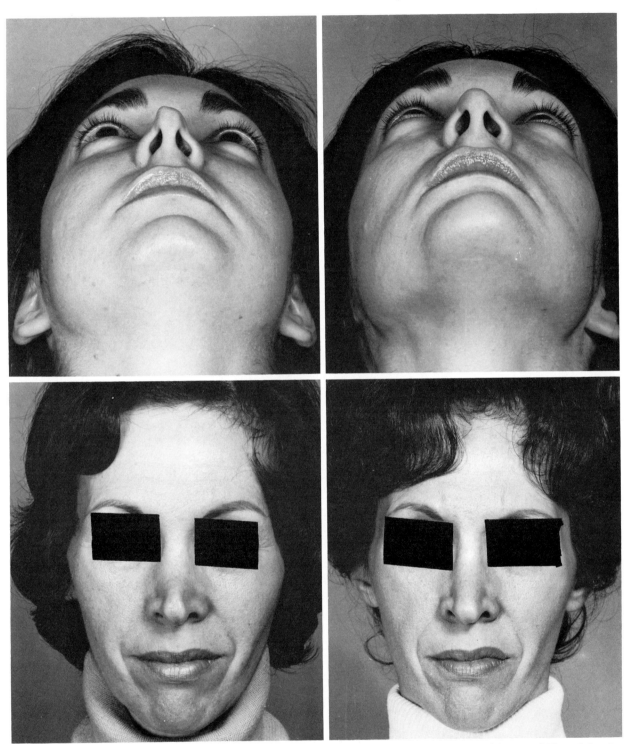

Figure 12–42.   Patients with marked asymmetry of the alar cartilages and knuckling corrected by remodelling of the alar cartilages utilizing a technique similar to that described by Williams. The entire alar cartilage remnant must be reshaped and evened from side to side. Postoperative splinting of the new shape with a small intravestibular prosthesis helps to maintain the relationships until fibrous fixation has occurred.

In the one patient (bottom) an infracture was also necessary. In most secondary rhinoplasty problems, there are multiple complications to cope with, rarely one.

alar cartilage is done, it is important to resect an accurately measured and symmetrical piece from both sides at the very height of the domes, or to transect the cartilages just on the medial side of the domes through the medial crus. Resecting on the medial side decreases the likelihood of sharpened cartilaginous points appearing postoperatively.

Knuckling or acute angulation of the alar domes can occur as a sequela of the primary operation. It is often seen when the cartilages are attenuated to this region and when the transition area between the medial and lateral crura at the dome is exceptionally narrow, but knuckling is much more apt to occur as a result of overly ambitious excision of the cephalic portion of the lateral crus and extending into the domes (Figure 12–40). In this event, the remaining portion of the dome may be represented by a narrow rim of cartilage, perhaps 2 to 3 mm in width, which can be brought into an acute angulation from the forces of postoperative contracture of the undermined soft tissues. Dissection of the lining from the vestibular surface of the cartilage is more likely to produce such a deformity than when such lining is left attached. Cross hatching of the alar cartilages — which is carried completely through the width of the cartilage in multiple locations such as the original Lipsett technique — can lead to postoperative knuckling and is one of the inherent drawbacks of this procedure. Correction of knuckling resulting from the Lipsett procedure was described by Williams (1977) and is illustrated in Figure 12–41. This Williams technique involves recreating the original deformity, resecting the offending pieces of cartilage, and accurately approximating the correction. The knuckling deformity can be an integral part of the primary problem in the unoperated nose; it should be recognized as such. Correction requires accurately measured total resection of the sharply angulated domes (Figure 12–42). Resection of the domes is contraindicated when projection of the tip is limited.

The Plunging Tip.

The plunging or drooping tip is frequently related to excessive lowering of the dorsal profile of the nose and is often associated with overshortening of the caudal septum. The older patient is particularly prone to such a problem postoperatively since loss of skin contractility contributes to excessive skin, which tends to flow in the direction of gravitational pull. Inexpert trimming and suturing of the upper lateral and alar cartilages in their new and adjusted anatomic relationships to the shortened caudal margin of the septum also can contribute to postoperative plunging of the tip. Unusual angulation between the medial and lateral crura in a caudal direction is a difficult primary deformity to correct, and when it is coupled with a short columella, postoperative plunging of the tip is almost assured. Correction of the deformity under these circumstances is more easily prevented than treated. Shortening of the upper lateral cartilages or approximating and suturing them to the cephalic margins of the alar cartilages at a second operation will help correct the problem in some patients.

Fixation of the medial crura of the alar cartilages to the denuded caudal septal border by an "orthopedic suture" may help to retain the tip in an elevated position. This is often referred to as the "tongue-in-groove" maneuver. Complete transection of the domes in patients with a plunging dome angle to reposition the medial and lateral crura in a new relationship is sometimes helpful.

It is ironic that the plunging tip deformity following a primary rhinoplasty often occurs because of specific efforts on the part of the surgeon to elevate the tip at the primary operation. Overremoval of the dorsum and overshortening of the nose can result in a plunging tip as well as in an overly shortened nose. Again, the young surgeon is admonished to underoperate rather than overoperate.

Overshortening.

Excessive shortening of the nose with excessive exposure of the nostrils ("pig snout") usually results from overresection of the caudal septum and/or the upper lateral and alar cartilages (Figures 12–43 and 12–44). In many such patients, the entire membranous septum has been resected, making correction exceedingly difficult.

The nasal spine is removed too often, in the author's opinion. Removal of this structure sometimes creates the illusion of lengthening the nose and other times results in overshortening, although often at the expense of an unwanted lengthening of the upper lip, which may hang like a curtain.

Correction of the overshortened nose is exceedingly difficult when there is a shortage of soft tissues (the membranous septum). After the nose is skeletonized, it can sometimes be stretched caudally and fixed with sutures in a more inferior position to maintain length. If sufficient lateral crus of the alar cartilage is present, it can be used for turnover flaps to fill the gap between the caudal septum and the columella (Millard, 1972) (see Figure 10–20). Dingman and Walter (1969) described composite grafts from the ear to reconstruct the membranous septum. Usually, saddling of the dorsum is associated with overshortening, since the surgeon who is apt to overshorten the nose is also apt to overcorrect the dorsal profile. Accordingly, bone grafts or cartilage grafts to restore the dorsum are often required and help

Text continued on page 384.

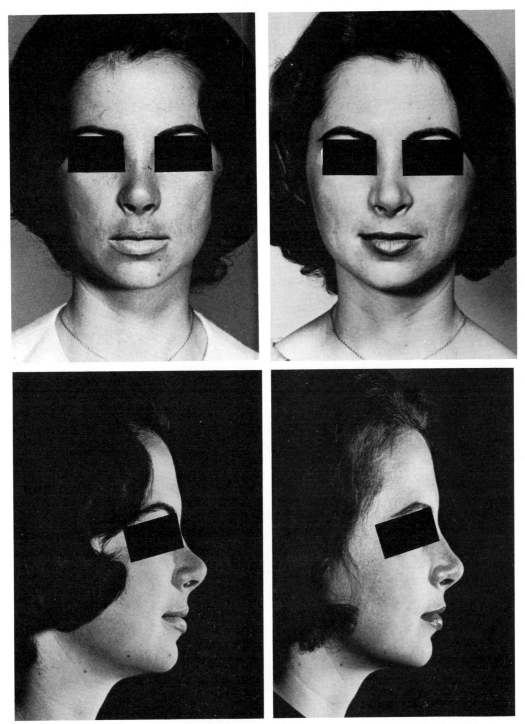

Figure 12–43. The preoperative views demonstrate the result of overexcision of the caudal border of the septum combined with total removal of the nasal spine— an overshortened nose. Separation of the soft tissues from the bony and cartilaginous skeleton of the nose, and their displacement caudally, achieved the lengthening shown in the postoperative photographs. Mattress sutures fix the soft tissues in their corrected position. The inferior displacement is further aided by lowering the septal angle. It must be emphasized that this not the sort of result that can usually be achieved; frequently, there is little that can be done for these unfortunate patients.

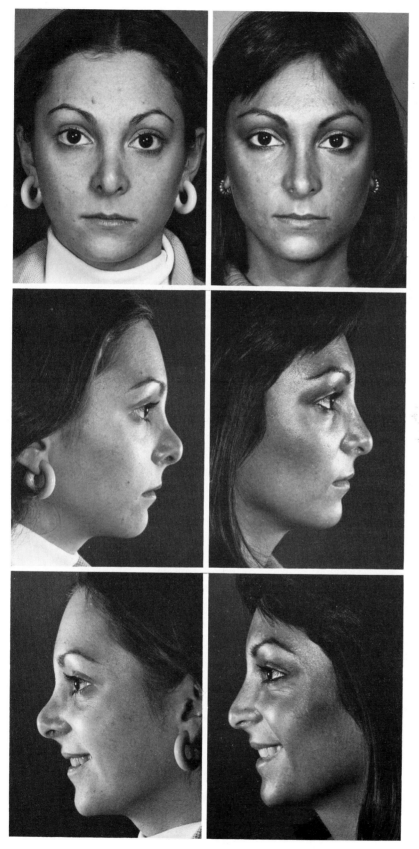

Figure 12–44. When too much dorsum has been resected, and too much removed from the caudal septum, the nose can resemble a pig's snout.

This patient has a "pig's snout" deformity that was the result of overresection of the dorsum and caudal septum that left a supratip deformity because the septal angle was left too high, but the domes of the alar cartilages were resected so that the forward projection of the tip was lost.

Improvement was obtained by lowering the septal angle and stretching the degloved nose. (Courtesy of Dr. C. Guy.)

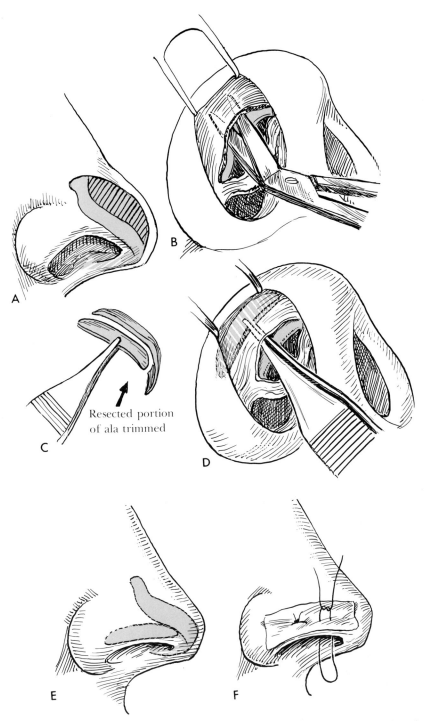

Resected portion
of ala trimmed

Figure 12–45. Caudal arching of the nostril can occur as a primary deformity, but it is more often the result of too much primary surgery with resection of lining, alar cartilage, and sometimes the upper lateral cartilages. Provided there is cartilage available from either the septum or perhaps a remnant of the alar cartilages, an implant can be fashioned that will aid in extending the retracted nostril rim in a more caudal direction.

A, The alar cartilage is present in some patients as demonstrated. The retracted nostril rim is shown.

B, The lining and the alar cartilage, or remnant of it, are undermined in a retrograde manner.

C, A cartilaginous plate is fashioned as a strut. This cartilage can also come from the septum or even the ear. Some surgeons have used preserved sclera.

D, The graft is inserted into the alar margin.

E, The graft is shown in position with the nostril deformity improved.

F, The graft is held in position with mattress sutures tied over stents. (After Meyer and Kesselring, 1977.)

immensely in the overall effect. In isolated cases, if the septum has not been unduly sacrificed, a septal flap can be developed and advanced in a caudal direction to gain length.

Correction of the Arching Nostril.   The arching nostril can be improved in some cases with rim implants of alar cartilage when and if the lateral crus has not been previously sacrificed (Figure 12–45). If the lateral crus is insufficient, implants of septal cartilage or vomer bone may be helpful (Figure 12–46).

Correction of the Amorphous Tip.   For want of a better term, a tip that has lost virtually all its normal landmarks that are generally formed by the underlining cartilaginous architecture can be called "amorphous." Such tips result from excessive or total resection of the alar cartilages, scar tissue formation in the subcutaneous planes, and loss of lining with cicatrix formation. The delicate faceting of the cartilages so important in defining a "normal" nose are frequently lost, as are anatomic definitions of the domes and both cephalic and

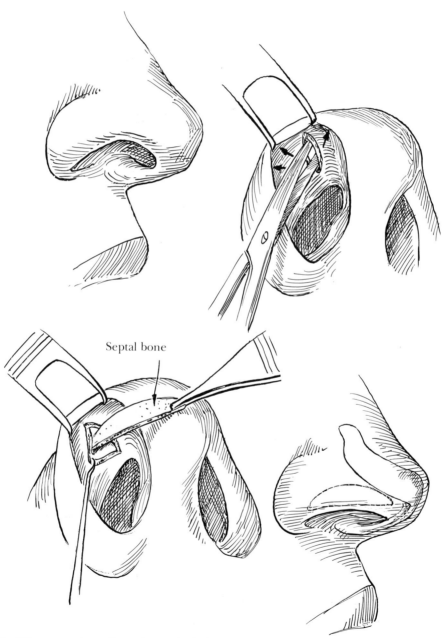

Septal bone

Figure 12–46.   The retracted nostril margin can also be improved with a bone plate as the graft. This technique has been suggested by Sheen and others. Bone is often available from the vomer or the ethmoid plate, although the latter is usually too thin and fragile to provide a strong graft.

The surgical technique is almost identical to that described in Figure 12–41 for insertion of cartilage implants.

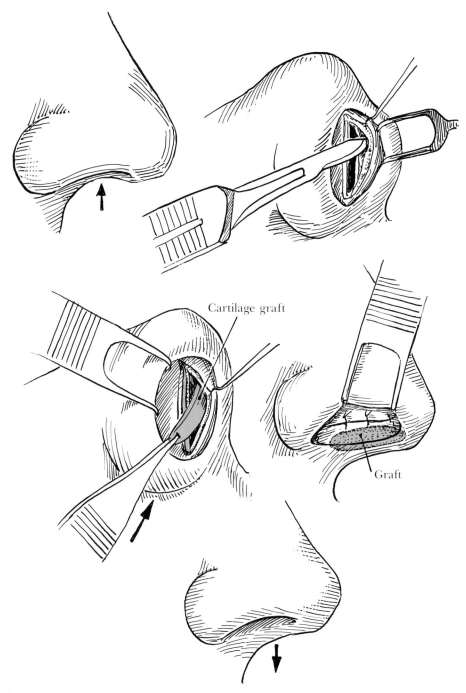

Figure 12–47. Retraction of the columella is a most distressing deformity following rhinoplasty or traumatic destruction of the nasal septum. It is *very difficult to correct.* When sufficient soft tissue is present — that is, when the membranous septum has not been destroyed — it is sometimes possible to improve the contour by an implant of bone or cartilage placed within the columella as a strut. The technique is illustrated here.

When extensive soft tissue and cartilage are missing, composite grafts to the region of the membranous septum from the ear, or flaps of nasal lining and alar cartilage from the side walls of the nose, can sometimes fill the gap, provided these structures too have not been mutilated or excised.

caudal margins of the lateral crura. Some contouring of such scarified tips can be gained by sculpting dissection of thick subcutaneous scar. Sheen (1976) has improved such tips with the use of bone and cartilage implants (Figure 12–46). There is often some bone and cartilage remaining in the septum along the floor of the vomer that can be utilized. Sheen (1975) originally recommended the implantation of a carefully carved double-notched piece of bone to produce projection of the tip; however, long-term results indicated that correction was best maintained by the use of septal cartilage.

Hanging Columella.   A hanging columella — a convexity or roundness of the caudal margin of the medial crura of the alar cartilages — may first become significant after rhinoplasty. This can be corrected by marginal incisions in the columella and trimming of the rounded cartilage and sometimes of the lining.

Retraction of the Columella.   This may result from excessive removal of the inferior or caudal margin of the septum and sometimes from resection of the membranous septum and/or medial crura. Correction of this deformity is difficult and often impossible. For minor deformities, a septal cartilage implant may be effective if sufficient lateral crus of alar cartilage is present (Figure 12–47). A retracted columella can be improved by Millard's alar turnover flap; however, rarely is there sufficient cartilage remaining after rhinoplasty. A composite graft can also be used in place of the missing membranous septum in severe retraction. Bone and alloplastic implants are generally disappointing because of insufficient soft tissue coverage.

(For references, see pages 450 to 453.)

Chapter 13

Problems in Rhinoplasty

THOMAS D. REES, M.D., F.A.C.S.

THE PROBLEM

This wide, flattened nose required narrowing throughout its length, extending from the bony root of the nose to and including the tip, where there was a diastasis of the alar cartilages.

Hypertrophy of the upper lateral cartilages as well as of the alars existed. Both paired cartilages formed nearly a 90 degree angle; the upper laterals with the septum and the medial with the lateral crura of the alar cartilages. There was no clearly defined dome, and the dorsal surface of the alars formed a large flat surface.

The intercanthal distance appeared increased because of the wide nasal root. The hump deformity on profile was minimal — an important consideration since overly ambitious reduction would unquestionably result in a relative saddle deformity.

The overall surgical plan was to excise the necessary amount of cartilage, connective tissue, and bone from the region of the midline to allow for narrowing and to reduce and narrow the tip.

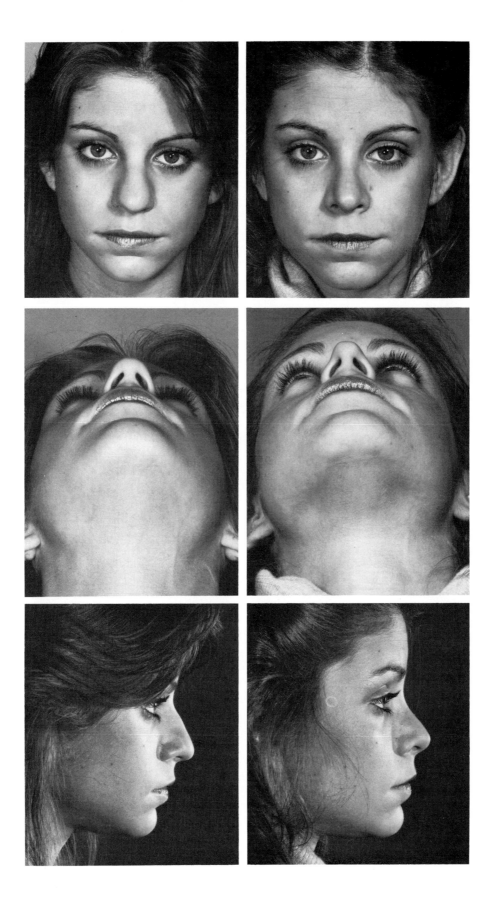

THE SURGICAL PLAN

A,B: The preoperative anatomy. The red area in *B* represents the bone and
              cartilage excised by rasp and osteotome (from the midline) and sharp
              cartilage dissection.

C,D: Postnarrowing result. Arrows in *D* indicate medial shifting of all elements
              permitted by *B*.

E,F,G: The small hump was removed by rasping and the nose was shortened very
              slightly by resecting a portion of the cephalic excess of alar cartilage and
              lifting the tip.

H,I: The rounded, almost box-like tip was remodelled. Diastasis was improved
              by resection of soft tissue and approximating suture of the medial crura.
              Cleansing the medial crura of intervening soft tissue and suturing the feet
              aided in increasing tip projection. The columella is lengthened slightly by
              this maneuver.

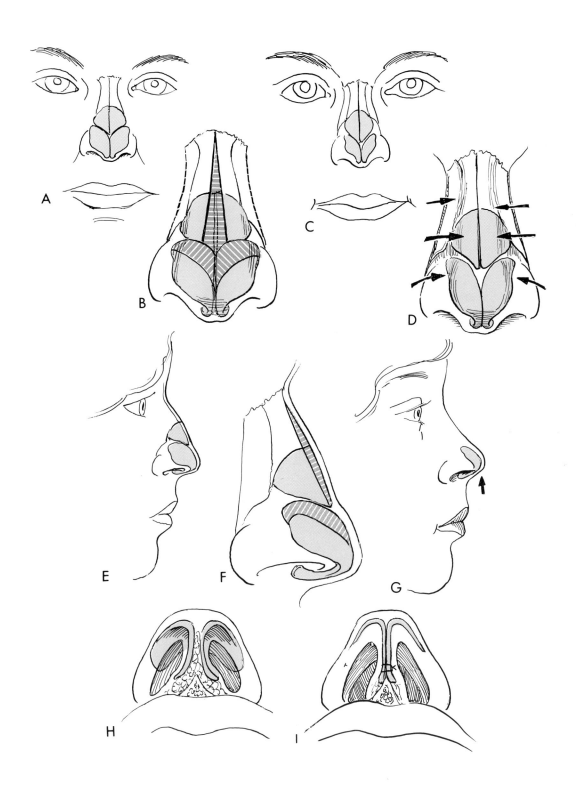

THE PROBLEM

The preoperative photographs show a relative box-tip deformity with a flat dorsal surface on front face. The bony nasal pyramid was wide, but the actual bony hump was only of moderate size. The lower septal dorsum and septal angle were high, clearly shown on the lateral animated view. The minor hump was accentuated by the absence of frontal bone "bossing" and, therefore, the lack of a nasion. A sloping forehead added to the profile problem. The upper lip appeared shortened because of a prominent caudal septal border and nasal spine.

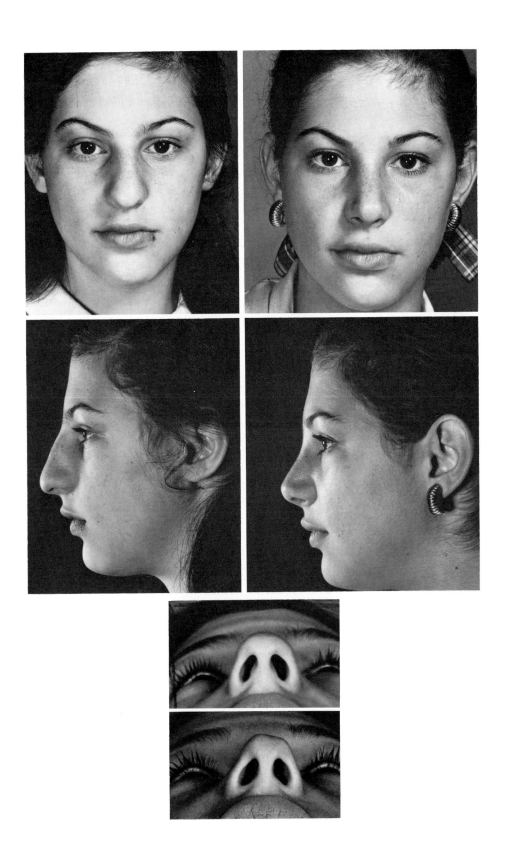

THE SURGICAL PLAN

A: Normal profile showing relationships of forehead to nose and chin. The frontal bone ordinarily projects forward.

B: Profile of patient: no frontal bossing was present. Nose projects forward. Correction required gouging out a nasion with a chisel and reducing the profile.

C,D: Front and "worm's eye" views show excessively large alar cartilages with an oblique transition angle (box-tip) and a wide bony pyramid.

E: Surgical plan of resection of alar cartilage indicated. The remaining alar rim was weakened enough so that increased angulation at the dome area occurred.

F,G: Plunging of the nose on animation.

H: Indicates portion of lateral crus resected.

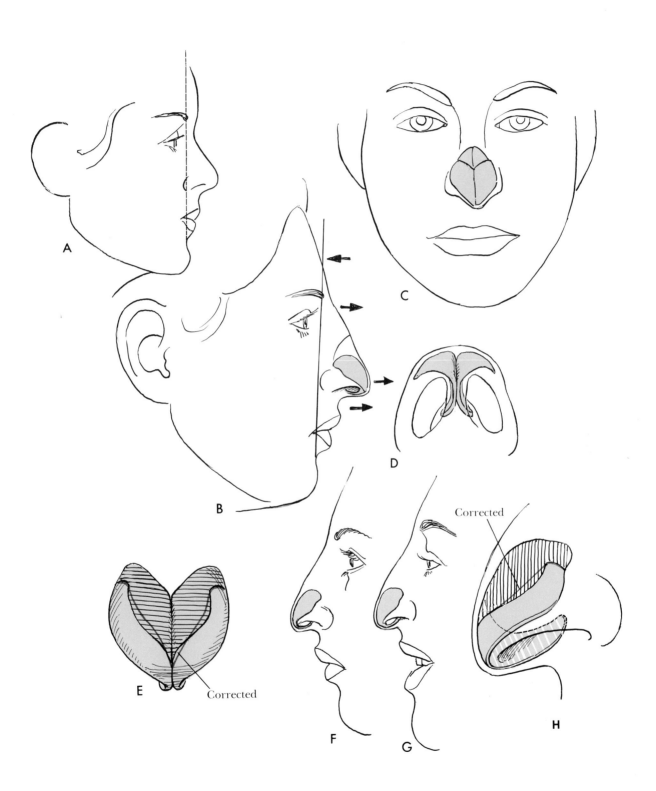

E —————— Corrected

Corrected —————— H

THE PROBLEM

Aside from a very small dorsal hump, this patient had a pleasing osteocartilaginous pyramid.

The principal problem was hypertrophied and bulbous alar cartilages with a slight diastasis at the tip. The skin was thicker than usual, but not exceptionally so.

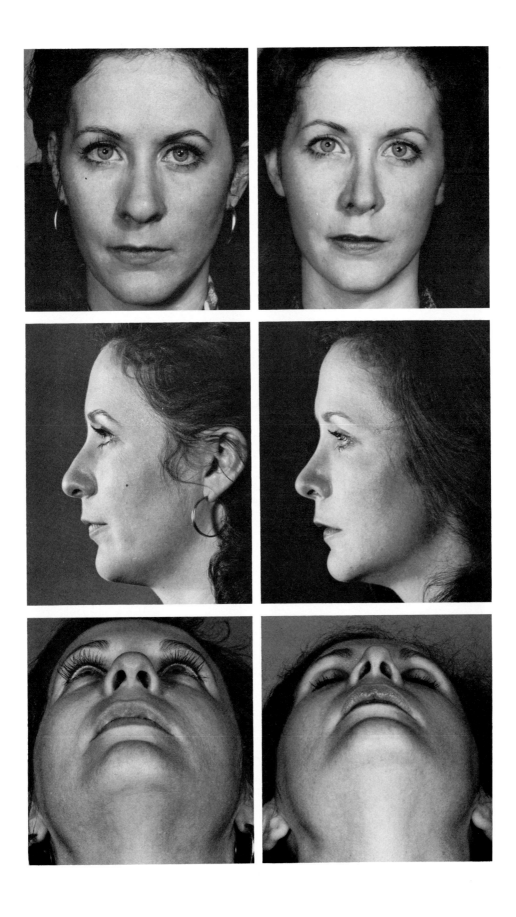

THE SURGICAL PLAN

The dorsal hump was rasped and a lateral osteotomy with infracture was accomplished.

A: The bulky configuration of the alar cartilages. Note the diastasis.

B: The planned amount of resection of the cephalic portion of the alar cartilage is indicated. Simple excision of the redundant cartilage resulted in a more acute angulation and triangulation of the tip from the action of natural wound contraction.

C,D: The forces of wound contraction are indicated by the arrows. Note that the medial crura were fixed together with mattress sutures.

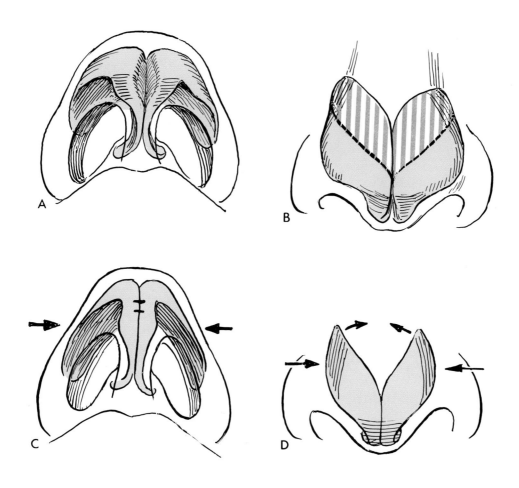

THE PROBLEM

The entire length of the nose was exceptionally wide in this patient but there was no hump to speak of. The nasal bones formed a wide pyramid almost "splayed" laterally as in a direct frontal injury. The tip and alae were broad, flat, and flared. The alar domes were large.

Also note the preoperative tendency for the tip to plunge on animation.

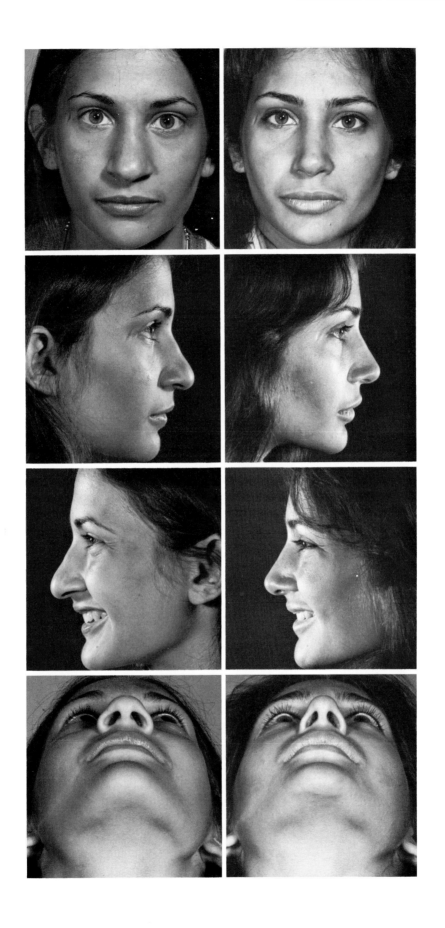

THE SURGICAL PLAN

A,B: Profile representation of the minimal profile reduction that was required. A
            rasp was used. Approximately two thirds of the cephalic portions of the
            lateral crura was excised by the intracartilaginous approach.
C,D: Frontal view showing reduction of cartilage and narrowing.
E–H: Correction of the lobule included resection of redundant lateral crus (*E* and
            G) and weakening of the still strong lateral crus by small cross-hatch inci-
            sions to provide for remodelling of the tip in a more triangular form.
I,J: Inferior representation of refinement of tip achieved by resection of excess
            lateral crus and a generous alar base resection.

The preoperative tendency for the nose to plunge on animation was overcome by
the operative steps illustrated plus *very conservative* trimming of the caudal septum. Had
the dorsal profile been reduced excessively, the plunging tendency would have been
greatly increased. Likewise, overzealous cutting back of the dorsal septum would
increase the plunging.

The tip was maintained as a separate entity to provide normal projection.

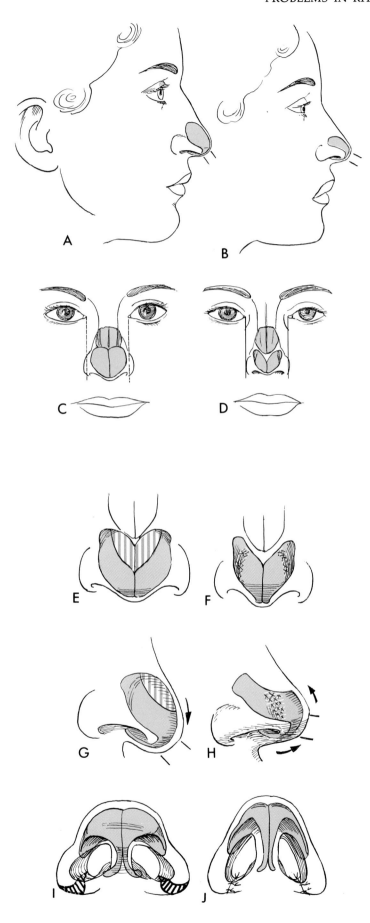

THE PROBLEM

The primary problem was that of large bulbous alar cartilages with quite thick skin. The osteocartilaginous vault was acceptable. The thick skin limited the result appreciably. A minor micrognathia was also present.

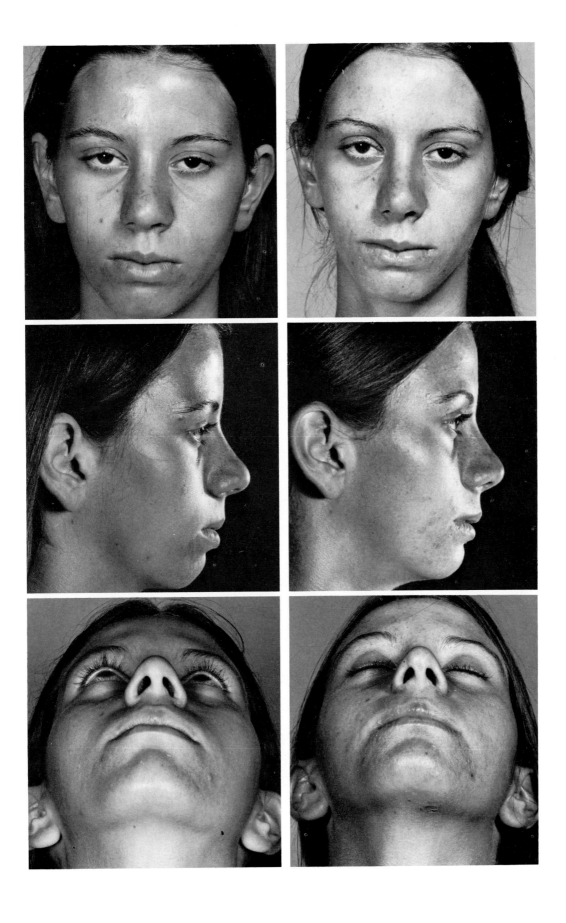

THE SURGICAL PLAN

A,B: The bulbous, box-like tip cartilages are illustrated.
C,D: Resection of all but a small 3 mm rim of the caudal portion of the lateral crura was done.
E: Front view of tip reduction.
F,G: Profile representation of tip reduction and small chin augmentation. A small chin implant helped.

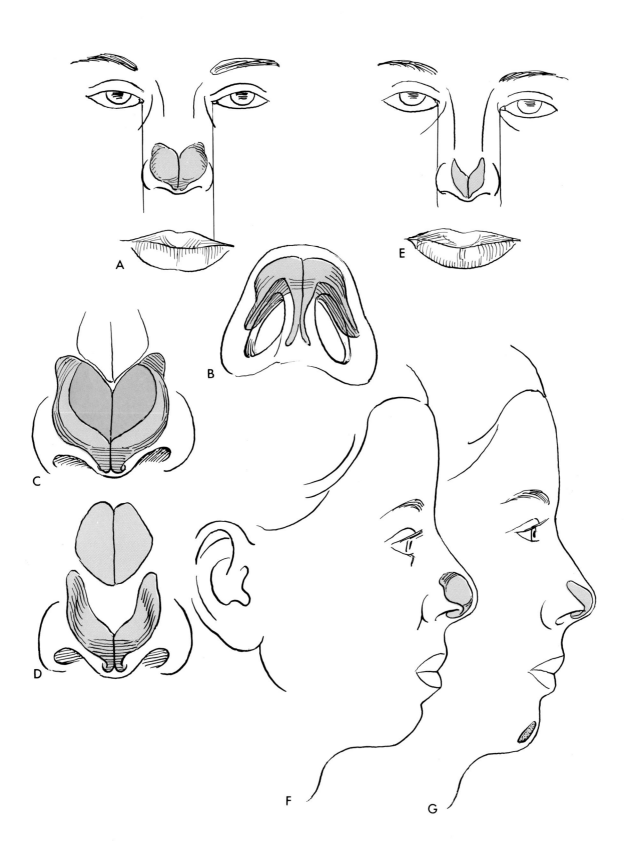

THE PROBLEM

A wide nasal pyramid with no hump and a relative saddle deformity on profile. The tip was very bulky with thick skin and subcutaneous tissue. The preoperative size and shape of the cartilages were difficult to assess because of the thickness of the soft tissue. The prognosis for the operative result was very guarded.

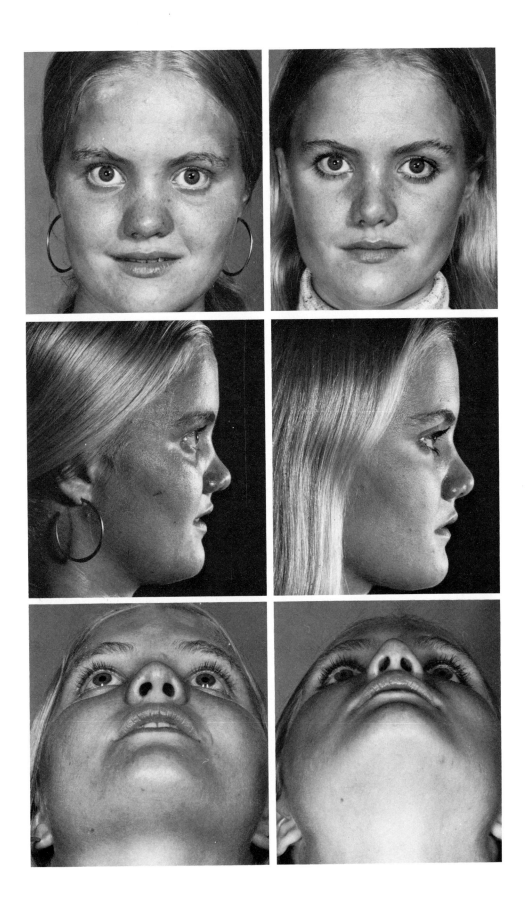

THE SURGICAL PLAN

The bony vault correction was limited to simple lateral osteotomy and infracture. Nothing was removed from the dorsum.

A,B: Preoperative and postoperative profiles represented.

C: Considerable subcutaneous fat and connective tissue were present over the alar cartilages and throughout the tip.

D,E,F: Most of the lateral crus of the alar cartilage along with its overlaying fat was excised through an intracartilaginous incision. As much extra fat was removed as was safe and possible (*F*) without injuring the dermis.

G-J: Excision of the lateral alar cartilages is represented. The excision through the dome transition zone between the medial and lateral crus was complete except for a very small interior rim.

K,L: Further refinement of the tip was accomplished by excising soft tissue wedges from the nostrils (Millard) and defatting the base of the medial crura, which were then sutured together.

M,N: The preoperative and postoperative cartilage mass is represented.

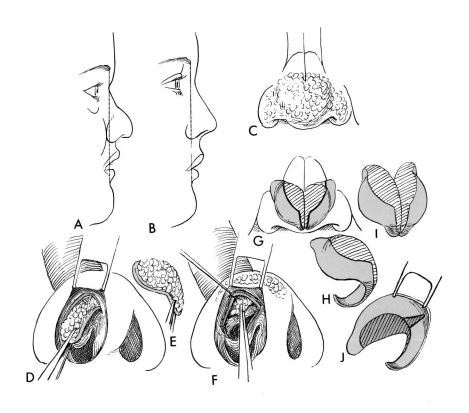

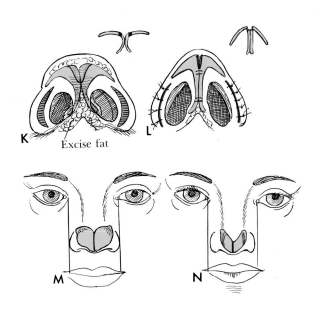

Excise fat

THE PROBLEM

The "parakeet" nose was represented in this patient by a lack of dorsal bony prominence of the cartilaginous septum with a high septal angle and hypertrophied alar cartilages. Note in the lateral view that the marked anterior projection of the septal angle overshadows any projection of the alar cartilages and, in fact, has displaced the alar cartilages caudally.

The "worm's eye" views show a caudal dislocation of the septum to the left, which is not evident on the front view.

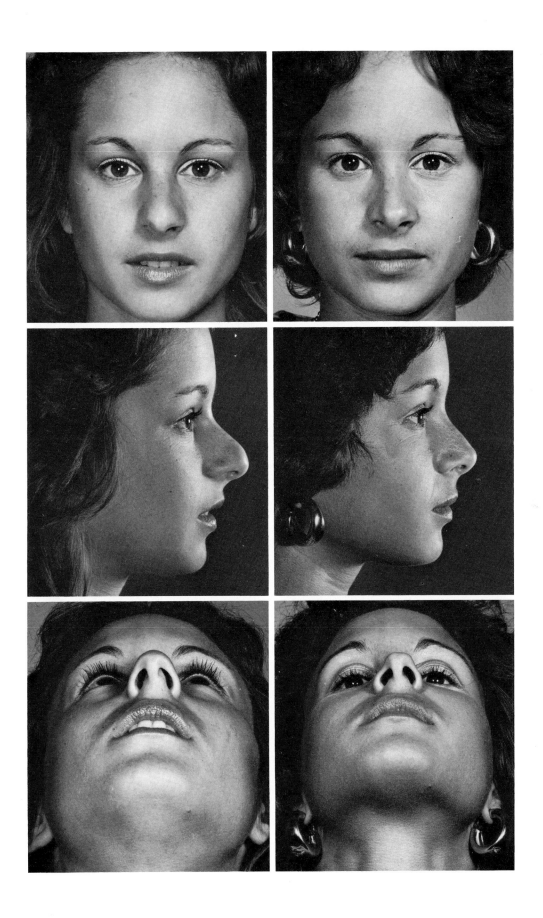

THE SURGICAL PLAN

A-E: The foreward projection was reduced piecemeal by first trimming the dorsal septum (*B*) and then cautiously trimming the curving caudal borders (*C*). The bony dorsum was essentially untouched except for minor raspings, and care was taken to maintain the tip projection.

F: The plan of excision of the alar cartilages is indicated.

G–J: Preoperative and postoperative representation of the remodelling of the tip cartilages. A rim was maintained intact.

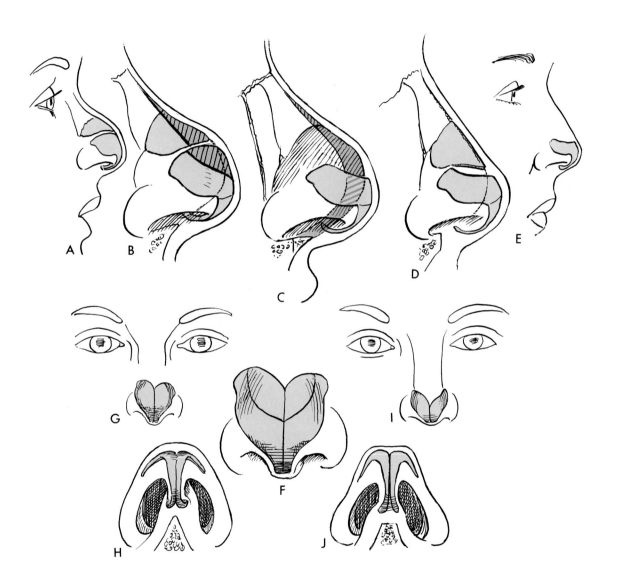

THE PROBLEM

A wide based nasal pyramid with arching hypertrophied alar cartilages. The caudal borders of the alar cartilages were clearly defined because the skin was thin. The inferior border of the medial crus was rounded, but not exaggeratedly so. From below, the tip was box-like with slightly flaring alae.

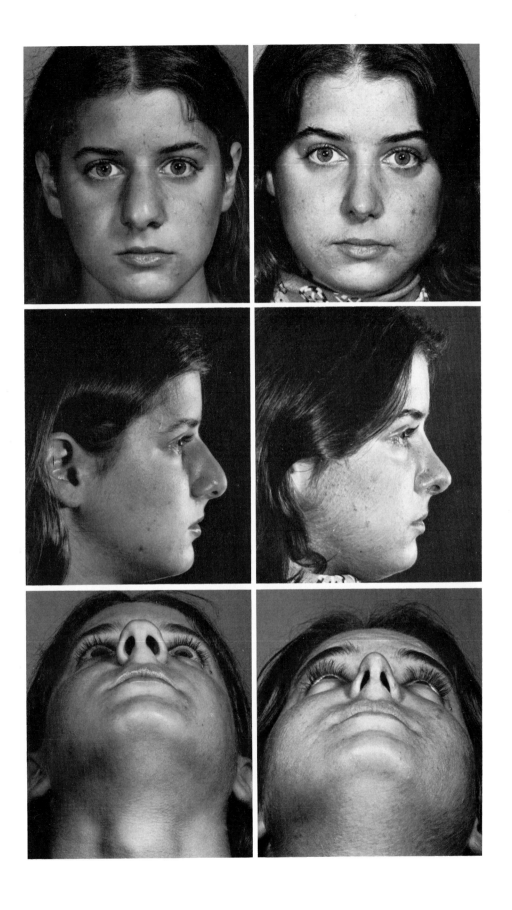

THE SURGICAL PLAN

A,C: Sliver of dorsal midline resection and alar cartilage excision indicated to narrow the framework.

B,D: The result.

E,F: Plan of excision of the huge flaring alar cartilages and weakening of the remaining intact rim. The cartilaginous arch can be weakened by cross cutting using any system of partial incisions that do not totally transect the cartilage, such as the modified Lipsett technique. Morcellizing also will weaken the cartilage, but it is unnecessarily harsh on the mucous membranes.

G,H: The alar cartilages are frequently separated in the midline in such tip configurations, adding to the box-like effect. Cleaning away the connective tissue and suturing them helps to alleviate this.

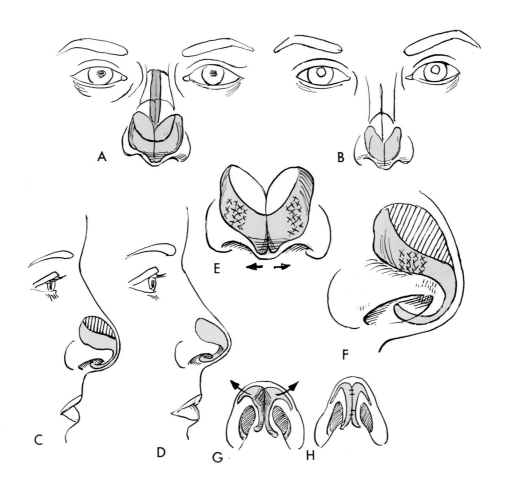

THE PROBLEM

No bony hump to speak of, but a wide based nose. The tip was strong, projecting forward with rounded, bulbous domes. The nostrils were thick and moderately enlarged. The angle between the medial and lateral crura was wide and arching.

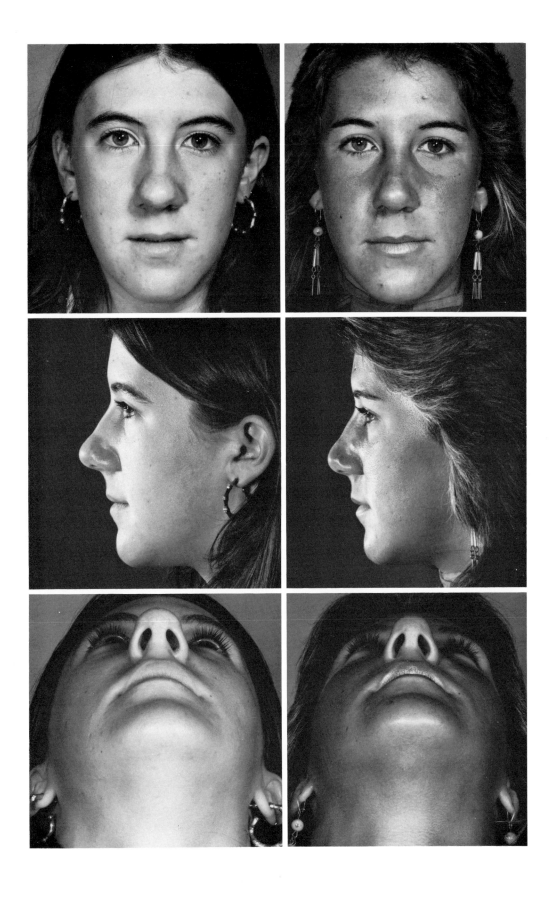

THE SURGICAL PLAN

A,B,C: The tip deformity and the plan of excision of alar cartilage.

D,E: The dorsum and caudal septum must be trimmed very conservatively; otherwise, the strong tip would accentuate any tendency toward saddling or postoperative dropping.

F,G,H: The tip was further recessed by resecting the lateral and superiormost extensions of the lateral crus. This technique is the exact opposite of resecting the domes or a piece of medial crus. It also allowed the lateral crura to settle toward the midline.

I: The nostrils were thinned by the "piece of pie" excision.

J,K,L: The results.

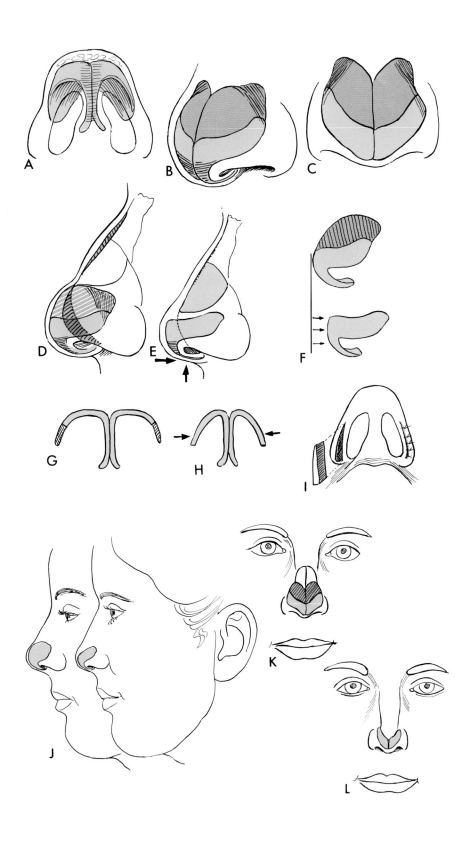

THE PROBLEM

Moderate hump at the junction of the bony and cartilaginous vaults. The alar cartilages were strong with visible facets. The junction of medial and lateral crura formed an angle that accentuated the slight plunging; note the prominence of the "soft triangle." The alar cartilages were separated by considerable soft tissue (diastasis). The inferior (caudal) margins of the inferior crura were rounded, suggesting a hanging columella.

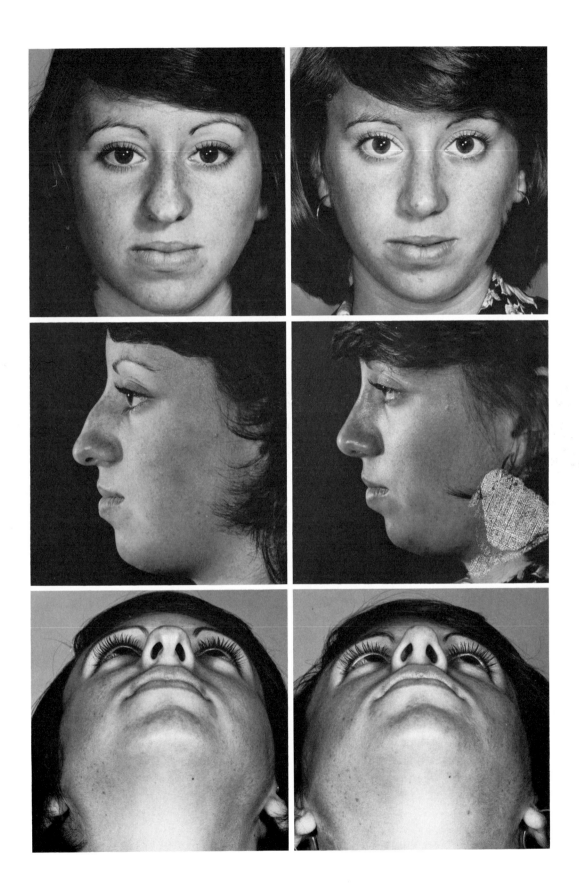

THE SURGICAL PLAN

A,B,C: The anatomic problems depicted.

D,E: Removal of the dorsal hump with a sharp osteotome and excision of a portion of the alar cartilages. The remaining struts were also weakened.

F: The tip was shifted to form a new labial-columella angle. Slight overcorrection was performed to allow for natural "settling."

G,H,I: Steps in tip reconstruction illustrated from below. Removing soft tissue or fat from between the medial crura and bringing the crura together by suture is an important step in converting the wide tip to a more refined triangular shape.

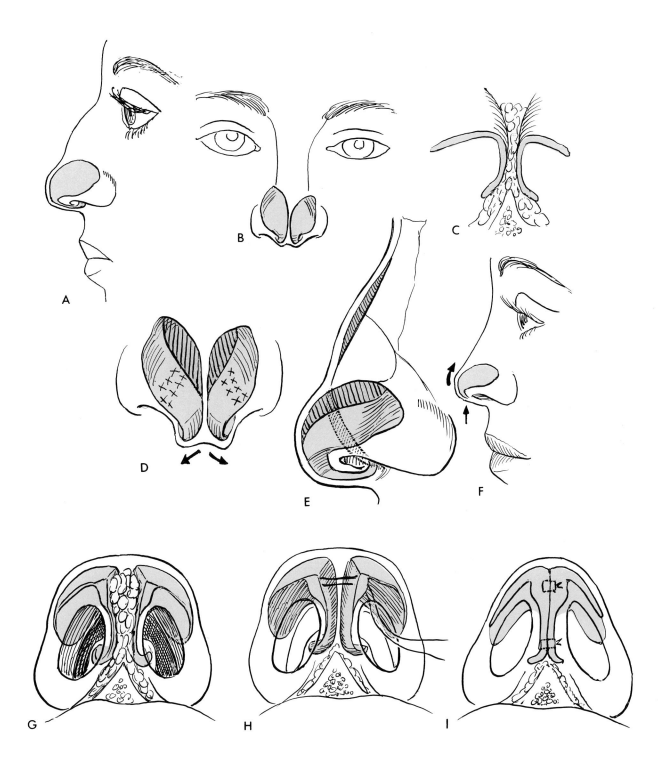

THE PROBLEM

The rounded tip with large domes and increased width of the entire lateral crura. There was also a small dorsal hump.

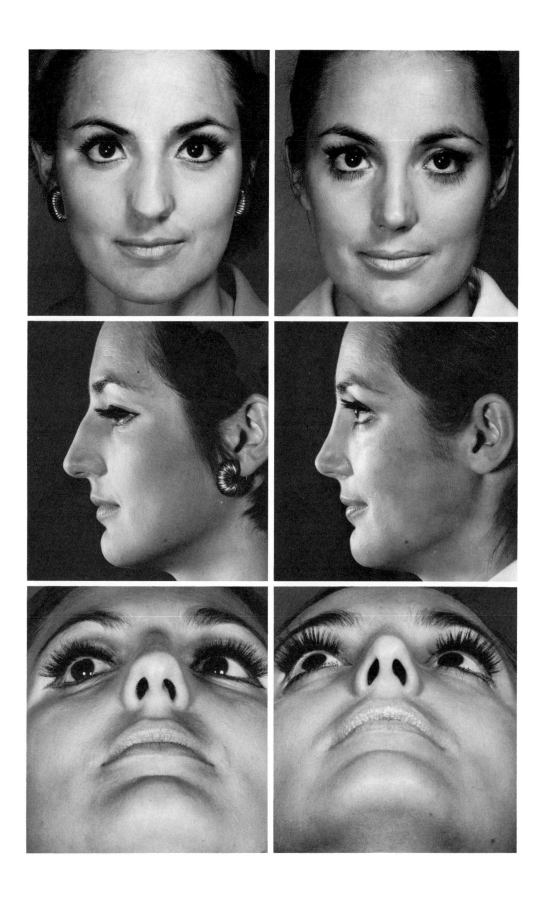

THE SURGICAL PLAN

A: Excision of redundant alar cartilage, leaving the rims intact but weakening
            them with cross cuts.
B,C: A slight diastasis of the alars was corrected with mattress sutures.
D–G: Preoperative and postoperative illustrations representing surgical plan.

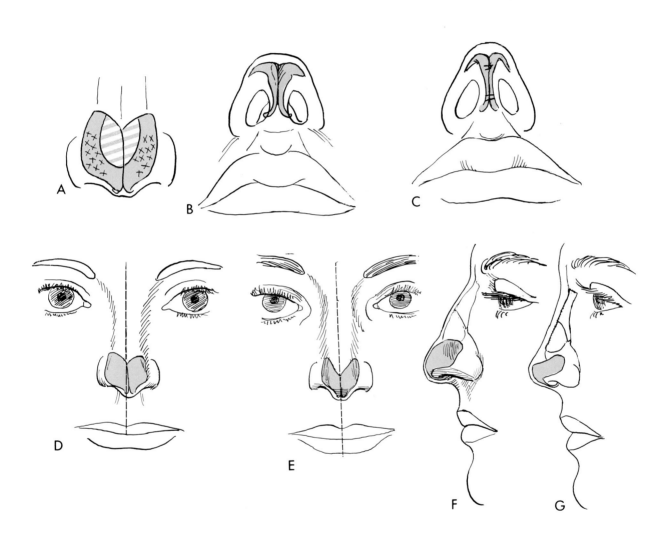

THE PROBLEM

The tip in this patient was somewhat broad and flattened on the dorsum of the nose. The angle formed between the medial and lateral crura was almost 90 degrees, giving the impression from below almost of a box-tip deformity.

The cartilages were quite thick and strong and the skin was thin, so that any defect of the underlying cartilages would be seen clearly through the skin. In addition, there was a definite plunging type of deformity, which was related to the downward angulation formed at the domes of the alar cartilages. The caudal septum also contributed slightly to the plunging deformity.

There was a very slight dorsal hump that required caution in reduction.

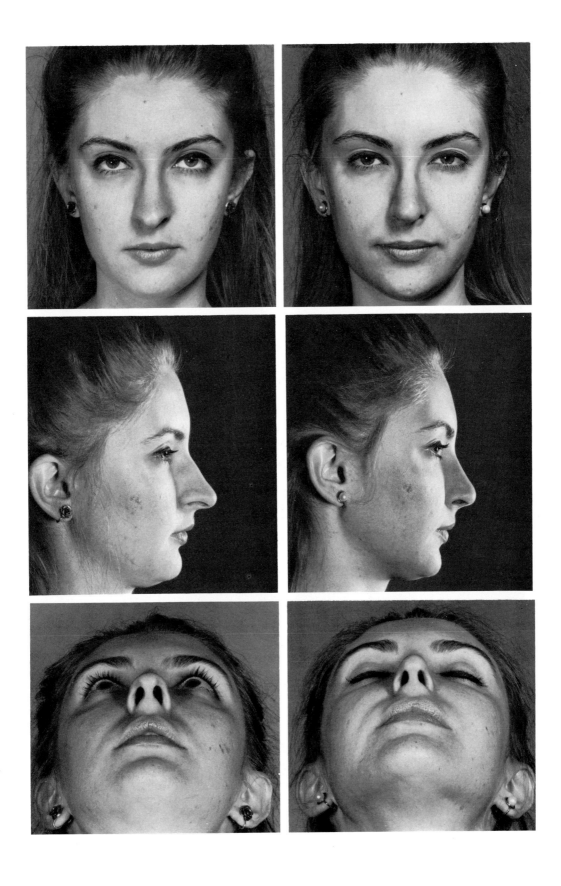

THE SURGICAL PLAN

A: The planned cartilage resection of the lateral crus is indicated in red. A slight separation of the caudal borders of the cartilage is shown by the arrows.

B: The dorsal profile was reduced slightly by rasping. The plunging tendency of the tip is indicated by the direction of the arrows. This must be corrected not only with cartilage resection but with a counter cephalic rotation of the tip and fixation at a higher level buttressed against the denuded caudal end of the septum.

C: The open angle of the alar cartilage anatomy is indicated by the arrows.

D: Front view after resection of the cephalic portion of the lateral crura and weakening of the remaining cartilage by small cross cuts.

E: The plunging tip was overcome by the surgical maneuvers indicated: elevation of the tip, resection of excess cartilage, recession of the tip, and fixation to the septum.

The bipedicle alar flap was ideal for this patient.

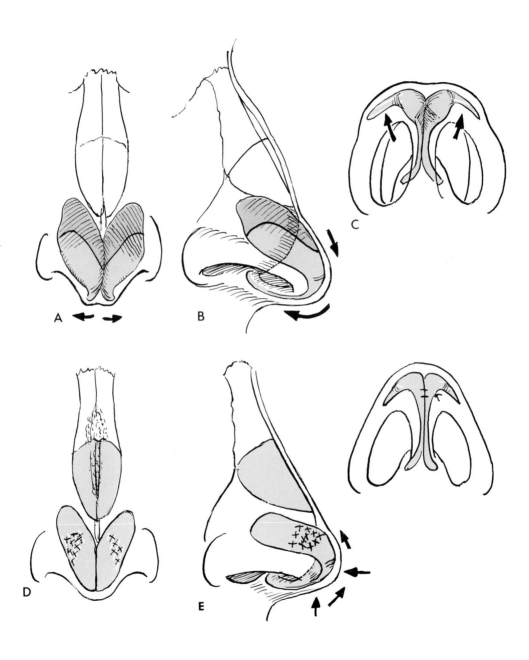

THE PROBLEM

This patient had one of the most difficult problems imaginable in rhinoplasty: a minimal skeletal hump and a strongly projecting caudal septal border with large alar cartilages.

The angle formed between the medial and the lateral crura projected downward, with an exaggerated curve to the inferior (caudal) margin of the medial crus that, together with the caudal septum, formed a plunging tip and a hanging columella.

The hanging columella is a function of all three of these anatomic problems, making it difficult to correct. In the front view, the increase in width of the alar cartilages can be seen. Part of this is because of diastasis of the cartilages and part because of the innate thickness of the cartilage and soft tissues.

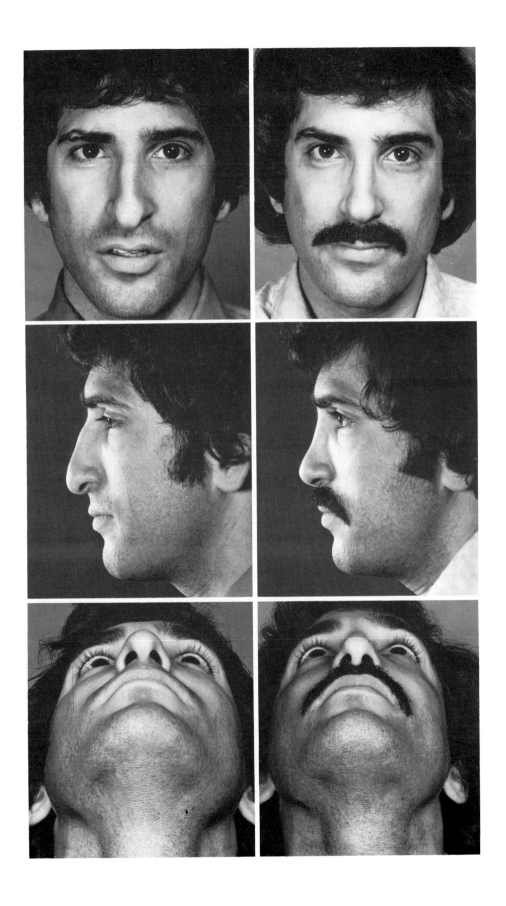

THE SURGICAL PLAN

A: The deformity viewed from the front. The alar cartilages were very large. The lateral crura also sweep in a cephalic direction. The transition between medial and lateral crura was elongated and exaggerated, accounting for much of the columellar overhang. There was also a slight twist to the dorsum.

B: The planned result.

C: The hanging tip rotated inferiorly on animation. The curvature was mostly due to the formation of the alar cartilages.

D: The plan was to excise the excess alar cartilage and reshape the inferior margins of the medial crura.

E,F: Inferior views showing plan to reverse the plunging forces and to gain length on the columella by bringing together the feet of the medial crura.

G: Amount of resection of cephalic portion of lateral crus is indicated.

H: Resection shown from front view.

I: Excessive resection of the caudal septum would accentuate plunging. Support for the tip on elevation would be eliminated.

J: Conservative trimming of the caudal septum was a must.

K: Desired cephalic rotation of alar cartilage shown by arrow.

L: Generous trimming of the caudal curving margins of the medial crura is indicated by red area.

M: "Tongue-in-groove" fixation of the denuded caudal septum between the medial crura is helpful in such problems to maintain tip elevation.

N: Front view after resection of lateral and medial crural elements.

O: The tip elevated into position and fixed with mattress sutures.

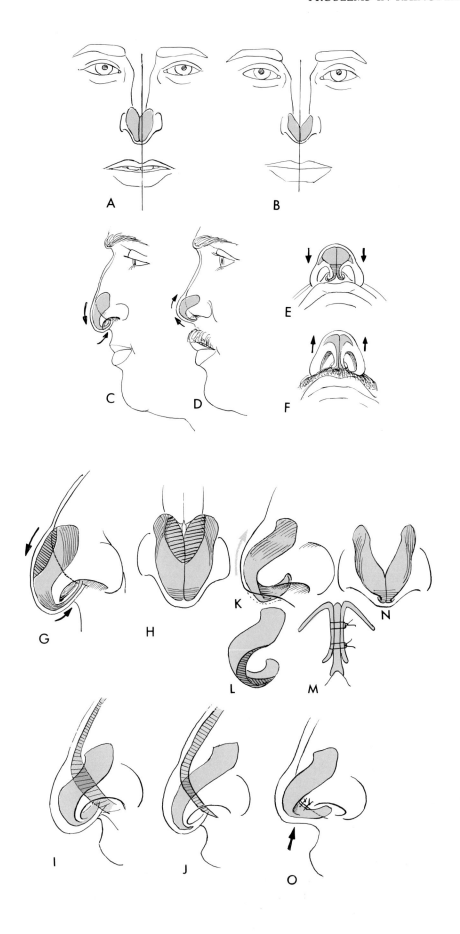

Chapter 14

The Non-Caucasian Nose

Thomas D. Rees, M.D., F.A.C.S.

The desire for a more perfect nose is by no means limited to the Caucasian race. Increasing numbers of people of Asian, African, and Indian extraction are undergoing rhinoplasty because of social, economic, and personal pressures.

Reports of rhinoplastic surgery in blacks are uncommon, although there are indications that the number of blacks seeking cosmetic surgery is increasing.

Rees (1969), Falces et al. (1970), Snyder (1971), Ortiz-Monasterio and Olmedo (1977), Stucker (1976), and de Alvelar (1976) discussed many of the special problems associated with rhinoplasty in the non-Caucasian nose, primarily in patients of black descent. Because of his unique and vast clinical experience with patients of Indian (Mestizo) extraction in Mexico, Dr. Ortiz-Monasterio has developed specialized techniques for dealing with these thick, difficult problem noses. Included in his armamentarium is the use of external dermabrasion and external incisions when required in order to affect a suitable overall reduction in the size of the Mestizo nose, as well as to acquire some degree of delicacy. The reader is urged to review his article on the subject in Clinics in Plastic Surgery (Vol. 4, 1977). The author has had minimal experience in treating the unique problems of the Indian nose.

Pitanguy (1965) described a "dermocartilaginous ligament" often associated with the flared, wide-tipped nose of mixed or Indian extraction in Brazil. Careful dissection of this ligament or thickened connective tissue is helpful in reducing the bulk of such tips and supratip areas quite considerably. (See Figure 9–49.)

The typical black nose is flattened and broad and often shows some degree of "saddle" deformity. The tip tends to be flat and rounded, and there is an increase in the angle between the medial and lateral crura at the alar dome. The alae are often flared and the nostrils are usually large.

There is frequently a low angle between the anterior and inferior border of the septum. This cartilaginous angle provides much of the tip projection of the nose. Whereas the projection of the septal angle must often be lowered in nasoplasty of Caucasians, in blacks it is generally desirable for it to be increased. This is best done by inserting a graft or implant. The inferior septal margin of the black nose is usually somewhat concave or receded, much like the retracted columella that may result from radical submucous resection with removal of the lower edge of the cartilaginous septum. It is rarely necessary to shorten the nose or to resect any of the inferior margin of the septum during rhinoplasty in blacks, but frequently it is necessary to insert a cartilage graft into the caudal border of the medial crura and the anterior aspect of the nasal spine.

The pyriform aperture is usually wide, with an increased distance between the nasal bones where they join the face. This may resemble the Caucasian nose after a direct blow to the dorsum has "splayed out" the bones. This increased distance between the facial attachments of the nasal bones gives the black nose a wide frontal appearance.

Text continued on page 450.

440

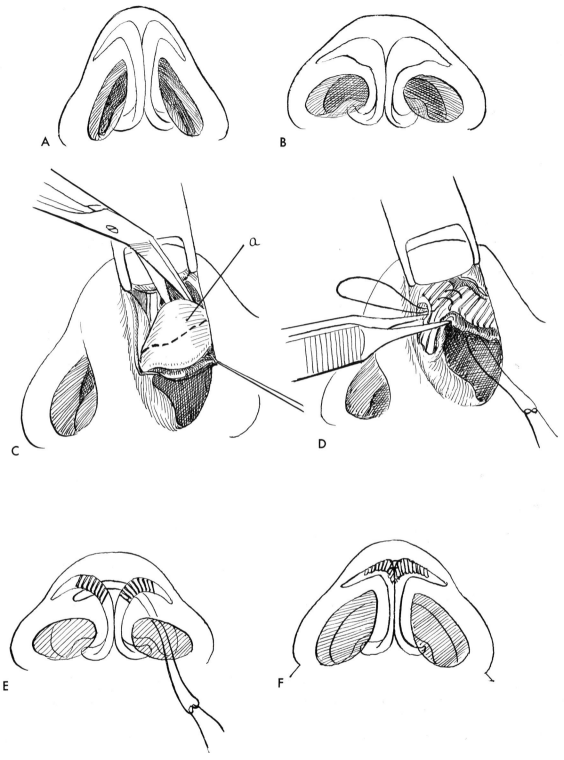

Figure 14–1. Rhinoplasty in the non-Caucasian nose requires a series of steps designed to alter those anatomic features that are different from those of the Caucasian. A prolonged and projecting tip with acute angulation of the alar crura and elliptical nares characterize the Caucasian nose *(A)*, while the non-Caucasian nose generally shows obtuse angulation of the alar domes, a short columella, flaring of the alae, and a low septal angle *(B)*.

The Lipsett maneuver used in reverse to achieve forward projection of the tip by suturing the scored alar cartilages has proved helpful. *C,* Exposure of the tip cartilages through a rim incision; "a" denotes the upper portion of the cartilage, which is to be removed (Safian, 1934). *D,* Weakening of the cartilage as in the Lipsett technique and "rolling in" of the lateral crura to form a new medial crus. *E,* A 4–0 plain catgut suture used to maintain the new medial crura in position. *F,* The medial crura in place (Rees, Guy, and Converse, 1966).

Illustration continued on the following page.

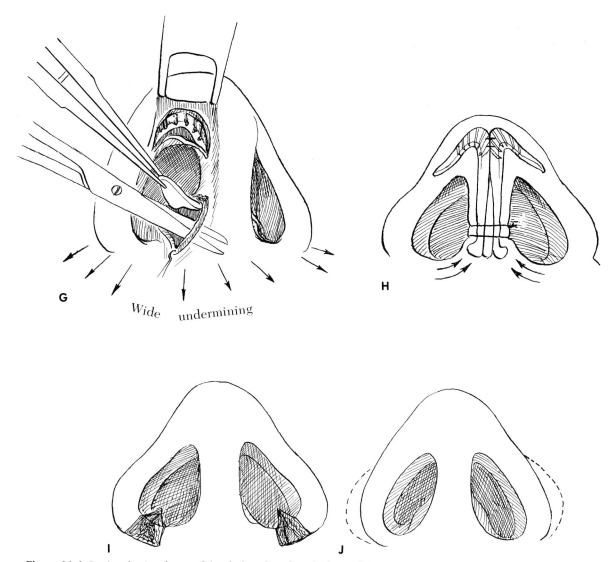

Figure 14–1 *Continued.*   Another useful technique is to free the base of the columella and suture the feet of the medial crura together. *G,* Wide undermining of the base of the columella and adjacent lip, to allow for sweeping of these soft tissues into a new columella to increase tip projection. *H,* After removal of the soft tissues lying between the feet of the medial crura, a 4–0 plain catgut suture approximates the crura and gains further tip projection.

Finally, alar base resections can reduce flaring. *I,* In this instance the resection mainly involves the floor of the nostril. *J,* The alar base resection completed, achieving both reduction of flaring and increase of projection.

(From Rees, T. D.: Plast. Reconstr. Surg. *43*:13, 1969. Reproduced with permission.)

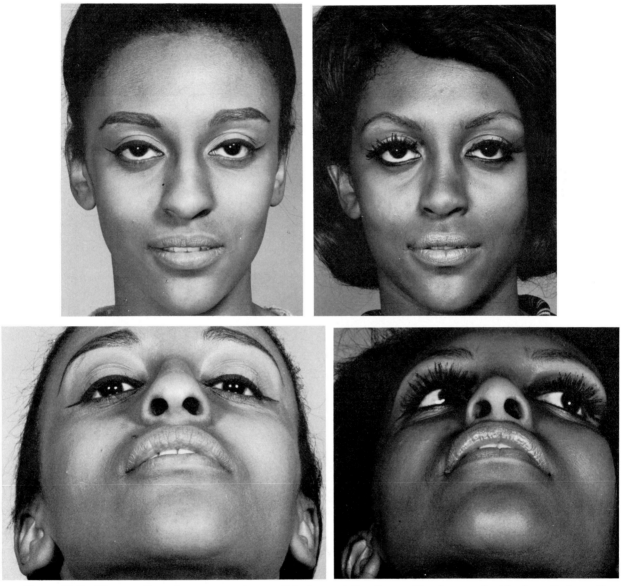

Figure 14–2.   The non-Caucasian nose may have a slight hump deformity, resulting from a mixed heritage. Postoperative views show the results of hump removal, narrowing osteotomy, and tip plasty.

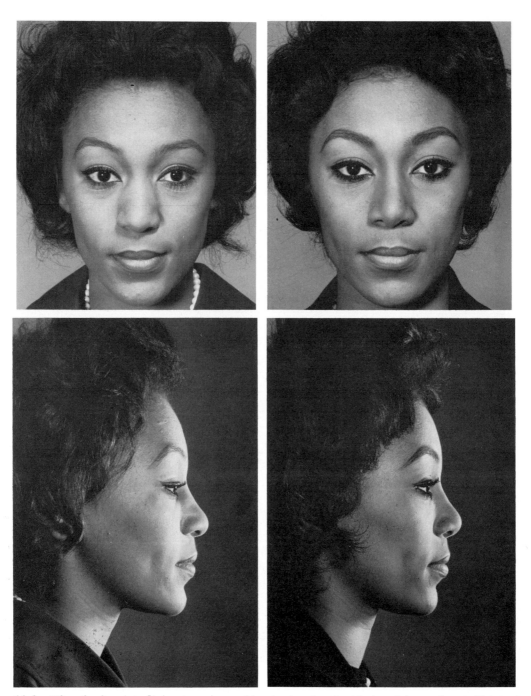

Figure 14–3. When the dorsal profile is not a major consideration but there is widening of the nasal pyramid, lateral osteotomy with infracture will not only narrow the nose but also result in a slight elevation of the nasal dorsum. This will often obviate the need for a dorsal implant. Osteotomy is done flush with the anterior surface of the maxilla to avoid "stair stepping" and is facilitated by the use of 3- or 4-mm. osteotomes.

(From Rees, T. D.: Plast. Reconstr. Surg. *43*:13, 1969. Reproduced with permission.)

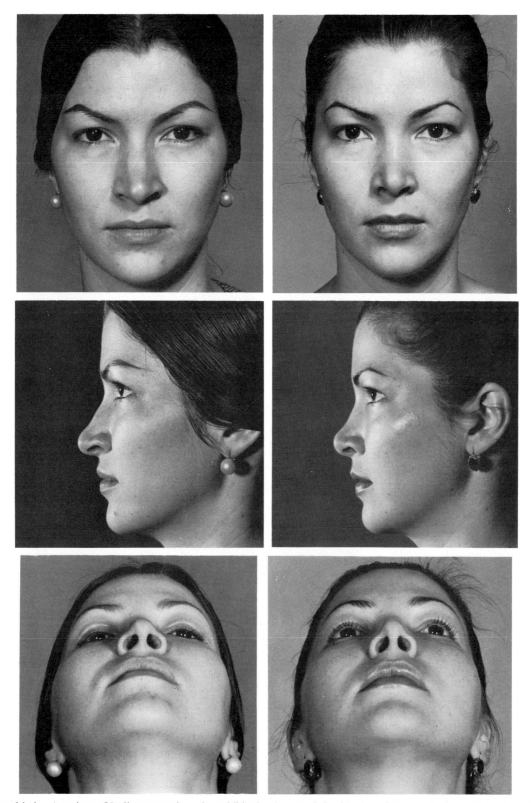

Figure 14–4. A patient of Indian extraction who exhibited a characteristic widening of the nasal base and flattening of the dorsum with a moderate degree of alar flare. The operative procedure consisted of lateral osteotomy, infracture, and a slight tip elevation. Flaring of the nostrils was diminished by alar base resection, and the supratip region was built up by inserting a small portion of septal cartilage under the dorsal skin.

In any patient with a significant degree of saddle deformity, a dorsal implant will be required. It may be inserted initially or secondarily. If the dissection has opened the nasal cavity into free communication with the submucous dissection, as is usual when the upper lateral cartilages are freed from the septum, a delay is advisable. This is especially true when alloplastic implants are being used for the correction.

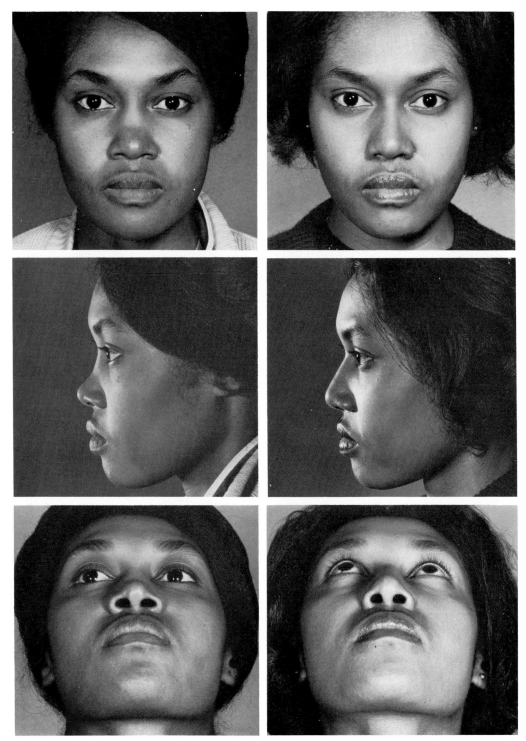

Figure 14–5. Correction of the supratip depression of a typical Negro nose. Correction in this patient was achieved in two stages: infracture with lateral osteotomy, followed after six weeks by insertion of a carved silicone dorsal implant.

Sometimes it is possible to infracture without disturbing the nasal lining, allowing dissection of a dorsal pocket for the graft with no connection to the airways except at the intercartilaginous incisions. In such instances the upper lateral cartilages are not freed from the septum, and the graft or implant is inserted through the intercartilaginous incision.

The choice between an autogenous bone graft and a prosthetic implant rests with the surgeon. The author prefers shaped silicone implants to correct natural saddle deformities in Negro or Asian noses, if the soft tissue is ample and unscarred. On the other hand, to repair a traumatized nose, with which there is often considerable scarring, contraction, and even loss of tissue, cancellous iliac bone is preferred, as it is less likely to be extruded or to cause skin breakdown.

The graft or implant should extend well up into the nasofrontal angle and downward to the supratip area. It should be so shaped that it does not pivot on an underlying bony fulcrum. Iliac bone grafts can be secured to the nasal bones by wire, an option that is not available when alloplastic implants are used.

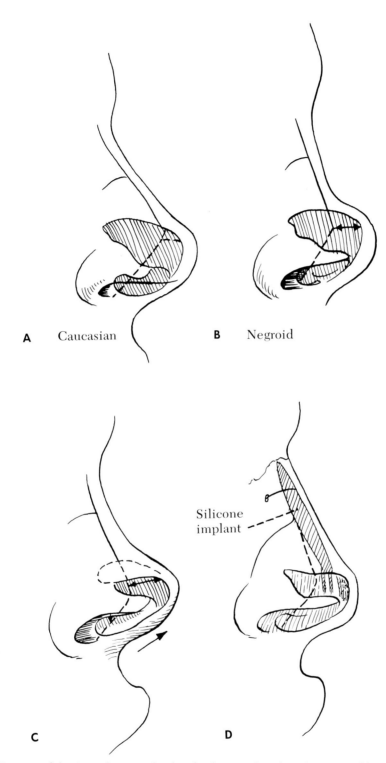

Figure 14–6. *A*, Features of the Caucasian nose showing the sharp angle and good support achieved by the nostril rims from the lateral crura of the alar cartilages. *B*, The typical Negroid nose, illustrating a relative saddle deformity, the obtuse septal angle and poor support achieved by the tip. There is usually a relative smallness of the alar cartilages and poor support of the nostril rim.

The non-Caucasian nose may be corrected. *C*, Projection of the nasal tip achieved by "rolling" of the lateral crus into the medial crus and removal of the upper border of the lateral crura. *D*, A silicone implant is placed along the nasal dorsum to correct the relative saddle deformity made more apparent by the tip projection. It is usually not desirable to fix a silicone implant in position with circumferential wire.

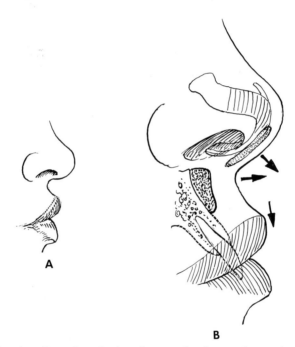

Figure 14–7. *A,* The acute lip-columella angle and columella retraction frequently seen in a non-Caucasian nose.

B, Improvement by a columella implant and an implant in the region of the nasal spine. These implants may be of silicone, cartilage, or bone.

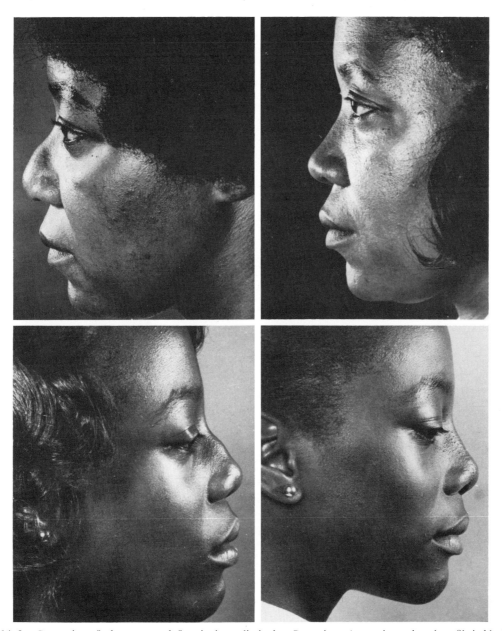

Figure 14–8. Correction of a hump nose deformity is not limited to Caucasians. A prominent dorsal profile in black patients is often accentuated by the relative shortness of the columella and lack of projection of the tip. A relative saddle deformity is more common in the black nose as well as all non-Caucasian noses. Correction of a hump nose deformity in the non-Caucasian is the same as in the Caucasian. The dorsal bone and cartilage should be lowered to achieve a natural and attractive line in connection with the tip projection.

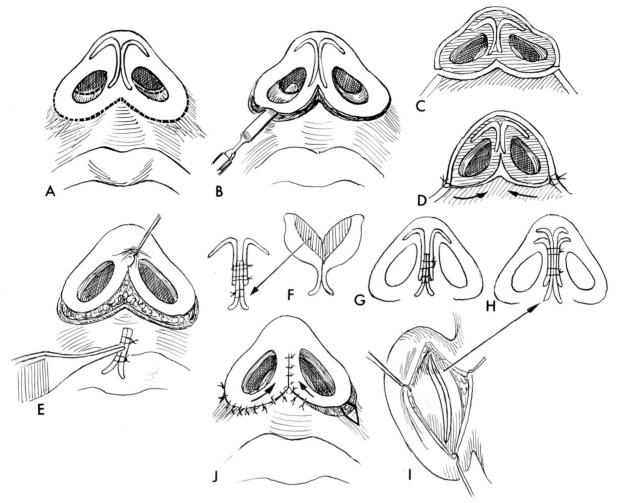

Figure 14–9.   The technique described by J. M. de Avelar (1976) is an adaptation of Cronin's technique for correcting nasal deformities in the bilateral cleft lip-nose problem. It is useful in gaining tip projection in the non-Caucasian nose, one of the major technical problems in rhinoplasty. A combination of the fine technical points of de Avelar and Cronin are illustrated above.

A, An incision is made around the base of the nostrils to the midline.

B, The soft tissues are freed with blunt and sharp dissection.

C, The dissection is completed. The base of the nose is detached.

D, Columellar length is obtained by medial rotation of the nostril flaps.

E–I, Grafts of autogenous cartilage are inserted to gain length and provide strength to the columella. These are obtained from the cephalic portion of the alar cartilages (*F*). They can be single or multi-tiered (*G* and *H*) and can be obtained from the concha of the ear (*I*).

J, The incisions are closed after rotation.

There are many minor anatomic variations in the "typical" black nose; intermarriage with other groups has produced structural differences that require special consideration when·performing nasal surgery. For example, blacks from the West Indies or the northern regions of Africa often have dorsal hump deformities of the nose, probably because of Indian or Arabic genetic influences. Such patients require reduction of this hump as part of the overall correction.

Figures 14–1 through 14–9 illustrate some of the common problems in non-Caucasian noses and the rhinoplastic procedures used to correct them.

REFERENCES

Anderson, J. R.: Straightening the crooked nose. Trans. Am. Acad. Ophthalmol. Otolaryngol. *76*:945, 1972.
Aston, S. J., and Guy, C. L.: The nasal spine. Clin. Plast. Surg. *4*:153, 1977.

Aufricht, G.: Combined nasal plastic and chin plastic; Correction of microgenia by an osteocartilaginous transplant from a large hump nose. Am. J. Surg. *25*:292, 1934.

Aufricht, G.: A few hints and surgical details in rhinoplasty. Laryngoscope *53*:317, 1943.

Aufricht, G.: Surgery of the radix and bony nose; Preliminary report of a new type of nasal clamp. Plast. Reconstr. Surg. *22*:315, 1958.

Aufricht, G.: Rhinoplasty and the face. Plast. Reconstr. Surg. *43*:219, 1969.

Aufricht, G.: Joseph's rhinoplasty with some modifications. Surg. Clin. North Am. *51*:299, 1971.

Baker, D. C., and Strauss, R. B.: The physiologic treatment of nasal obstruction. Clin. Plast. Surg. *4*:121, 1977.

Becker, O. J.: Problems of the septum in rhinoplastic surgery. Trans. Am. Acad. Ophthalmol. Otolaryngol. *55*:244, 1951.

Beekhuis, G. J.: Nasal obstruction after rhinoplasty: Etiology and techniques for correction. Laryngoscope *86*:540, 1976.

Bernstein, L.: The basic technique for surgery of the nasal lobule. Otolaryngol. Clin. North Am. *8*:599, 1975.

Berson, M. I.: Prevention of deformities in corrective rhinoplasty. Laryngoscope *53*:276, 1943.

Boo-Chai, K.: Augmentation rhinoplasty in the Oriental. Plast. Reconstr. Surg. *34*:81, 1964.

Brent, B.: Conchal cartilage. *In* Sheen, J.: Aesthetic Rhinoplasty. St. Louis, C. V. Mosby Co., 1978.

Brown, J. B., and McDowell, F.: Plastic Surgery of the Nose. Springfield, Ill., Charles C Thomas, 1965.

Buttler, J.: Work of breathing through the nose. Clin. Sci. *19*:55, 1960.

Calzolari, L.: Rhinoplastica correttiva. Minerva Chir. *20*:14, 1965.

Champion, R.: Anosmia associated with corrective rhinoplasty. Br. J. Plast. Surg. *19*:182, 1966.

Cinelli, J. A.: Correction of the combined elongated nose and recessed naso-labial angle. Plast. Reconstr. Surg. *21*:139, 1958.

Cinelli, J. A.: Lengthening of the nose by a septal flap. Plast. Reconstr. Surg. *43*:99, 1969.

Cohen, S.: Postrhinoplastic intranasal adhesions. Arch. Otolaryngol. *54*:683, 1951.

Cohen, S.: Complications following rhinoplasty. Plast. Reconstr. Surg. *18*:213, 1956.

Cole, P.: Further observations on the conditioning of respiratory air. J. Laryngol. *67*:669, 1953.

Conroy, W. C.: Simple nasal tip setback. Plast. Reconstr. Surg. *33*:564, 1964.

Converse, J. M.: Corrective surgery of nasal deviations. Arch. Otolaryngol. *52*:671, 1950.

Converse, J. M.: Maxillofacial deformities and maxillofacial prosthetics. J. Prosthet. Dent. *13*:511, 1963.

Converse, J. M., Wood-Smith, D., Wang, M. K. H., Macomber, B., and Guy, C. L.: Deformities of the nose. *In* Converse, J. M. (ed.): Plastic Reconstructive Surgery. Philadelphia, W. B. Saunders Company, 1964, pp. 869–948.

Cottle, M. H.: Concepts of nasal physiology as related to corrective nasal surgery. Arch. Otolaryngol. *72*:11, 1960.

de Avelar, J. M.: Personal contribution for the surgical treatment of the Negroid nose. Aesth. Plast. Surg. *1*:81, 1976.

Denecke, H. J., and Meyer, R.: Plastic Surgery of Head and Neck. New York, Springer Verlag, 1967.

Diamond, H.: Rhinoplasty techniques. Surg. Clin. North Am. *51*:317, 1971.

Dieffenbach, J.: Die operative Chirurgie. Leipzig, 1845.

Dingman, R.: Corrections of nasal deformities due to defects of the septum. Plast. Reconstr. Surg. *18*:291, 1956.

Dingman, R., and Walter, C.: Use of composite ear grafts in correction of the short nose. Plast. Reconstr. Surg. *43*:117, 1969.

Dufourmentel, C., and Mouly, R.: Chirurgie Plastique. Paris, Flammarian et Cie, 1959.

Dupont, C., Cloutier, G. E., and Prevost, Y.: Autogenous vomer bone graft for permanent correction of the cartilagenous septal deviations. Plast. Reconstr. Surg. *38*:243, 1966.

Eitner, E.: Kosmetische Operationen. Berlin, Springer Verlag, 1932.

Falces, E., Wesser, D., and Gorney, M.: Cosmetic surgery of the non-Caucasian nose. Plast. Reconstr. Surg. *45*:317, 1970.

Farina, R.: Plastica de navig; Tratamento do dorso esteo cartilaginosoe perfil nasal. Rev. Paul. Med. *64*:23, 1964.

Flowers, R. S., and Anderson, R.: Injury to the lacrimal apparatus during rhinoplasty. Plast. Reconstr. Surg. *42*:577, 1968.

Fomon, S.: Cosmetic Surgery, Principles and Practice. Philadelphia, J. B. Lippincott Company, 1960.

Fomon, S., and Bell, J. W.: Rhinoplasty — A fine art. Arch. Otolaryngol. *85*:685, 1967.

Fomon, S., and Bell, J. W.: Rhinoplasty — New Concepts: Evaluation and Application. Springfield, Ill, Charles C Thomas, 1970.

Fomon, S., Bell, J. W., Lubart, J., Schattner, A., and Syracuse, V. R.: The nasal hump problem. Arch. Otolaryngol. *79*:164, 1964.

Fomon, S., Bell, J. W., Schattner, A., and Syracuse, V. R.: Postoperative elongation of the nose. Arch. Otolaryngol. *64*:456, 1956.

Fomon, S., Sayad, W. Y., Schattner, A., and Neivert, H.: Physiological principles in rhinoplasty. Arch. Otolaryngol. *53*:256, 1951.

Fred, G. B.: Postoperative dropping of the nasal tip after rhinoplasty. Arch. Otolaryngol. *67*:177, 1958.

Fredericks, S.: Tripod resection for "Pinocchio" nose deformity. Plast. Reconstr. Surg. *53*:531, 1972.

Fry, H.: Nasal skeletal trauma and the interlocked stresses of the nasal septal cartilage. Br. J. Plast. Surg. *20*:146, 1967.

Gibson, T., and Davis, W. B.: The distortion of autogenous cartilage grafts: Its causes and prevention. Br. J. Plast. Surg. *10*:257, 1958.

Gnudi, M. T., and Webster, J. P.: The Life and Times of Gasparé Tagliacozzi, Surgeon of Bologna (1545–1599). New York, Reichner, 1950.

Goldman, I. B.: Rhinoplasty: Its surgical complications and how to avoid them. J. Int. Coll. Surg. *13*:285, 1950.

Goldman, I. B.: The importance of the medical crura in nasal-tip reconstruction. Arch. Otolaryngol. *65*:143, 1957.

Goldwyn, R. M., and Shore, S.: The effects of submucous resection and rhinoplasty on the sense of smell. Plast. Reconstr. Surg. *41*:427, 1968.

González-Ulloa, M.: Quantitative principles in cosmetic surgery of the face (profileplasty). Plast. Reconstr. Surg. *29*:186, 1962.

Gordon, H. L., and Baker, T. J.: Primary cosmetic rhinoplasty. Clin. Plast. Surg. *4*:9, 1977.

Grignon, J. L.: Les eches des rhinoplasties. Ann. Otolaryngol. (Paris) *80*:51, 1963.

Hage, J.: Collapsed alae strengthened by conchal cartilage; The butterfly cartilage graft. Br. J. Plast. Surg. *18*:92, 1964.

Hilding, A.: Experimental surgery of the nose and sinuses. I. Changes in the morphology of epithelium following variations in ventilation. Arch. Otolaryngol. *16*:9, 1932.

Inoue, S., and Harashima, H.: Rhinomanometry. Otologia (Fukuoka) *24*:445, 1952.

Kazanjian, V. H., and Converse, J. M.: The Surgical Treatment of Facial Injuries. Baltimore, The Williams & Wilkins Co., 1972.

Klabunde, E. H., and Falces, E.: Incidence of complications in cosmetic rhinoplasties. Plast. Reconstr. Surg. *34*:192, 1964.

Konno, A.: Air flow and resistance in the nasal cavity. Part I. Observation on nasal airflow, using the model made from nasal and nasopharyngeal casts of the human body. Part 2. Bilateral rhinometry using a pneumotachometer. Its principles and clinical application. J. Otolaryngol. Jap. *72*:36–48; 49–65, 1969.

Levignac, J.: Des petitis et des gros ennuis dans la rhinoplastie. Ann. Otolaryngol. (Paris) 75:560, 1958.

Lewis, M. L.: Prevention and correction of cicatricial intranasal adhesions in rhinoplastic surgery. Arch. Otolaryngol. 60:215, 1954.

Lillie, J. C.: Methods in Medical Research, Vol. 2, edited by J. H. Comroe. Chicago, The Year Book Publishing Co., 1950.

Lipsett, E. M.: A new approach to surgery of the lower cartilaginous vault. Arch. Otolaryngol. 70:42, 1959.

Maliniac, J. W.: Prevention and treatment of sequelae in corrective rhinoplasty. Am. J. Surg. 50:84, 1940.

McIndoe, A., and McLaughlin, C. R.: Advances in plastic surgery. Practitioner 169:427, 1952.

McIndoe, A.: Personal communication, 1955.

Meyer, R., and Kesselring, U. K.: Sculpturing and reconstructive procedures in aesthetic and functional rhinoplasty. Clin. Plast. Surg. 4:15, 1977.

Millard, D. R.: External excisions in rhinoplasty. Br. J. Plast. Surg. 12:340, 1960.

Millard, D. R.: The triad of columella deformities. Plast. Reconstr. Surg. 31:370, 1963.

Millard, D. R.: Adjuncts in augmentation mentoplasty and corrective rhinoplasty. Plast. Reconstr. Surg. 36:48, 1965.

Millard, D. R.: Secondary corrective rhinoplasty. Plast. Reconstr. Surg. 44:545, 1969.

Millard, D. R.: Congenital nasal tip retrusion and three little composite ear grafts. Plast. Reconstr. Surg. 48:501, 1971.

Millard, D. R.: The versatility of a chondromucosal flap in the nasal vestibule. Plast. Reconstr. Surg. 50:580, 1972.

Natvig, P., Sether, L. A., Gingrass, R. P., and Gardner, W. D.: Anatomical details of the osseo-cartilaginous framework of the nose. Plast. Reconstr. Surg. 48:528, 1971.

O'Connor, G. B., and McGregor, M. W.: Secondary rhinoplasties: Their cause and prevention. Plast. Reconstr. Surg. 15:404, 1955.

O'Connor, G. B., McGregor, M. W., Shapiro, L., and Tolleth, H.: The bulbous nose. Plast. Reconstr. Surg. 39:278, 1967.

Ogura, J. H., Togawa, K., Dammkoehler, K., Nelson, J. R., and Kawasaki, M.: Nasal obstruction and the mechanics of breathing. Physiologic relationship and effects of nasal surgery. Arch. Otolaryngol. 83:135, 1966.

Ogura, J. H., Unno, T., and Nelson, J. R.: Nasal surgery. Physiological considerations of nasal obstruction. Arch Otolaryngol. 88:288, 1968.

Ortiz-Monasterio, F., Lopez-Mas, J., and Araico, J.: Rhinoplasty in the thick-skinned nose. Br. J. Plast. Surg. 27:19, 1974.

Ortiz-Monasterio, F., and Olmeda, A.: Rhinoplasty on the mestizo nose. Clin. Plast. Surg. 4:89, 1977.

Peck, G.: Rhinoplasty surgery. In Millard, D. R. (ed.): Symposium on Corrective Rhinoplasty. St. Louis, C. V. Mosby Co., 1976, p. 8.

Pitanguy, I.: Surgical importance of a dermacartilaginous ligament in bulbous noses. Plast. Reconstr. Surg. 36:247, 1965.

Planas, H.: The twisted nose. Clin. Plast. Surg. 4:55, 1977.

Pollet, J., and Baudelot, S.: Séquelles de la chirurgie esthétique de la base du nez. Ann. Chir. Plast. (Paris) 12:185, 1967.

Pollet, J.: Three autogenous struts for nasal tip support. Plast. Reconstr. Surg. 49:527, 1972.

Pollet, J., and Weikel, A. M.: Some technical considerations in primary rhinoplasty. Aesth. Plast. Surg. 1:25, 1976.

Pollet, J., and Weikel, A. M.: Revision rhinoplasty. Clin. Plast. Surg. 4:47, 1977.

Proetz, A. W.: Respiratory air currents and their clinical aspects. J. Laryngol. 67:1, 1953.

Rees, T. D.: Nasal plastic surgery in the Negro. Plast. Reconstr. Surg. 43:13, 1969.

Rees, T. D., Guy, G. L., and Converse, J. M.: Repair of the cleft-lip nose; Addendum to the synchronous technique with full-thickness skin grafting of the nasal vestibule. Plast. Reconstr. Surg. 37:47, 1966.

Rees, T. D., Krupp, S., and Wood-Smith, D.: Secondary rhinoplasty. Plast. Reconstr. Surg. 46:322, 1970.

Rees, T. D.: An aid in the treatment of supratip swelling after rhinoplasty. Laryngoscope 81:308, 1971.

Rees, T. D.: Current concepts of rhinoplasty. Clin. Plast. Surg. 4:131, 1977.

Rees, T. D.: Rhinoplasty in the older adult. Ann. Plast. Surg. 1:27, 1978.

Rethi, A.: Right and wrong in rhinoplastic operations. Plast. Reconstr. Surg. 3:361, 1948.

Rode, B.: Zur Technik des Gipsverbandes in der Behandlung der Nasenbein-frakturen und Deformitäten. Z. Hals. Nas. Ohrenheilk. 43:294, 1938.

Roe, J. O.: The deformity termed "pug nose" and its correction by a simple operation. Med. Rec. 31:621, 1887.

Roe, J. O.: The correction of angular deformities of the nose by subcutaneous operation. Med. Rec. New York 40:57, 1891.

Rogers, B. O.: Secondary and tertiary rhinoplasty. Transactions of the 4th International Congress of Plastic and Reconstructive Surgery, pp. 1065–1071. Amsterdam, Excerpta Medica Foundation, 1969.

Rogers, B. O.: Rhinoplasty. In Goldwyn, R. M. (ed.): The unfavorable result in plastic surgery. Boston, Little, Brown and Co., 1972.

Rogers, B. O.: Early historical developments of corrective rhinoplasty. In Millard, D. R. (ed.): Symposium on Corrective Rhinoplasty. St. Louis, C. V. Mosby Co., 1976, p. 18.

Rogers, B. O.: Secondary and tertiary correction of postrhinoplastic deformities: Some Dos and Don'ts. In Millard, D. R. (ed.): Symposium on Corrective Rhinoplasty. St. Louis, C. V. Mosby Co., 1976, p. 23.

Rohrer, F.: Der Stromungsmiderstand in den menschlichen Ateurwegen und der Einfluss der unregelmässigen Verzweigung des Bronchialsystems auf den Atmungsveilauf in verschiedenen Lungenbeziken. Pfluger's Arch. J. Ges. Physiol. 162:255, 1915.

Safian, J.: Corrective Rhinoplastic Surgery. New York, Paul B. Hoeber, Inc., 1935.

Safian, J.: Fact and fallacy in rhinoplastic surgery. Br. J. Plast. Surg. 11:45, 1958.

Safian, J.: The split-cartilage tip technique or rhinoplasty. Plast. Reconstr. Surg. 45:217, 1970.

Seeley, R. D.: Reconstruction of the nasal tip: A new technique. Plast. Reconstr. Surg. 3:594, 1948.

Seltzer, A. P.: Cautions in rhinoplastic surgery. Eye Ear Nose Throat Monthly 32:35, 1953.

Seltzer, A. P.: The surgically induced saddle nose. Eye Ear Nose Throat Monthly 30:250, 1951.

Sheen, J. H.: Supratarsal fixation in upper blepharoplasty. Plast. Reconstr. Surg. 54:424, 1974.

Sheen, J. H.: Secondary rhinoplasty. Plast. Reconstr. Surg. 56:137, 1975.

Sheen, J. H.: Achieving more nasal tip projection by use of small autogenous vomer or septal cartilage grafts. Plast. Reconstr. Surg. 56:35, 1975. (Discussion by Horton, C. E.: Plast. Reconstr. Surg. 56:211, 1975.)

Sheen, J. H.: Absorption of small bone graft in nasal tip (letter to the ed.). Plast. Reconstr. Surg. 56:332, 1975.

Sheen, J. H.: Secondary rhinoplasty surgery. In Millard, D. R. (ed.): Symposium on Corrective Rhinoplasty. St. Louis, C. V. Mosby Co., 1976, p. 133.

Sheen, J. H.: A change in the technique of supratarsal fixation in upper blepharoplasty. Plast. Reconstr. Surg. 59:831, 1977.

Sheen, J. H.: Tarsal fixation in lower blepharoplasty. Plast. Reconstr. Surg. 62:24, 1978.

Ship, A. G.: Alar base resection for wide flaring nostrils. Br. J. Plast. Surg. 28:77, 1975.

Shulman, J.: Personal communication, 1977.

Silver, A. G.: Pitfalls in rhinoplasty. Eye Ear Nose Throat Monthly 31:556, 1952.

Skoog, T.: A method of hump reduction in rhinoplasty. Arch. Otolaryngol. 83:283, 1966.

Skoog, T.: Plastic Surgery. Philadelphia, W. B. Saunders Co., 1975.

Smith, T. W.: As clay in the potter's hand. Ohio Med. J. 63:1055, 1967.

Snyder, G. B.: Rhinoplasty in the Negro. Plast. Reconstr. Surg. 47:572, 1971.

Speizer, F., and Frank, R.: A technique for measuring nasal and pulmonary flow resistance simultaneously. J. Appl. Physiol. 19:176, 1964.

Steiss, C. F.: Errors in rhinoplasty and their prevention. Plast. Reconstr. Surg. 28:276, 1961.

Stokstead, P.: The physiological cycle of the nose under normal and pathological conditions. Acta Otolaryngol. 42:175, 1952.

Stucker, F. J.: Non-Caucasian rhinoplasty. Trans. Am. Acad. Ophthalmol. Otolaryngol. 82:417, 1971.

Takahashi, K.: Verläufige Mitteilungen über die Erfarochung. Z. Laryng. 11:203, 1922.

Takemiya, S., Togawa, K., Unno, T., and Konno, A.: Bilateral rhinomanometry using pneumotachometer. Japan. J. Otolaryngol. (Tokyo) 66:985, 1963.

Tonndorf, W.: Der Weg der Atemluft in der Menshclichen Nase. Arch. J. Orh-USW. H.K. 41:146, 1939.

Uchida, J.: The Practice of Plastic Surgery. Tokyo, Kinbara, 1958, p. 62.

Weir, R. F.: On restoring sunken noses without scarring the face. New York Med. J. 56:449, 1892.

Wexler, M.: Post-rhinoplastic complications. Eye Ear Nose Throat Monthly 31:553, 1969.

Willemot, J.: Correction of old nasal deviations. Plast. Reconstr. Surg. 43:430, 1969.

Williams, H. L.: Report of committee on standardization of definitions, terms, symbols in rhinometry of the American Academy of Ophthalmology and Otolaryngology. American Academy of Ophthalmology and Otolaryngology, 1970.

Williams, J. E.: The pinched nasal tip. Clin. Plast. Surg. 4:41, 1977.

Wright, W. K.: Study on hump removal in rhinoplasty. Laryngoscope 77:508, 1967.

Physiology

Abramson, M., and Harker, L. A.: Physiology of the nose. Otolaryngol. Clin. North Am. 6:623, 1973.

Baker, D. C., Jr.: Steroid therapy in otolaryngology. Trans. Am. Acad. Ophthalmol. Otolaryngol. 76:297, 1972.

Baker, D. C., Jr., and Strauss, R. B.: Intranasal injections of long-acting corticosteroids. Ann. Otol. Rhinol. Laryngol. 71:525, 1962.

Baker, D. C., and Strauss, R. B.: The physiologic treatment of nasal obstruction. Clin. Plast. Surg. 4:121, 1977.

Baran, M. L. R.: Le risque d'amaurose au cours du traitement local des alopécies par corticotherapie injectable. Bull. Soc. Fr. Derm. Syphiligr. 71:25, 1964. (Abstracted in Schoch, A. G., and Alexander, L. J.: The Schoch Letter: Current News in Dermatology. Dallas, The Penicillin Research Center, January 1965.

Barelli, P. A.: The anatomy and surgery of the lower lateral cartilage. In The American Rhinologic Society: Rhinologic Lectures from the Kansas City Courses, 1977.

Barelli, P. A.: Personal communication, 1978.

Beekhuis, G. J.: Nasal obstruction after rhinoplasty: etiology and techniques for correction. Laryngoscope 86:540, 1976.

Blaxter, P. L., and Britten, M. J. A.: Transient amaurosis after mandibular nerve block. Br. Med. J. 1:681, 1967.

Blue, J. A.: Rhinitis medicamentosa. Ann. Allergy 26:425, 1968.

Bridger, P.: Physiology of the nasal valve. Arch. Otolaryngol. 92:543, 1970.

Brown, E. A.: Nasal function and nasal neurosis. Ann. Allergy 9:563, 1951.

Chervinsky, P.: Dexamethosone aerosol in perennial allergic rhinitis. Ann. Allergy 24:150, 1966.

Cinelli, A. A.: Physiologic rhinoplastic principles. In Maloney,

W. H. (ed.): Otolaryngology. New York, Harper and Row, 1971.

Cockcroft, D. W., MacCormick, D. W., Newhouse, M. T., and Hargreave, F. E.: Beclomethasone dipropionate aerosol in allergic rhinitis. Can. Med. Assoc. J. 115:523, 1976.

Cole, P.: Further observations on the conditioning of respiratory air. J. Laryngol. 67:669, 1953.

Cottle, M. H.: The structure and function of the nasal vestibule. Arch. Otolaryngol. 62:173, 1955.

Cottle, M. H.: Concepts of nasal physiology as related to corrective nasal surgery. Arch. Otolaryngol. 72:11, 1960.

Cottle, M. H.: Personal communication, 1978.

Courtiss, E. H., Goldwyn, R. M., and O'Brien, J. O.: Resection of obstructing inferior nasal turbinates. Plast. Reconstr. Surg. 62:249, 1978.

Dolowitz, D. A.: Drug treatment in allergic disorders. Otolaryngol. Clin. North Am. 4:591, 1971.

Dutrow, H. V.: Conservative surgical treatment of hypertrophic rhinitis. Arch. Otolaryngol. 21:59, 1935.

Ersner, M. S.: Rhinoplastic procedures to establish normal physiologic function. Penn. Med. J. 51:749, 1948.

Fomon, S., Silver, A. G., Gilbert, J. G., and Syracuse, V. R.: Physiologic surgery of the nares. Arch. Otolaryngol. 47:608, 1948.

Fry, H. J. H.: Judicious turbinectomy for nasal obstruction. Aust. N.Z. J. Surg. 42:291, 1973.

Fry, H. J. H.: The fractured nose. In Calnan, J. (ed.): Recent Advances in Plastic Surgery. London, Churchill Livingstone, 1976.

Gibson, G. J., Maberly, D. J., Lal, S., et al.: Double-blind crossover trial comparing intranasal beclomethosone dipropionate and placebo in perennial rhinitis. Br. Med. J. 4:503, 1974.

Golding-Wood, P. H.: Observations on petrosal and vidian neurectomy in chronic vasomotor rhinitis. J. Laryngol. 75:232, 1961.

Golding-Wood, P. H.: Vidian neurectomy: its results and complications. Laryngoscope 83:1673, 1973.

Goldman, I. B.: Rhinoplastic sequelae causing nasal obstruction. Arch. Otolaryngol. 83:151, 1966.

Goode, R. L.: Diagnosis and Treatment of Turbinate Dysfunction. American Academy of Otolaryngology, 1977.

Goodman, L. S., and Gilman, A. (eds.): The Pharmacological Basis of Therapeutics. New York, MacMillan Company, 1975.

Gorney, M.: The septum in rhinoplasty: form and function. In Millard, D. R. (ed.): Symposium on Corrective Rhinoplasty. St. Louis, C. V. Mosby Co., 1977.

Hager, G., and Heise, G.: Uber eine schwere Komplikation mit bleibender praktischer Erblindung eines Auges nach intranasaler injektion. H. N. O. 10:325, 1962.

Hasegawa, M., and Kern, E. B.: The human nasal cycle. Mayo Clin. Proc. 52:28, 1977.

Heetderks, D. R.: Observations on the reaction of normal nasal mucous membrane. Am. J. Med. Sci. 174:231, 1927.

Hinderer, K. H.: Diagnosis of anatomic obstruction of the airways. Arch. Otolaryngol. 78:660, 1963.

Hinderer, K. H.: Anatomy and physiology of the valve. In The American Rhinologic Society: Rhinologic Lectures from the Kansas City Courses, 1977.

Holmes, T. H., Goodell, H., Wolf, S., and Wolff, H. G.: The nose, an experimental study of reactions within the nose in human subjects during varying life experiences. Springfield, Ill., Charles C Thomas, 1950.

Horton, C. E.: Combined septoplasty and rhinoplasty. In Symposium on Aesthetic Surgery of the Nose, Ears, and Chin. St. Louis, C. V. Mosby Co., 1973.

House, H. P.: Submucous resection of the inferior turbinal bone. Laryngoscope 61:637, 1951.

Hurd, L. M., and Holden, W. A.: A case of paraffin injection into the nose followed immediately by blindness from embolism of the central artery of the retina. Med. Rec. 64:53, 1903.

Jaffe, B. F.: Diseases and surgery of the nose. Clin. Symp. 26:1, 1974.

Joseph, G.: Preliminary discussion of the thick septum problem. Rev. Laryngol. Otol. Rhinol. 5:111, 1967.

Kabaker, S. S.: The collected letters of the International Correspondence Society of Ophthalmogists and Otolaryngologists, October 30, 1975.

Kayser, R. L.: Uber den Weg der Atmungluft durch die nase. Arch. Laryngol. 3:101, 1895.

Kern, E. B.: Rhinomanometry. Otolaryngol. Clin. North Am. 6:863, 1973.

Kern, E. B.: Surgery of the nasal valve. In Sisson, G. A., and Tardy, M. E. (eds.): Plastic and Reconstructive Surgery of the Face and Neck. Stuttgart, Georg Thieme Verlag, 1975.

Konno, A.: Surgical physiology of the nose. In Rees, T. D., and Wood-Smith, D. (eds.): Cosmetic Facial Surgery. Philadelphia, W. B. Saunders Company, 1973.

Lichtenstein, L. M., and Norman, P. S.: Pathogenesis of allergic rhinitis. In Samter, M. (ed.): Immunological Diseases. Boston, Little, Brown and Co., 1971.

Little, S. W.: Management of enlarged turbinates. Va. Med. Monthly 90:484, 1963.

Mabry, R. L.: Intranasal Steroid Injection. Poster Presentation at the American Academy of Otolaryngology, September, 1978.

Mabry, R. L.: Intraturbinal steroid injection: indications, results, complications. South. Med. J. 71:789, 1978.

MacKenzie, J. N.: Irritation of the sexual apparatus as an etiological factor in the production of nasal disease. Am. J. Med. Sci. 87:360, 1884.

Markham, J. W.: Sudden loss of vision following alcohol block of the infraorbital nerve. J. Neurosurg. 38:655, 1973.

May, M., and West, J. W.: The "stuffy" nose. Otolaryngol. Clin. North Am. 6:655, 1973.

McCleve, D. F., and Goldstein, G. C.: Treatment of allergic and vasomotor rhinitis with corticosteroid injections of the turbinates. Read Before the American Academy of Opthalmology and Otolaryngology, October 1, 1977.

McGrew, R. N.: Sudden blindness secondary to injections of common drugs in the head and neck: I. Clinical experiences. Trans. Am. Acad. Ophthalmol. Otolaryngol. 86:147, 1978.

McGrew, R. N.: Sudden blindness secondary to injections of common drugs in the head and neck. II. Animal studies. Trans. Am. Acad. Opthalmol. Otolaryngol. 86:152, 1978.

Mink, P. J.: Physiologie der obern Luftwege. Leipzig, F.C.W. Vogel, 1920.

Mygind, N.: Intranasal beclomethasone dipropionate. ORL Digest, August, 1977, pp. 19–30.

Natvig, P., Sether, L. A., Gingrass, R. P., and Gardner, W. D.: Anatomical details of the osseous-cartilaginous framework of the nose. Plast. Reconstr. Surg. 48:528, 1971.

Naumann, H. H.: On the physiology of the nasal cavity. In Conley, J., and Dickinson, J. T. (eds.): Plastic and Reconstructive Surgery of the Face and Neck. Stuttgart, Georg Thieme Verlag, 1972.

Negus, V. E.: The comparative anatomy and physiology of the nose and paranasal sinuses. London, E. and S. Livingstone Ltd., 1958.

Norman, P. S., Winkenwerder, W. L., Abayani, B. F., and Migeon, C.: Adrenal function during the use of dexamethasone aerosols in the treatment of ragweed hayfever. J. Allergy 40:57, 1967.

Norman, P. S.: Allergic rhinitis and sinusitis. Postgrad. Med. 54:94, 1973.

Ogura, J. H., Togawa, K., and Dammkoehley, K.: Nasal obstruction and the mechanics of breathing. Physiologic relationship and effects of nasal surgery. Arch. Otolaryngol. 83:135, 1966.

Ogura, J. H., Unno, T., and Nelson, J. R.: Nasal surgery. Physiological considerations of nasal obstruction. Arch. Otolaryngol. 88:288, 1968.

Ozenberger, J. M.: Cryosurgery in chronic rhinitis. Laryngoscope 80:723, 1970.

Ozenberger, J. M.: Cryosurgery for the treatment of chronic rhinitis. Laryngoscope 83:508, 1973.

Piesel, Jones, and Richmond: The collected letters of the International Correspondence Society of Ophthalmologists and Otolaryngologists. December 30, 1975.

Proctor, D. F.: The upper airways. Nasal physiology and defense of the lungs. Am. Rev. Respir. Dis. 115:97, 1977.

Proetz, A. W.: Applied Physiology of the Nose. St. Louis, Annals Publishing Co., 1941.

Proetz, A. W.: Physiology of the nose from the standpoint of the plastic surgeon. Arch. Otolaryngol. 39:514, 1944.

Reed, G. F.: Nasal obstruction: causes and treatment. Postgrad. Med. 54:464, 1963.

Remington, J. S., Vosti, K. L., Lietze, A., et al.: Serum proteins and antibody activity in human nasal secretions. J. Clin. Invest. 43:1613, 1964.

Richardson, J. R.: Turbinate treatment in vasomotor rhinitis. Laryngoscope 58:834, 1948.

Ritter, F. N.: The vasculature of the nose. Ann. Otol. Rhinol. Laryngol. 79:468, 1970.

Ritter, F. N.: The Paranasal Sinuses. St. Louis, C. V. Mosby Co., 1973.

Rogers, B. O.: The role of physical anthropology in plastic surgery today. Clin. Plast. Surg. 1:439, 1974.

Romanes, G. J. (ed.): Cunningham's Textbook of Anatomy. London, Oxford University Press, 1964.

Rooker, D. W., and Jackson, R. T.: The effects of certain drugs, cervical sympathetic stimulation and section on nasal patency. Ann. Otol. Rhinol. Laryngol. 78:403, 1969.

Rowe, R. J., Desalter, T. W., and Kinkella, A. M.: Visual changes and triamcinolone. J.A.M.A. 201:117, 1967.

Rundcrantz, H.: Postural variations of nasal patency. Acta Otolaryngol. (Stockh.) 68:435, 1969.

Sanders, S. H.: Allergic rhinitis and sinusitis. Otolaryngol. Clin. North Am. 4:565, 1971.

Schaeffer, J. P.: The Nose, Paranasal Sinuses, Nasolacrimal Passageways, and Olfactory Organ in Man. Philadelphia, P. Blakiston's Son and Co., 1920.

Schmalix, J.: Die knorpeligen Strukturen der Nasenspitze und ihre Verbindung. Arch. klin. exper. Ohr. Nasen-Kehlkopfheilk. 190:146, 1968.

Schwarz, M., and Becker, P. E.: Anomalien, Missbildungen und Krankheiten der Ohren, der Nase und des Halses. In Becker, P. E. (ed.): Humangenetik. Stuttgart, Georg Thieme Verlag, 1964.

Selmanowitz, V. J., and Orentreich, N.: Cutaneous corticosteroid injection and amaurosis: analysis for cause and prevention. Arch. Dermatol. 110:729, 1974.

Sidi, E., and Tardiff, R.: Treatment of allergic rhinitis associated with eczema and hydrocortisone acetate injected into the nasal mucous membranes. Sem. Hop. Paris 35:1922, 1955.

Simmons, M. W.: Intranasal injection of corticosteroids. Calif. Med. 92:155, 1960.

Spector, M.: Indications for a submucous resection. Arch. Otolaryngol. 70:334, 1959.

Stahl, R. H.: Allergic disorders of the nose and paranasal sinuses. Otolaryngol. Clin. North Am. 7:703, 1974.

Stoksted, P.: The physiological cycle of the nose under normal and pathological conditions. Acta Otolaryngol. (Stockh.) 42:175, 1952.

Stoksted, P.: Rhinometric measurements for determination of the nasal cycle. Acta Otolaryngol. (Stockh.) (Suppl.) 109:159, 1953.

Taylor, M.: The nasal vasomotor reaction. Otolaryngol. Clin. North Am. 6:645, 1973.

Taylor, M.: The origin and functions of nasal mucous. Laryngoscope 84:612, 1974.

Thompson, S., and Negus, V. E.: Diseases of the Nose and Throat. New York, Appleton-Century-Crofts, 1948.

Tonndorf, W.: Der Weg der Atemluft in der Menschlichen Nase. Arch. J. Orh-USW. H.K. 41:146, 1939.

Wall, J. W., and Shure, N.: Intranasal cortisone; preliminary study. Arch. Otolaryngol. 56:172, 1952.

Walsh, F. B., and Hoyt, W. F.: Clinical Neuro-opthalmology,

Ed. 3. Baltimore, Williams and Wilkins Co., 1969, Vol. 3, pp. 2501–2510.

Walter, C.: Composite grafts in nasal surgery. Arch. Otolaryngol. *90*:622, 1969.

Walter, C.: The nasal septum. *In* Paparella, M. M., and Shumrick, D. A. (eds.): Otolaryngology, Vol. 3. Philadelphia, W. B. Saunders Company, 1973.

Webster, R. C., Davidson, T. M., and Smith, R. C.: Curved lateral osteotomy for airway protection in rhinoplasty. Arch. Otolaryngol. *103*:454, 1977.

Williams, R. I.: Functions of the nasal septum as related to septal reconstructive surgery. Laryngoscope *63*:212, 1953.

Williams, R. I.: Physiology of the nose in reconstructive surgery. Rocky Mt. Med. J. *51*:352, 1954.

Williams, R. I.: The nasal index: anthropological and clinical. Ann. Otol. Rhinol. Laryngol. *65*:171, 1956.

Williams, R. I.: Nasal physiology. *In* Paparella, M. M., and Shumrick, D. A. (eds.): Otolaryngology, Vol. 1. Philadelphia, W. B. Saunders Company, 1973.

Wolfe, S. G., Jr.: Causes and mechanisms in rhinitis. Laryngoscope *62*:601, 1952.

Wright, J.: A History of Laryngology and Rhinology. Philadelphia, Lea and Febiger, 1914.

INDEX

Note: Page numbers in *italics* refer to illustrations.
Page numbers followed by (t) refer to tables.

Abdomen, excess skin of, abdominoplasty in, 1013
  plastic surgery of. See *Abdominoplasty.*
Abdominal wall
  asymmetry of, abdominoplasty and, 1038
  deformities of, correction of. See *Abdominoplasty.*
  muscle of, plication of, 1018, *1021, 1022*
  musculoaponeurotic laxity of, abdominoplasty in,
    1013, *1032–1034*
Abdominoplasty, 1007–1038
  combination procedures in, 1011, *1012*
  complications of, 1035
  drains in, 1026, *1027*
  history of, 1007–1008
  informed consent for, 1013
  minilift, 1011
  patient selection and preoperative evaluation in,
    1011–1014
  postoperative care of, 1035–1038
  preoperative preparation for, 1015, *1016*
  surgical technique in, 1015–1035, *1017, 1019–1034*
    choice of, 1014
  transverse incisions in, 1008–1011, *1009*
  vertical incisions in, 1011
Acne pits, dermabrasion in, 764, *765*
Adipectomy, plastic, 1007
Adornment, self, 1
Age, for rhinoplasty, 105–107
  anatomic considerations in, 106
Aging
  of eyelid skin, *472, 477*
    premature, *513, 514*
  of skin, 464
    and results of rhytidectomy, *630–631*
    and secondary rhytidectomy, 722
Air, processing of, nose and, 67
Airflow, nasal, 68–70, *69*
  nasal structures and, 70–79
  obstruction of. See *Obstruction, nasal.*
Airway
  management of, 44
  nasal, infracture and, 172, *173*
    resistance of, and nasal obstruction, 69
      rhinoplasty and, 82, *83*
  obstruction of, 44
Ala(e) of nose
  and nostrils, 269, *276*
  collapse of, 75, *75*
    evaluation of, 85, *85*
Ala-columella angle, 247, *247*
Alar base resection, 269–283, *275, 276*
  ancillary techniques with, 269
  in non-Caucasian nose, *442*
  incision in natural crease in, *278, 279,* 283
  Millard, *238,* 242
  variations in design of, *280,* 283

Alar cartilage. See *Cartilage(s), alar.*
Alar crease, 186, *186, 187*
Alar domes
  knuckling of, 222, *223*
    rhinoplasty and, *377,* 380
    correction of, *378, 379,* 380
  resection of, 207, *208, 209*
Alar flap technique
  bipedicle, 199, *203–205*
    modified, *206,* 207, *207*
  Lipsett, 213, *214–217*
    modification of, 213, *218–222*
    with alar base resection, 269, 277
  Millard, in retracted columella, *264–267,* 268
Allergy, and rhinitis, 87
Alopecia
  acquired, 866
  androgenetic, 865
  classification of, 865–867
  dermatologic, 867
  hormonal, 866
  infectious, 866
  lateral scalp flaps and, 884
  male pattern, 865
    lateral scalp flaps in, 875, *881–883*
    strip grafts in, 885
  neoplastic disorders with, 865
  neurogenic and psychiatric, 866
  nutritional, 867
  toxic (pharmacologic or occupational), 866
  traumatic, 866
  treatment of, 867–868
Amastia, 980
Analgesia, local, principles of, 41
  reasonable premedication for, 41
  safe, principles of, 41–43
Analgetics, adverse reactions to, 42
  dose concentration of, 42, 42(t)
  inadvertent intravenous injection of, 42
Anesthesia, 40–48
  attention to detail during, 44–46
  equipment for, reduction in bulk of, 44
  for augmentation mammaplasty, 960–961
  for blepharoplasty, 470
  for nasal tip surgery, 181, *182*
  for rhinoplasty, 108, *111, 112*
    special techniques of, 46
  for surgery of turbinates, 91
  premature recovery from, 45
  premedication for, 40
  preoperative evaluation for, 40
  special techniques of, 46–47
Anesthetic agents, 43–44
Anosmia, rhinoplasty and, 336
Antibiotics, prophylactic, in rhytidectomy, 598

Antihelix, unfurled, 834, *840*
Antihistamines, in turbinate disorders, 89
Antisepsis, prior to rhytidectomy, 598
Areola
   free transplantation of, 934
      technique for, 934, *935–937, 939–941*
   malposition of, reduction mammaplasty and, 952
   reconstruction of, after mastectomy, 1005, *1005*
Aries-Pitanguy technique, of mastopexy, *946*
   of reduction mammaplasty and mastopexy, 910, *911,
     912*
Artery, ophthalmic, branches of, 94(t)
Aspirin-containing compounds, 732
Atropine sulfate, preoperative, 41
Auricular nerve, injury to, rhytidectomy and, 719

Baldness, treatment of, 863–899. See also *Alopecia;* and
   Hair transplantation.
Barbiturates, preoperative, 40
Beauty, concepts of, 1–15
Becker, rocker effect of, *162,* 164, *164*
Belladonna alkaloids, preoperative, 41
Bell's palsy, and rhytidectomy, *720,* 721
Belt lipectomy, 1009, *1010*
Bichat's fat pad, *636, 640*
Biesenberger technique, of reduction mammaplasty,
   904
Bifid nose, modification of, 222, *232, 235*
Bimaxillary protrusion, *774, 782*
Bite, anterior open, ramus osteotomy and, 794
Bleeding. See also *Hematoma.*
   augmentation mentoplasty and, 806
   lateral scalp flaps and, 880
   rhinoplasty and, 334
   tendencies to, evaluation of prior to rhytidectomy,
     596
Blepharitis, chronic, blepharoplasty and, 564
Blepharochalasis, 464, *465*
   definition of, 461
   history of, 460
Blepharoplasty, 457–580
   anesthesia for, 470
   background of, 459–460
   complications of, 526–564
     prevention of, 467
   history of, 459–462
   incision in, 470
   morphologic considerations in, 464–467
   of lower eyelids, 484–518
     incision in, 485, *486–488*
     Silver technique of, 503, *503*
   of Oriental eyelid, 565–577
   of upper eyelids, 470–484
     incision in, 470, *479, 480*
     Lewis Z-plasty technique of, *483,* 484, *484*
     previous, and forehead lift, 747
     Silver technique of, *482,* 483
     with forehead lift, 732, *733, 734,* 741
   postoperative considerations in, 525–580
   secondary, 565
   surgical procedures for, 470–524
     technique for, 470, *471–474*
       history of, 461–462
   systemic and ophthalmologic considerations in,
     467–469
   terminology of, 460–461
Blindness, blepharoplasty and, 534
   intranasal steroid injection and, 93
Blood pressure, elevation of, and hematoma formation,
   712
Blood supply, nasal, anatomy of, 64–65, *64, 65*
Blood vessels, of external ear, *837*
   superficial temporal, in forehead lift, 741, *743*

Body, contouring of, 901–1072
Bone(s)
   absorption of, augmentation mentoplasty and, 806,
     807
   graft of, to dorsum, in overshortened nose, *341, 342,*
     360
   hyoid, and cervicomental angle, 644, *644*
   iliac, graft of, in overresection of osteocartilaginous
     hump, *341*
     in saddle nose deformity, technique of, 348,
       350–357
   nasal, anatomy of, 53–55
   surgical cutting of. See *Osteotomy.*
   turbinate. See *Turbinates.*
Boo-Chai procedure, in Oriental eyelid, 572, *576, 577*
Box-tip deformity. See *Tip of nose, box (square).*
Breast(s)
   absence of, 980
   asymmetry of, 978–987, *979*
     indications for surgery in, 979
   augmentation of, 954–990. See also *Mammaplasty,
     augmentation.*
   carcinoma of, and mastectomy, 996
     mammaplasty and, 988
     risk of, and subcutaneous mastectomy, 988
   cysts of, augmentation mammaplasty and, 975
     reduction mammaplasty and, 952
   developmental abnormalities of, 978–987
   excision of. See *Mastectomy.*
   firmness of, augmentation mammaplasty and, 975
   hypertrophy of, 903
     correction of. See *Mammaplasty, reduction.*
   hypertrophy and ptosis of
     Aries-Pitanguy technique in, 910, *911, 912*
     free nipple-areolar transplantation in, 934,
       935–937, 939–941
     McKissock technique in, 913, *913–916, 919–921*
     Strömbeck technique in, 918, *922–926, 928, 929*
   hypoesthesia of, augmentation mammaplasty and,
     978
   opposite, management of, after mastectomy,
     1005–1006
   plastic surgery of. See *Mammaplasty.*
   ptosis of, correction of. See *Mastopexy.*
     classification of, 938
     without hypertrophy, correction of, 938–950,
       943–949
   reconstruction of, after mastectomy. See *Mastectomy,
     breast reconstruction after.*
   reduction of, 903–953. See also *Mammaplasty,
     reduction.*
   skin of, in breast reconstruction after mastectomy,
     998
   supernumerary, 980
   tuberous, 980
     augmentation mammaplasty in, *981–983,* 982
     surgical correction of, *981,* 982, *983–985*
   tuberous ptotic, 982
     augmentation mammaplasty in, 985, *986, 987*
     surgical correction of, 985, *985–987*
Brevital, 43
   in rhinoplasty, 46
Buttocks
   asymmetry of, postoperative, 1066
   plastic surgery of, 1039–1072
     complications of, 1065
     indications for, 1039–1041
     informed consent for, 1040
     postoperative care of, 1065–1066
     preoperative preparation for, 1040
   ptosis and redundancy of, 1054
     technique for, 1054, *1054–1056*
   reduction of, 1039
     history of, 1039

Callus, formation of, rhinoplasty and, 337
Cancer, breast, and mastectomy, 996
    mammaplasty and, 988
    risk of, subcutaneous mastectomy and, 988
Canthus, lateral, elevation of, in blepharoplasty, *483*, 484, *484*
Capsules, fibrous, augmentation mammaplasty and, 975
Capsulotomy, closed ·compression, 976
  open, 977
Carbon dioxide, retention of, 44
Carcinoma, breast, and mastectomy, 996
    mammaplasty and, 988
    risk of, subcutaneous mastectomy and, 988
Cartilage(s)
  alar
    anatomy of, 57, *58*, *59*
    arching, *416–417*
      surgical plan for, *418–419*
    bulbous, *396–397*, *404–405*
      surgical plan for, *398–399*, *406–407*
    reduction of, 207, *211*
    remodeling of, 199, *203*
  conchal, excess, 834, *840*
  dorsal, excess, *139*, 144
  ear, chondritis of, rhytidectomy and, 717
    tubing of, *846*
  elasticity of, Fry theory of, 300, 304, *304*
  lateral, anatomy of, *54*, 57
    lower. See *Cartilage(s), alar.*
    upper, removal of, in rhinoplasty, 320, *321*
  nasal, anatomy of, *54*, 55–60
    rhinoplasty and, 348
    separation of from septum, 120
  quadrangular, anatomy of, 55, *55*, *56*
    autograft of, in deviated nose, 287, *297*, *312*, *313*
    preoperative physical evaluation of, 104
  septal, anatomy of, 55, *55*, *56*
    autograft of, in deviated nose, 287, *297*, *312*, *313*
    preoperative physical evaluation of, 104
Castanares technique, of correction of cheek overhang deformity, *703–705*
  of double chin excision, *695–697*
Casts, dental, 776
    equipmen for. 779, *780*
    in prognathism, 780, *781*
Cautery, chemical, 95
Cellulite, 1057
Cephalograms, 771, *772*
  analysis of, 773
  evaluation of, 776, 776(t)
    cut-out technique of, 776, *777–778*
Cervicomental angle, correction of, 591
  hyoid bone and, 644, *644*
  loss of, *666–667*
Cheek(s)
  dimple of, *707*
  dissection of SMAS in, *636*, *637*, *640*
  skin undermining over, 592
  swelling of, blepharoplasty and, *569*
Cheek overhang deformity, correction of, Castanares technique of, *703–705*
Cheekbone, reconstruction of, 822
Cheiloplasty, 828, *829*
Chemabrasion, 749–764
  anesthesia for, special techniques of, 46
  complications of, 763
  in pigmentation of eyelid skin after blepharoplasty, *529*, 530
  indications for, 749
  postoperative care of, 762
  precautions in, 759
  procedure for, 759, *760–761*
  repeat, 764
  systemic reaction to, 756
  with dermabrasion, 768–769

Chemical(s), and alopecia, 866
  in chemabrasion, 756
Chemical cautery, 95
Chemical skin peel. See *Chemabrasion.*
Chin
  asymmetry of, horizontal osteotomy in, *814*, *815*, 816
  augmentation of. See *Mentoplasty, augmentation.*
  dimple of, 822, *827*, *828*
  ·double, augmentation mentoplasty in, *824*
    excision of, Castanares technique of, *695–697*
    rhytidectomy in, 592
  horizontal osteotomy of, 806–817, *808–815*
    complications of, 816
    postoperative care of, 816
    technique for, 816
  reduction of, 795
    complications of, 795
  role of, 770
  soft tissue of, 822
Chin implants. See also *Mentoplasty, augmentation.*
  extrusion of, 806
  malposition of, 806
  rhytidectomy with, 587, *591*, *699–701*
  silicone, *775*, 796
  types of, 796
Chisel, in hump reduction, 132, *135*
Chondritis of ear cartilage, rhytidectomy and, 717, *717*
Cocaine, in rhinoplasty, 111, *111*
  reactions to, 108
Columella of nose, 243–269, *247*, *256*
  anatomy of, 57
  hanging, 255, *258–262*
    rhinoplasty and, 386
  retracted, 258, *263–267*
    rhinoplasty and, *385*, 386
Columella-alar angles, 247, *247*
Columella-lip angle, in non-Caucasian nose, *448*
Compazine, preoperative, 40
Concha, deeply cupped, Furnas technique in, *854–857*
Conchal cartilage, excess, 834, *840*
Conchal rim, excess, *840*
  inadequate removal of, 835, *841*
Consultation, first, prior to rhinoplasty, *101–102*, 103
  prior to surgery, 19, *20–22*, 25
Contracture, spherical fibrous capsular (SFCC), augmentation mammaplasty and, 975 ·
Converse–Wood-Smith technique, of otoplasty, *838–839*, *841*, *843*, *848–849*
Cornea, injury to, blepharoplasty and, 528
Corrugator muscle, resection of, *686*, *687*
Corticosteroids. See *Steroids.*
Cottle sign, 86
Coughing, 45
Crease
  alar, 186, *186*, *187*
  gluteal, *1042*
  inframammary, 908, *909*
    incision in, in augmentation mammaplasty, 961, *962–968*
  nasolabial, correction of, 592, *593*, *628–629*
  palpebral, construction of, in Oriental eyelid, 565, 572, *573–577*
  supratarsal, 470, *478*
    construction of, in Oriental eyelid, 565, 572, *573–577*
Croton oil, in chemabrasion, 756
Crow's feet, 518, *518*
Crus, medial, in hanging columella, 255, *258–262*
  resection of, in Pollett technique, 207, *210*, 222, 230
Cryosurgery, 95
Cut-out technique, of cephalometric evaluation, 776, *777–778*
Cyclopropane, 43
Cysts, augmentation mammaplasty and, 975
  reduction mammaplasty and, 952

Darwin's tubercle, large, 835, *843*
Demerol, preoperative, 41
Dental compound splint, in rhinoplasty, 325, *331*
Dental models, 776
  equipment for, 779, *780*
  in prognathism, 780, *781*
Depression, after rhytidectomy, 711
Dermabrasion, 764–766
  indications for, 764, *765*
  operative procedure for, 768
  postoperative care of, 768
  with chemabrasion, 768–769
Dermachalasis, 464, *466*
  definition of, 461
Dermatologic alopecia, 867
Dermolipectomy, in trochanteric lipodystrophy, 1041, *1041–1048*
Diastasis recti abdominis, abdominoplasty in, 1013, *1031, 1032*
Diazepam, preoperative, 41
  prior to rhinoplasty, 198
Dimple, cheek, *707*
  chin, 822, *827, 828*
Dorsum of nose
  cartilage of, excess, *139*, 144
  deviation of, camouflage of, 295, *296–299*
  graft of, 145, *146–148*
    in overshortened nose, *341, 342*, 360
  hump in. See *Nose, hump in.*
  rhinoplasty and, 348
Drains, in abdominoplasty, 1026, *1027*
  in rhytidectomy, 708, *710*
Dressings, eye, 525–526, *526*
  in augmentation mentoplasty, 806
  in rhytidectomy, 708, *709*
Droperidol, preoperative, 41
Drugs. See *Medication.*
Dry eye syndrome, blepharoplasty and, 527, *527*

Ear
  anatomy of, 834, *836, 837*
  cartilage of, chondritis of, rhytidectomy and, 717, *717*
    tubing of, *846*
  external, anatomy of, *836*
    musculature and vascular supply of, *837*
    nerve supply of, *836*
  lop or protruding, 833, *838–839, 848–849*
    analysis of, *844*
    Converse–Wood-Smith technique of correction of, *838–839, 841, 843, 848–849*
    Furnas technique of correction of, *854–857*
    Mustardé technique of correction of, *850–853*
    pathology of, *834–835*
  machiavellian, 835, *842*
  perforation of, 1, *4, 5, 11*
  plastic surgery of. See *Otoplasty.*
  telephone, 835, *858*
Earlobe, correction of, *847*
  in rhytidectomy, 609, *613–614*
Ecchymosis, rhinoplasty and, 335
Ectropion
  blepharoplasty and, 545, *546*
    Mustardé repair of, 553, *560, 561*
    secondary blepharoplasty in, 565, *571*
  cicatricial, blepharoplasty and, 550, *551*
    graft in, 550, *552–554, 556–559*
  in blepharoplasty, 473
  in dry eye syndrome, blepharoplasty and, *527*
  permanent, blepharoplasty and, 550, *551*
  senile, 553, *560–562*
  temporary, blepharoplasty and, 550, *550*
Edema, malar, blepharoplasty and, *569*
  periorbital, 468, *469*
  rhinoplasty and, 335

Electrocautery, 95
Embolus, pulmonary, abdominoplasty and, 1038
Endocrine therapy, for alopecias, 867
Endotracheal tube, 44
Enflurane, 43
Enophthalmos, blepharoplasty and, 534, *535–537*
Epinephrine, 42, 42(t)
Epiphora, blepharoplasty and, 528
Epistaxis, rhinoplasty and, 334
Epithelial tunnels, eyelid sutures and, 530, *530*
Ethnic group, and nasal physiology, 79, *80*
Ethrane, 43
Eversion technique, of nasal tip surgery, 222–243, *224–229*
Exophthalmos, 468
  in blepharoplasty, 473
  in dry eye syndrome, blepharoplasty and, *527*
Eye(s)
  asymmetry of, blepharoplasty and, *537–540*, 541
    correction of, *540, 541*
  dark circles under, 466, *467*
  dressings for, 525–526, *526*
  dry, blepharoplasty and, 527, *527*
  edema of, 468, *469*
  examination of, before blepharoplasty, 467
  muscles of, *464*
Eyebrow
  aesthetic surgery of, 731–748
  natural elevation of, forehead lift and, 747
  ptosis of, *684, 685*
    forehead lift in, 732, *734*
    secondary blepharoplasty in, 565, *567, 568*
Eyebrow lift, direct, vs. forehead lift, 747
Eyelashes, loss of, blepharoplasty and, 564
Eyelid(s)
  baggy, 463–469
    etiology of, 463–464
  lower
    blepharoplasty of, 484–518
    fat of, familial, *495, 505, 506*
      removal of, 485, *486–488, 494, 495*
    skin of
      excess, *474*
        excision of, 485, *486–488, 497, 501, 553, 555*
      pigmentation of, *474*
      undermining of, *504, 510, 511*
  Oriental
    blepharoplasty of, 565–577
    Boo-Chai procedure in, 572, *576, 577*
    Fernandez procedure in, 572, *573–575*
    levator muscle in, 572, *573*
  plastic surgery of. See *Blepharoplasty.*
  senile, blepharoplasty in, 504, *517*
  skin of, aging of, *472, 477*
    premature, *513, 514*
    pigmentation of, blepharoplasty and, chemabrasion in, *529, 530*
  sutures of, and epithelial tunnels, 530, *530*
  upper
    blepharoplasty of. See *Blepharoplasty, upper eyelid.*
    ptosis of, forehead lift in, 732, *734*
    recurrence of skin fold in, secondary blepharoplasty in, 565, *566*
    redundant skin of, elliptical excision of, 470, *475, 476, 480*
      forehead lift in, 732, *733*
    suture of, *479, 480, 483*

Face
  aesthetic surgery of, 581–727
    history of, 583–586
    physical considerations in, 587–595
  analysis of, 771
  chemical peel of. See *Chemabrasion.*
  contouring of, 770

Face (*Continued*)
  curves of, 773, *773*
  framework and integument of, 770
  mechanical or surgical abrasion of. See *Dermabrasion.*
  pigmentation of, rhytidectomy and, 715
  skin of, 770
  soft tissues of, balance of, 773
    considerations of, 822–832
  subcutaneous fat of, 634, *638*
  superficial muscular aponeurotic system of. See *SMAS.*
Face lift. See *Rhytidectomy.*
Facial nerve. See *Nerve, facial.*
Facial plane, 776, *779*
Fat
  dissection of, in platysma surgery, *654–655, 659*
  lower eyelid, familial, *495, 505, 506*
    removal of, 485, *486–488, 494, 495*
  necrosis of, reduction mammaplasty and, 951
  periorbital, 464
    asymmetrical, 472
    familial, *507, 508*
    removal of, and enophthalmos, 534, *535–537*
      and scleral show, 545, *547–549*
  subcutaneous, facial, 634, *638*
Fat hernia, definition of, 461
Fat pad, Bichat's (buccal fat pad), *636, 640*
Femoral nerve, lateral cutaneous, injury to, abdominoplasty and, 1038
Fentanyl, operative, 41
Fernandez procedure, in Oriental eyelid, 572, *573–575*
Filtration, nose and, 67
Flow limiting segment. See *Valve, internal nasal.*
Fold. See *Crease.*
Forehead, aesthetic surgery of, 731–748
  ptosis of, forehead lift in, 732, *734*
Forehead flap, 736, *738*
  trimming of, 741, *744*
Forehead lift
  and exposure for ancillary procedures, 747
  and previous upper eyelid blepharoplasty, 747
  complications of, 744–747
  duration of, 744, *745, 746*
  history of, 731–732
  in male, 748
  incisions in, 736, *737, 738*
    alternative, 747–748
  indications for, 732
  postoperative care of, 744
  preoperative preparation for, 732
  surgical technique for, 736–744
  vs. direct eyebrow lift, 747
  with rhytidectomy, 741, *742*
  with upper eyelid blepharoplasty, 732, *733, 734,* 741
Fracture, greenstick, 153, *160–161, 171*
Frontalis muscle, in forehead lift, excision of, 736, *740*
  history of, 731
Frown lines, glabellar, 592
  vertical, *686, 687*
Fry theory of cartilage elasticity, 300, 304, *304*
Furnas technique, of otoplasty, *854–857*

Genioplasty. See *Mentoplasty.*
Gigantomastia, free nipple-areolar transplantation in, 934, *935–937, 939–941*
Glabellar frown lines, 592
Glatzel's mirror test, 86
Gluteal crease, *1042*
Gluteal depressions, lateral, postoperative, correction of, 1048, *1049–1053*
Graft(s). See also *Implant.*
  bone, to dorsum, in overshortened nose, *341, 342,* 360
  cartilage, in deviated nose, *287, 297, 312, 313*

Graft(s) (*Continued*)
  iliac bone, in overresection of osteocartilaginous hump, *341*
    in saddle nose deformity, technique of, 348, *350–357*
  in cicatricial ectropion after blepharoplasty, 550, *552–554, 556–559*
  of dorsum, 145, *146–148*
  punch, 865–874, *888, 889*
    with strip grafts, *886, 887, 896, 897*
  scalp. See *Graft(s), strip;* and *Scalp flaps, lateral.*
  strip, 885–899, *888, 889, 896*
    complications of, 896
    linear, technique for, 887, *890–892*
    postoperative course of, 896–897
    punch grafts with, *886, 887, 896, 897*
    running-W, technique for, 894, *894, 895*
Grave's disease, 541
Greenstick fracture, 153, *160–161, 171*
Guerrero-Santos technique, for platysma flap, *657, 658, 659*
Gynecomastia, 990–995
  reduction mammaplasty in, 990, *991–994*
    history of, 903
  treatment of, 990, *991–994*

Hair
  autograft of, 865
  loss of, forehead lift and, 747
    rhytidectomy and, 717
  trimming of, prior to rhytidectomy, 598, *598*
Hair transplantation
  at hairline, *870, 873*
  autograft and homograft techniques of, 868–874
    preliminary trials of, 874
  criteria for refusing patients for, 885
  lateral scalp flaps in. See *Scalp flaps, lateral.*
  postoperative care of, 872
  punch grafts in, 865–874, *888, 889*
    with strip grafts, *886, 887, 896, 897*
  recipient dominance in, 869, *869*
  selection of patients for, 885–887
  strip grafts in. See *Graft(s), strip.*
  technique for, 869, *870, 871,* 887–896
Hairline
  hair transplantation at, *870, 873*
  location of, 877
  reconstruction of, 887
    lateral scalp flaps in. See *Scalp flaps, lateral.*
  strip grafts in, 885
Halothane, 43
Healing, delayed, lateral scalp flaps and, 880
Heart, chemabrasion and, 759
Heating, of air, nose and, 67
Hematoma
  abdominoplasty and, 1035
  augmentation mammaplasty and, 977
  blepharoplasty and, 530, *531, 532*
  forehead lift and, 744
  lateral scalp flaps and, 880
  otoplasty and, 835
  plastic surgery of buttocks and thighs and, 1065
  postoperative, 47
  prognathism correction and, 794
  reduction mammaplasty and, 951
  retrobulbar, blepharoplasty and, 531, *533*
  rhinoplasty and, 335
  rhytidectomy and, 712, 713(t)
    removal of, 714, *714*
Hemorrhage. See *Bleeding.*
Hernia, fat, definition of, 461
History
  of abdominoplasty, 1007–1008
  of aesthetic surgery of neck and face, 583–586

History (*Continued*)
  of augmentation mammaplasty, 955–959
  of blepharoplasty, 459–462
  of breast reconstruction after mastectomy, 996–997
  of forehead lift, 731–732
  of mastopexy, 902–905
  of nasal obstruction, 284
  of nasal physiology, 66–67
  of otoplasty, 833–834
  of patient, 103–104
  of psychiatric treatment, and rejection of patient, 34
  of reduction mammaplasty, 903–905
  of rhinoplasty, 51–52
  of rhytidectomy, 583
Hockey stick incision, 187, *190–193*
Hormones, and alopecia, 866
  and postoperative bleeding, 596
Humidification, of air, nose and, 67
Hyoid bone, and cervicomental angle, 644, *644*
Hyperpigmentation, chemabrasion and, 763
Hypoesthesia. See also *Sensory changes.*
  breast, augmentation mammaplasty and, 978
  lip, augmentation mentoplasty and, 806
  prognathism correction and, 793
Hypomastia, correction of. See *Mammaplasty, augmentation.*
Hypotension, induced, 45

Immunotherapy, in turbinate disorders, 90
Implant. See also *Graft(s).*
  breast. See also *Mammaplasty, augmentation.*
    after subcutaneous mastectomy, 987
    choice of, 959
    in augmentation mammaplasty, history of, 957
    in reconstruction after mastectomy, 998, *1000, 1004*
    inflatable, *966, 971–974, 973*
      deflation and rupture of, augmentation mammaplasty and, 978
    location of, 960
    malposition of, augmentation mammaplasty and, 978
  chin. See *Chin implants.*
  in deformities of nasal tip, 371, *372*
  in non-Caucasian nose, 440, *445–450*
  in retracted columella, 262, *263*
  in saddle nose deformity, 348, *350–357*
Inapsine, preoperative, 41
Incision(s)
  across temple, *706*
  hockey stick, 187, *190–193*
  in bipedicle alar flap, 199, *204*
  in blepharoplasty, 470
    lower eyelid, 485, *486–488*
    upper eyelid, 470, *479, 480*
  in forehead lift, 736, *737, 738*
    alternative, *747–748*
  in natural crease, in alar base resection, *278, 279, 283*
  in radical submucous resection, in nasal obstruction, *294*
  in rhinoplasty, 114, *117–119*
    first, *117,* 118
    transfixion, *124–125*
  inframammary fold, in augmentation mammaplasty, 961, *962–968*
  periareolar, in augmentation mammaplasty, 965, *969–974*
  in reduction mammaplasty, in gynecomastia, 991, *992*
  preauricular, in rhytidectomy, 609, *612*
  submental, in augmentation mentoplasty, 801, *802–805*
  in platysma surgery, *647*

Incision(s) (*Continued*)
  T, of neck, *698*
  transverse, in abdominoplasty, 1008–1011, *1009*
  transverse and vertical, in abdominoplasty, 1011, *1012*
  vertical, in abdominoplasty, 1011
Incisor, lower, in facial plane, 776, *779*
Inderal, preoperative, 41
Indian nose, 440, *445*
Infection
  abdominoplasty and, 1037
  and alopecia, 866
  and rhinitis, 87, *87*
  augmentation mammaplasty and, 977
  augmentation mentoplasty and, 806
  blepharoplasty and, 564
  horizontal osteotomy and, 816
  lateral scalp flaps and, 880
  reduction mammaplasty and, 952
  rhinoplasty and, 335
  rhytidectomy and, 717
  scalp, treatment of, 867
  wound, plastic surgery of buttocks and thighs and, 1066
Infracture, and lateral osteotomy, 153–176, *154–161, 169, 170*
  results of, 172, *173, 175*
  and nasal airway, 172, *173*
Innovar, 46
  preoperative, 41
Intercartilaginous technique, of nasal tip surgery, 181–187, *183–184*
  dangers of, 181, *185*
  results of, 187, *188, 189*
Intuition, in patient selection, 24
Itching, forehead lift and, 747
Ivalon, in augmentation mammaplasty, 957

Jaw, surgery of, 770
Joseph, 51
Joseph saw, in reduction of large hump, *142–145,* 145
Joseph tip plasty, 187, *194–198*
Jowls, and rhytidectomy, 587, *590*
Jugular vein, external, *646*

Kazanjian maneuver, in deviated nose, *311*
Keloids, otoplasty and, 859
Keratoconjunctivitis sicca, blepharoplasty and, 527, *527*
Keratosis, superficial, chemabrasion in, 749, *753*
Ketamine hydrochloride, 44

Lacrimal apparatus, injury to, rhinoplasty and, 336
Lagophthalmos, blepharoplasty and, 564
Laminar airflow, in nasal cavity, 68
Latissimus dorsi musculocutaneous island flap, in breast reconstruction after mastectomy, 998, *999–1004*
LeGarde maneuver, 231, *233*
Levator muscle, fixation of, *481,* 483
  in Oriental eyelid, 572, *573*
Lewis Z-plasty technique, of upper eyelid blepharoplasty, *483,* 484, *484*
Light, for rhinoplasty, 108, *109, 110*
Limen nasi. See *Valve, internal nasal.*
Limen vestibuli. See *Valve, internal nasal.*
Liminal chink. See *Valve, internal nasal.*
Lip, 243–269
  augmentation of, 832
  contouring of, 828, *829*
  hypoesthesia of, augmentation mentoplasty and, 806
  perforation of, 1, *6, 12, 13*

Lip (*Continued*)
    posture of, competent, 773
        incompetent, 773, *774, 775*
    reduction of, *829–832,* 832
    tethered, 247, *252–255*
Lip-columella angle, in non-Caucasian nose, *448*
Lip-tip-columella complex, 243–269
Lipectomy, abdominal, 1007
    belt, 1009, *1010*
Lipodystrophy, trochanteric, 1041–1065
    evaluation and treatment of, 1041, *1041–1048,
        1063–1064*
Lipoma, submental, *689–692*
    subplatysmal, *670–672*
Lipomatosis, trochanteric, 1041
Lipsett alar flap technique, 213, *214–217*
    modification of, 213, *218–222*
    with alar base resection, 269, *277*
Litigation, by patient, 24, 30
    possibility of, and rejection of patient, 35
Lobule, nasal, anatomy of, 65
    correction of, 177–180

MacGregor's patch, 592
Machiavellian ear, 835, *842*
Macrogenia, correction of, 795
    complications of, 795
Macromastia, 903
    correction of. See *Mammaplasty, reduction.*
Makeup, 2, *8, 9*
Malar. See *Cheek(s).*
Malarplasty, 822
Male
    forehead lift in, 748
    loose neck skin in, *681*
    rhytidectomy in, *678–681*
        and hematoma, 713, 713(t)
    turkey gobbler neck in, *682*
Male pattern alopecia, 865
    lateral scalp flaps in, 875, *881–883*
    strip grafts in, 885
Malpractice suits, 24, 30
    possibility of, and rejection of patient, 35
Mammaplasty
    and breast carcinoma, 988
    and mammograms, 989
    augmentation, 954–990
        anesthesia for, 960–961
        complications of, 975–978
        history of, 955–959
        in ptotic tuberous breast, 985, *986, 987*
        in tuberous breast, *981–983,* 982
        incision in, inframammary fold, 961, *962–968*
            periareolar, 965, *969–974*
        indications for, 954–955, 959–960
        informed consent for, 960
        postoperative care of, 974–975
        silicone in, reaction to, 976
        silicone gel in, *958,* 961, *964*
        silicone liquid in, 955, *956, 957*
        subcutaneous mastectomy and, 987–990
        techniques for, 961–974
    reduction
        complications of, 950
        free nipple-areolar transplantation in, 934,
            935–937, 939–941
        history of, 903–905
        in gynecomastia, 990, *991–994*
            history of, 903
        indications for, 907–908
        informed consent for, 908
        new nipple site in, 908–910, *909*

Mammaplasty (*Continued*)
    reduction, postoperative care of, 950–953
        technique for
            Aries-Pitanguy, 910, *911, 912*
            McKissock, 913, *913–916, 919–921*
            modern, 905–907
            Pitanguy, 927, *930–933*
            Schwartzmann, 904
            selection of, 910–938
            Strömbeck, 905, 918, *922–926, 928, 929*
    social and psychologic considerations in, 32
Mammary. See *Breast(s).*
Mammograms, and mammaplasty, 989
Mandible
    contouring of, 817–821
    dissection of SMAS over, *637*
    osteotomy of, 791
        in bimaxillary protrusion, 782
        in mandibular retrognathia, 796
Mandibular prognathism, definition of, 785
Mandibular retrognathia, 795–796
    correction of, complications of, 796
Mastectomy
    breast carcinoma and, 996
    breast reconstruction after, 996–1006
        history of, 996–997
        selection of patients for, 997
        technique of, 998–1005
        timing of, 997–998
    management of opposite breast after, 1005–1006
    subcutaneous, and augmentation mammaplasty,
        987–990
Mastoid area, dissection of SMAS in, 637
Mastopexy, 903–953
    free nipple-areolar transplantation in, 934, *935–937,
        939–941*
    history of, 902–905
    indications for, 907–908
    new nipple site in, 908–910, *909*
    postoperative care of, 950–953
    technique for
        Aries-Pitanguy, 910, *911, 912,* 946
        McKissock, 913, *913–916, 919–921*
        selection of, 910–938
        Strömbeck, 918, *922–926, 928, 929*
    without reduction mammaplasty, 938, *943–949*
Maxilla, osteotomy of, in bimaxillary protrusion, 782
Maxillary prognathism, 817, *818–821*
McKissock technique, of reduction mammaplasty and
    mastopexy, 913, *913–916, 919–921*
Medial crus, in hanging columella, 255, *258–262*
    resection of, in Pollett technique, 207, *210,* 222, 230
Medication. See also names of specific drugs.
    after rhytidectomy, 710
    and nasal obstruction, 88(t)
    aspirin-containing, 732
    prior to anesthesia, 40
    prior to rhinoplasty, 108
    reasonable, prior to local analgesia, 41
Mental nerves, injury to, horizontal osteotomy and, 816
Mentoplasty, 770–832
    augmentation, 796–806, *797–799*
        and rhytidectomy, 587, *591, 699–701, 823, 825,
            826*
        in bimaxillary protrusion, *774*
        complications of, 806
        dressings and postoperative care of, 806
        in double chin, *824*
        intraoral approach to, 798, *800, 801*
        submental (external) approach to, 801, *802–805*
        technique for, 798
    diagnosis and treatment planning in, 771
Meperidine, preoperative, 41
Mestizo nose, 440

Methohexital, 43
  in rhinoplasty, 46
Methoxyflurane, 43
Microgenia, *591*
  rhytidectomy and augmentation mentoplasty in, *823,*
    825
Micrognathia, horizontal osteotomy in, *812, 813,* 816
Millard alar base resection, *238, 242*
Millard alar flap technique, in retracted columella,
  264–267, 268
Millard retractor, in nasal tip surgery, 180, *181*
Minilift, history of, 583, *584*
Minilift abdominoplasty, 1011
Morphine sulfate, preoperative, 41
Müller's smooth muscle, 541, *541, 542*
Muscle
  abdominal wall, plication of, 1018, *1021, 1022*
  corrugator, resection of, *686, 687*
  extraocular, imbalance of, 562, *563*
  frontalis, in forehead lift, excision of, 736, *740*
    history of, 731
  inferior oblique, imbalance of, blepharoplasty and,
    562, *563*
  latissimus dorsi, in breast reconstruction after
    mastectomy, 998, *999–1004*
  levator, fixation of, *481, 483*
    in Oriental eyelid, 572, *573*
  Müller's smooth, 541, *541, 542*
  nasal, anatomy of, 60, *61, 62*
  of external ear, *837*
  of eye, *464*
  orbicularis oculi. See *Orbicularis oculi muscle.*
  pectoralis major, in breast reconstruction after
    mastectomy, 998
  platysma. See *Platysma muscle.*
  procerus, resection of, *686, 687*
  rectus, separation of, abdominoplasty in, 1013, *1031,*
    1032
  sternocleidomastoid, dissection of SMAS over, *642*
Muscle-skin flap, in lower eyelid blepharoplasty, 485,
  489–496, 507
Mustardé technique, of ectropion repair after
  blepharoplasty, 553, *560, 561*
  of otoplasty, *850–853*
Mutilation, self, 1

Narcotics, preoperative, 41
Nares. See *Nostril(s).*
Nasal airway resistance, and nasal obstruction, 69
  rhinoplasty and, 82, *83*
Nasal cycle, 70
Nasal index, 81
Nasal profile, reduction of, 128–137, *132*
Nasal sprays, in turbinate disorders, 90
Nasion, 776, *779*
Nasofrontal angle, *149–153,* 153
Nasolabial angle, 243, *244, 247*
Nasolabial folds, correction of, 592, *593, 628–692*
Neck
  aesthetic surgery of, 581–727. See also *Rhytidectomy.*
    history of, 583–586
    physical considerations in, 587–595
  chemabrasion of, *758, 759*
  deformities of, platysma in, preoperative
    photographs of, 596, *597*
  skin of, loose, in male, *681*
    redundant, *693, 694*
  structures of, *645–647*
  superficial muscular aponeurotic system of. See
    SMAS.
  T incision of, *698*
  turkey, *702*
  turkey gobbler, *664–665, 668–669, 674–675*
    in male, *682*

Negroid nose, 440, *447*
Nembutal, preoperative, 40
Neoplastic disorders, with alopecia, 865
Nerve(s)
  auricular, injury to, rhytidectomy and, 719
  facial
    and SMAS, *635, 636*
    in rhytidectomy, 592, 609
    injury to, forehead lift and, 747
      rhytidectomy and, 719
      SMAS surgery and, 717
  injury to, rhytidectomy and, 718
  lateral femoral cutaneous, injury to, abdominoplasty
    and, 1038
  mental, injury to, horizontal osteotomy and, 816
  supplying external ear, *836*
  supplying nose, anatomy of, 60–64, *63*
Neurectomy, vidian, 95
Neurogenic alopecia, 866
Neuroleptanalgesia, 46
Nipple(s)
  new site for, in reduction mammaplasty and
    mastopexy, 908–910, *909*
  slough of, reduction mammaplasty and, 951
  retraction of, reduction mammaplasty and, 952
  supernumerary, 980
  transposition of, history of, 904
Nipple-areolar complex
  free transplantation of, 934
    technique for, 934, *935–937,* 938, *939–941*
  malposition of, reduction mammaplasty and, 952
  reconstruction of, after mastectomy, 1005, *1005*
Nose
  airflow in, 68–70, *69*
    nasal structures and, 70–79
    obstruction of. See *Obstruction, nasal.*
  airway of, infracture and, 172, *173*
  airway resistance of, and nasal obstruction, 69
    rhinoplasty and, 82, *83*
  ala of. See *Ala(e) of nose.*
  anatomy of, 53–65, *54*
  blood supply of, anatomy of, 64–65, *64, 65*
  bony framework of, anatomy of, 53–55
  cartilages of. See *Cartilage(s).*
  columella of. See *Columella of nose.*
  deviated, 284–319. See also *Septum of nose, deviated.*
  dorsum of. See *Dorsum of nose.*
  final checking of, in rhinoplasty, 320, *322, 323*
  functions of, 67–68
  hump in, *424–425.* See also *Dorsum of nose.*
    cartilaginous, reduction of, *128–131*
    in non-Caucasian nose, *443, 449*
    large, reduction of, 144–153
      en bloc, *140, 141,* 145
    osteocartilaginous, overresection of, 339,
      340–342, 346, 347
    reduction of, 120, *128–137*
    replacement of, 145, *146–148*
    surgical plan for, *426–427*
  incision of, 114, *117–119*
  Indian, 440, *445*
  internal, anatomy of, 60
    rhinoplasty and, 361
  internal valve of. See *Valve, internal nasal.*
  lobule of, anatomy of, 65
    correction of, 177–180
  lower, correction of, 177–180
  Mestizo, 440
  muscles of, anatomy of, 60, *61, 62*
  narrowing of. See *Osteotomy, lateral.*
  Negroid, 440, *447*
  nerve supply of, anatomy of, 60–64, *63*
  non-Caucasian, 440–455
    dorsal hump in, *443, 449*
    lip-columella angle in, *448*

Nose (*Continued*)
  non-Caucasian, septal angle in, 440, *441, 447*
    supratip depression in, *446*
  obstruction of. See *Obstruction, nasal.*
  osteocartilaginous framework of, overresection of,
      339, *340–342, 346, 347*
    postoperative widening of, 345, *345*
    rhinoplasty and, 339
  overshortened, 348, *358, 359*, 380, *381, 382*
    rhinoplasty and, 348, *358, 359*
      correction of, *341, 342*, 360
  parakeet, *412–413*
    surgical plan for, *414–415*
  parrot, rhinoplasty and, 361, *363, 364*
  perforation of, 1, *3, 6*
  periosteum of, elevation of, 118, *118, 119*
    inflammation of, rhinoplasty and, 335
  physical evaluation of, 104–105
  physiology of, 66–98
    anthropologic considerations in, 79–82
    history of, 66–67
  Pinocchio, resection of, 207, *208–213*
    bipedicle alar flap technique in, 199, *205*
  plastic surgery of. See *Rhinoplasty.*
  preoperative evaluation of, 114, 115
  reconstruction of, history of, 51
  root of, wrinkle of, *688*
    forehead lift and, 747
  saddle, correction of, 348, *350–357*
    rhinoplasty and, 348
  skeletonizing, 114, *121–125*
  skin of, 53
    rhinoplasty and, 338
    undermining of, in forehead lift, 736, *739*
  soft tissues of
    anatomy of, 53
    in lateral osteotomy and infracture, *174*, 176
    rhinoplasty and, 338
    undermining of, 120, *120–125*
  structures of, and airflow, 70–79
  tension, 77
  tip of. See *Tip of nose.*
  upper, narrowing of, *154*
  vestibule of. See *Vestibule of nose.*
  wide and flattened, *388–389, 400–401, 408–409*
    surgical plan for, *390–391, 402–403, 410–411*
Nosedrops, in turbinate disorders, 90
Nostril(s)
  and airflow, 70, *71–73*
  and ala, 269, *276*
  arching, rhinoplasty and, correction of, *383*, 384,
      384
  flaring, correction of, 269, *276*, 282, 283, *283*
  reduction of, *237, 238*, 242
Nostril sill, natural crease at, *278, 279*, 283
Numbness, forehead lift and, 747
Nutrition, and alopecia, 867

Obesity, and heavy fat thighs, 1057
Obstruction
  airway, 44
  nasal
    drugs and, 88(t)
    evaluating patient for, 82–87, *84–86*, 84(t)
    history of, 284
    measurement of, 86
    nasal airway resistance and, 69
    postoperative, 332
    radical submucous resection in, *286, 288–291*, 292
      incision in, *294*
    rhinoplasty and, 336
    septum and, 284–319
Obwegeser, sagittal split of, 786, *792–794*

Occlusion, analysis of, 773
  anterior open, ramus osteotomy and, 794
  classification of, 779, 784
Oil, croton, in chemabrasion, 756
Olfaction, altered, rhinoplasty and, 336
  nose and, 68
Ophthalmic artery, branches of, 94(t)
Ophthalmologic considerations, in blepharoplasty,
    467–469
Orbicularis oculi flap, 518–524
  results of, *522–524*
  technique of, 518, *518–521*
Orbicularis oculi muscle
  in blepharoplasty, 461
  interaction of skin with, *515*, 518, *518*
  redundant, 485, *498–501*
    correction of, 485, *502*
Oriental eyelid. See *Eyelid(s), Oriental.*
Os internum. See *Valve, internal nasal.*
Osteocartilaginous framework of nose, overresection
    of, 339, *340–342, 346, 347*
  postoperative widening of, 345, *345*
  rhinoplasty and, 339
Osteocartilaginous vault of nose, 114–176
  reduction of, 128–137, *132*
Osteotome, in hump reduction, 132
Osteotomy
  body, in mandibular retrognathia, 796
  horizontal, of chin, 806–817, *808–815*
    complications of, 816
    postoperative care of, 816
    technique for, 816
  lateral
    and infracture, 153–176, *154–161, 169, 170*
      results of, 172, *173, 175*
    high, 153, *163*, 165, *166*
      rhinoplasty and, *343, 344*, 345
    saw technique of, 165, *167, 168*
  mandibular, 791
    in bimaxillary protrusion, 782
    in mandibular retrognathia, 796
  maxillary, in bimaxillary protrusion, 782
  medial, *160*, 164, *165*
  of ramus. See *Ramus, osteotomy of.*
Ostium internum. See *Valve, internal nasal.*
Otoplasty, 833–861
  complications and untoward results of, 835–859
  history of, 833–834
  inadequate correction in, 835
  technique for, *844–857*
    Converse–Wood-Smith, *838–839, 841, 843,*
      848–849
    Furnas, *854–857*
    Mustardé, *850–853*
Outfracture, *160–163*, 164, *165*
  of turbinates, 95
Overgrafting, dermabrasion in, 764, *766, 767*

Packings, in rhinoplasty, 325, *327*
Pain, augmentation mammaplasty and, 978
  rhytidectomy and, 721
Paints, in self-adornment, 1, *8, 9, 11*
Palpebral fold, construction of, in Oriental eyelid, 565,
    572, *573–577*
Paraffin, in augmentation mammoplasty, 955, *956*
Parakeet nose, *412–413*
  surgical plan for, *414–415*
Parotid area, dissection of SMAS in, 634
Parrot beak, rhinoplasty and, 361, *363, 364*
Patient
  behavior of, 23
  concept of success of, 37
  counseling of, for lateral scalp flaps, 876

Patient (*Continued*)
  education of, for rhinoplasty, 100–103, *101–102*
  evaluation of, for augmentation mammaplasty, 959
    for nasal obstruction, 83–87, *84–86*, 84(t)
    for plastic surgery of buttocks and thighs, 1040
    for reduction mammaplasty, 907
    psychiatric, 23, 30
    psychosocial, 25, 29–39
  first interview with, 19, 25
  history of, 103–104
  in- or ambulatory, rhinoplasty in, 107
  litigation by, 24, 30
    possibility of, and rejection of patient, 35
  motivation of, 30
  older, rhinoplasty in, 105
  perfectionist, 27
  position of, for abdominoplasty, 1018
    for rhinoplasty, 108, *109*
    for rhytidectomy, 599
  preconsultation letter for, *20–22*
  problem, 23
  rejection of
    criteria for, 34–36
      for hair transplantation, 885
    history of psychiatric treatment and, 34
    possibility of litigation and, 35
  relationship to doctor, in rhytidectomy, 710
  satisfaction of, 19–28
    after rhytidectomy, 711
  selection of, 19–28
    for abdominoplasty, 1011–1014
    for breast reconstruction after mastectomy, 997
    for chemabrasion, 749
    for hair transplantation, 885–887
    for lateral scalp flaps, 876
    for rhinoplasty, 100
    for rhytidectomy, 23, 587–595, *588, 589*
      special factors in, 587
    intuition in, 24
  self-image of, 24
  younger, rhinoplasty in, 105
Pectoralis major muscle, in breast reconstruction after
    mastectomy, 998
Pentazocine, preoperative, 41
Penthrane, 43
Pentobarbital, preoperative, 40
Pentothal, 43
Perichondritis, otoplasty and, 835
Periosteum, nasal, elevation of, 118, *118, 119*
    inflammation of, rhinoplasty and, 335
Periostitis, rhinoplasty and, 335
Perphenazine, preoperative, 41
Phenol, in chemabrasion, 756
Phenothiazine, preoperative, 40
Phonation, nose and, 68
Photographs, preoperative, 596, *597*, 782
Physical activity, after rhinoplasty, 332
Physician. See *Surgeon.*
Pig snout, 380, *382*
Pigmentation
  chemabrasion and, 763
  chemabrasion in, 749, *754, 755*
  of eyelid after blepharoplasty, chemabrasion in, *529,
    530*
  of lower eyelid, *474*
  rhytidectomy and, 715
Pinocchio nose, resection of, 207, *208–213*
  bipedicle alar flap technique in, 199, *205*
Pitanguy technique, of nasal tip surgery, *239*, 242
  of reduction mammaplasty, 927, *930–933*
Plaster of Paris splint, in rhinoplasty, 325, *329*
Plastic surgery, aesthetic. See also names of specific
    surgical procedures.
  general considerations in, 17–48

Plastic surgery (*Continued*)
  patient for. See *Patient.*
  popularity of, 29
  special problems in, 31
Platysma flap, Guerrero-Santos technique for, *657,
    658, 659*
  operative approach to, 645, *651–653*
  sequelae of, 716, *716*
Platysma muscle, 634–683, *643*
  evaluation of, 645
  in neck deformities, preoperative photographs of,
    596, *597*
  in rhytidectomy, 623, 634
  plication of, *656*, 659
  ptosis of, correction of, *661–663*, 683
  techniques of sectioning, 645
  transection of, *659–660*, 683
    partial, 673
Platysma surgery
  dissection of fat in, *654–655*, 659
  instruments for, *683*
  Skoog technique of, 645, *648*
    sequelae of, 716, *716*
  standard, 645, *649, 650*
  submental incision in, *647*
  variations of, 645
Pogonion, 776, *779*
Pollett technique, 207, *210*
  of medial crus resection, 207, *210*, 222, *230*
Polly tip, rhinoplasty and, 361, *363, 364*
Polymastia, 980
Polythelia, 980
Polyvinyl, in augmentation mammaplasty, 957
Procerus muscle, resection of, *686, 687*
Prochlorperazine, preoperative, 40
Profile, nasal, reduction of, *128–137*, 132
Prognathism, 782
  clinical assessment of, 785
  dental models in, 780, *781*
  mandibular, definition of, 785
  maxillary, 817, *818–821*
  sagittal split in, 786, *792–794*
  treatment of, complications of, 791
  vertical osteotomy of ramus in, 786, *787–790*
Propranolol, preoperative, 41
Prosthesis. See *Implant.*
Protection, nose and, 68
Psychiatric alopecia, 866
Psychiatric evaluation, of patient, 23, 30
  of surgeon, 28
Psychiatric treatment, history of, and rejection of
    patient, 34
Psychiatrist, surgeon and, 37
Psychologic considerations, in mammaplasty, 32
  in plastic surgery, 26, 29–39
Psychologist, surgeon and, 37
Psychosocial evaluation, of patient, 25, 29–39
Ptosis
  blepharoplasty and, 543, *543, 544*
  breast. See *Breast(s), hypertrophy and ptosis of,* and
    Breast(s), ptosis of.
  correction of. See *Mastopexy.*
  of buttocks, 1054
    technique for correction of, 1054, *1054–1056*
  of eyebrow, *684, 685*
    secondary blepharoplasty in, 565, *567, 568*
  of forehead, eyebrows, and upper eyelids, forehead
    lift in, 732, *734*
  of medial thigh, 1056, *1058*
    technique for correction of, 1057, *1058–1064*
  of platysma muscle, correction of, *661–663*, 683
Ptosis atonica, definition of, 460
Pulmonary embolus, abdominoplasty and, 1038
Punch, for hair transplantation, 869, *870*

Punch grafts, 865–874, *888, 889*
  with strip grafts, *886,* 887, *896, 897*
Pygmalion complex, 36

Race, and nasal physiology, 81, *81, 82*
Radiographs, 771
  cephalometric. See *Cephalograms.*
Ram's tip, rhinoplasty and, 361, *363, 364*
Ramus, osteotomy of
    and anterior open bite, 794
    sagittal, 786, *792–794*
      in mandibular retrognathia, 795
    vertical or oblique, 786, *787–790*
      in mandibular retrognathia, 796
Rasp, in hump reduction, 132, *133, 136–137*
Rectus muscle, separation of, abdominoplasty in, 1013, *1031, 1032*
Respiration, nose and, 67
Retractor of Millard, in nasal tip surgery, 180, *181*
Retrognathia, horizontal osteotomy in, *810, 811,* 816
    mandibular, 795–796
      correction of, complications of, 796
Rhinitis
    allergic, 87
    atrophic, 89
    hyperplastic or hypertrophic, 88
    infectious, 87, *87*
    postrhinoplasty, 89
    vasomotor, 88
Rhinitis medicamentosa, 88
Rhinomanometry, 87
Rhinoplasty, 49–455
    age for, 105–107
      anatomic considerations in, 106
    and rhinitis, 89
    anesthesia for, 108, *111, 112*
      special techniques for, 46
    complications of, 320–386, *342–344, 346–347, 358 359, 363–364. 366, 368–370, 374, 376–377, 381*
      classification of, 338–386
      early, 334
      general considerations in, 332
      late, 336
    final steps in, 320–325
    history of, 51–52
    incision in, 114, *117–119*
      first, *117,* 118
      transfixion, *124–125*
    minimal, 132, 144, *138*
    nature of, 99–100
    operative procedure in, 114–120, *116*
      history of, 52
    packings, dressings, and splints in, 325–332
    patients for, 24
      education of, 100–103, *101–102*
      selection of, 100
    postoperative care for, 332–337, *333*
    postoperative considerations in, 320–386
    preoperative considerations in, 99–113
    preparation and, 107–113
    problems in, 387–439
    secondary, 337–338
      evaluation of, 337
      timing of, 338
    sutures in, 320, *324*
Rhytidectomy
    ancillary techniques in, *684–707*
    and augmentation mentoplasty, 587, *591, 699–701, 823, 825, 826*
      in bimaxillary protrusion, *774*
    Bell's palsy and, *720,* 721

Rhytidectomy *(Continued)*
    classical technique of, 600–633, *601–603*
      procedure for, 600–622, *604–608*
      results of, 622–633, *624–633*
      technical details in, 609
    complications of, 712–721
    dressings and drains in, 708, *709, 710*
    facial nerve in, 592, 609
    history of, 583
    in male, *678–681*
      and hematoma, 713, 713(t)
    instruments for, *683*
    platysma muscle in, 623, 634
    postoperative care of, 708–712
    postoperative considerations in, 708–727
    preauricular incision in, 609, *612*
    preoperative preparation for, 596–599
    results of, aging and, *630–631*
    secondary, 721–724
      timing of, 722
    selection of patients for, 23, 587–595, *588, 589*
      special factors in, 587
    SMAS in, 623, 634
    sutures in, 600, *602, 608*
    upper, *620–621,* 622
    with chin implant, 587, *591, 699–701, 823, 825, 826*
    with forehead lift, 741, *742*
Riding breeches deformity, 1041, *1041.* See also *Trochanteric lipodystrophy.*
Rocker effect of Becker, *162,* 164, *164*
Roe, John Orlando, 51
Roentgenography, 771
    cephalometric. See *Cephalograms.*

Saddle nose deformity, correction of, 348, *350–357*
    rhinoplasty and, 348
Safian technique, of nasal tip surgery, 199, *200–202*
Sagittal split, 786, *792–794*
    in mandibular retrognathia, 795
Saw, Joseph, in reduction of large hump, *142–145,* 145
Saw technique, of lateral osteotomy, 165, *167, 168*
Scalp, fungal infections of, treatment of, 867
    grafts of. See *Graft(s), strip;* and *Scalp flaps, lateral.*
Scalp flaps, lateral, 875–884
    choice of procedures for, 876
    contraindications for, 876
    design of, 877, *877*
    experience and results of, 880–884, *881–883*
    history of, 875
    indications for, 876
    method for, 875–876
    pitfalls and complications of, 880
    postoperative care of, 880
    preoperative planning of, 876–878
    preparation for, 878
    surgery for, 878, *879*
    technique for, 878–880
Scar(s)
    abdominoplasty and, 1037
    augmentation mammaplasty and, 978
    blepharoplasty and, secondary blepharoplasty in, 565, *570*
    chemabrasion and, 763
    dermabrasion in, 764, *765*
    hypertrophic, otoplasty and, 835, *858*
    of nasal vestibule, rhinoplasty and, 361, *367*
    plastic surgery of buttocks and thighs and, 1065
    reduction mammaplasty and, 952
    rhytidectomy and, 718
    secondary, social and psychologic considerations in, 33
    umbilical, abdominoplasty and, 1037
    visible, absence of, forehead lift and, 747

Scarification, 1, *14, 15*
Schwartzmann technique, of reduction mammaplasty,
  904
Scleral show. See *Ectropion*.
Sclerosing solutions, 94
Scopolamine hydrobromide, preoperative, 41
Secobarbital, preoperative, 40
Seconal, preoperative, 40
Self-adornment, 1
Self-cleansing, nose and, 68
Self-image, 24
Self-mutilation, 1
Sensory changes. See also *Hypoesthesia*.
  abdominoplasty and, 1038
  augmentation mammaplasty and, 978
  forehead lift and, 747
  reduction mammaplasty and, 952
Septal angle, in non-Caucasian nose, 440, *441, 447*
Septal plasty, in septal deviation, 295, *300–301*
Septum of nose
  anatomy of, *305*, 319
  and airflow, 76, 77
  and nasal obstruction, 284–319
  cartilaginous, anatomy of, 54, *55, 56*
    autograft of, in deviated nose, 287, 297, *312, 313*
    preoperative physical evaluation of, 104
  cartilaginous caudal
    anatomic variants of, 245, *246*
    excision of, 120
    in hanging columella, 255, *258, 259, 262*
    projecting, *436–437*
      surgical plan for, *438–439*
    resection of, 247, *247–250*
    trimming of, 177, *179*
  deviated, 284, *285, 287, 305*
    autograft of septal cartilage in, 287, 297, *312, 313*
    correction of, 284–319, *306*
    high, correction of, *307–310*
    Kazanjian maneuver in, *311*
    repositioning of, *302, 303,* 304
    rhinoplasty and, *351,* 371
    Shulman technique in, *298, 299*
    swinging door technique in, *314–318*
  membranous, anatomy of, 59
  perforation of, rhinoplasty and, 336
  separation of cartilages from, 120
Seroma, abdominoplasty and, 1035
Sexual organ, secondary, nose as, 68
SFCC, augmentation mammaplasty and, 975
Shulman technique, in nasal deviation, *298, 299*
Sight, loss of, blepharoplasty and, 534
  intranasal steroid injection and, 93
Silicone, as chin implant, *775, 796*
  liquid, in augmentation mammaplasty, 955, *956,
    957*
  reaction to, in augmentation mammaplasty, 976
Silicone gel, in augmentation mammaplasty, 958, 961,
  964
Silver technique, of lower eyelid blepharoplasty, 503,
  503
  of upper eyelid blepharoplasty, *482,* 483
Sjögren's disease, blepharoplasty and, 527, *527*
Skin
  abdominal, excess, abdominoplasty in, 1013
  aging of, 464
    and results of rhytidectomy, *630–631*
    and secondary rhytidectomy, 722
  biomechanical properties of, 723
  blepharoplasty and, 529
  breast, in breast reconstruction after mastectomy,
    998
  changes in, chemabrasion and, 756, *757*
    dermabrasion and, 764
  chemical abrasion of. See *Chemabrasion*.
  color of, chemabrasion and, 763

Skin *(Continued)*
  eyelid, aging and, *472, 477*
    premature, *513, 514*
  lower. See *Eyelid(s), lower, skin of*.
  pigmentation of, blepharoplasty and,
    chemabrasion in, *529,* 530
  upper, redundant, elliptical excision of, 470, *475,
    476, 480*
    forehead lift in, 732, *733*
  facial, 770
    pigmentation of, rhytidectomy and, 715
  interaction of orbicularis oculi muscle with, *515, 518,
    518*
  mechanical or surgical abrasion of. See *Dermabrasion*.
  nasal, 53
    rhinoplasty and, 338
    undermining of, in forehead lift, 736, *739*
  neck, loose, in male, 681
    redundancy of, *693, 694*
  necrosis of, forehead lift and, 744
    lateral scalp flaps and, 884
  of buttocks, redundancy of, 1054
    technique for correction of, 1054, *1054–1056*
  of medial thigh, redundancy of, 1056, *1058*
    technique for correction of, 1057, *1058–1064*
  of submental area, redundant, *693, 694*
  pigmentation of. See *Pigmentation*.
  postauricular, removal of, *845*
  redistribution of, in rhytidectomy, 609, *616–619*
  rhinoplasty and, 336
  slough of
    abdominoplasty and, 1036
    blepharoplasty and, 562, *562*
    reduction mammaplasty and, 951
    rhytidectomy and, 715
  stretching and, 722
  undermining of, in rhytidectomy, 600, *604, 610–611*
    results of, 622, *624–625*
    over cheeks, 592
Skin flap, abdominal, 1018, *1019*
  resection of, 1024, *1025*
  in rhytidectomy, 600, *601, 604–608*
Skin-muscle flap, in lower eyelid blepharoplasty, 485,
  489–496, 507
Skin peel. See *Chemabrasion*.
Skoog technique
  of hump replacement, 145, *146–148*
  of orbicularis oculi flap, 518
  of platysma surgery, 645, *648*
  sequelae of, 716, *716*
SMAS, 634–683, *635–642*
  dissection of, *637*
    in cheek area, *636, 637, 640*
    in temporal area, *639, 641*
    over sternocleidomastoid muscle, *642*
  in rhytidectomy, 623, 634
  surgery of, sequelae and complications of, 716
Smell, altered sense of, rhinoplasty and, 336
  nose and, 68
Soap, liquid, in chemabrasion, 756
Social considerations, in plastic surgery, 29–389
Social worker, surgeon and, 37
Sodium methohexital, 43
  in rhinoplasty, 46
Spine of nose, 245
  anatomic variants of, 245, *246*
  repair of, *251*
Spherical fibrous capsular contracture (SFCC),
  augmentation mammaplasty and, 975
Splints, in rhinoplasty, 325, *329, 331*
Stair-step deformity, 153, *163,* 165, *166*
  rhinoplasty and, *343, 344,* 345
Staple gun, in rhytidectomy, *615*
Sternocleidomastoid muscle, dissection of SMAS over,
  642

Steroids
    in augmentation mammaplasty, 977
    in turbinate disorders, 90
    intralesional injection of, in alopecia, 867
    intranasal injection of, 91
        complications of, 93
        indications for, 91, 91(t)
        results of, 93
        technique for, 92, 92
Strömbeck technique, of reduction mammaplasty, 905
        of reduction mammaplasty and mastopexy, 918,
        922–926, 928, 929
Sublimaze, preoperative, 41
Submucous resection, 121, 126–127
    in nasal tip surgery, 240, 241, 242
    radical, in nasal obstruction, 286, 288–291, 292
        incision for, 294
Succinylcholine chloride, 44
Sun, protection from, after chemabrasion, 763
        after dermabrasion, 768
Superficial muscular aponeurotic system (SMAS). See
        SMAS.
Supratarsal fold, 470, 478
    construction of, in Oriental eyelid, 565, 572, 573–577
Supratip deformity, rhinoplasty and, 360, 360,
        362–366
Supratip depression, in non-Caucasian nose, 446
Surgeon
    concept of success of, 37
    intuition of, in patient selection, 24
    motivation of, 36–37
    psychologic evaluation of, 28
    relationship to patient, in rhytidectomy, 710
    reliance of, on other professionals, 37
Surgery. See names of specific surgical procedures.
Sutures
    eyelid, and epithelial tunnels, 530, 530
        upper, 479, 480, 483
    in rhinoplasty, 320, 324
    in rhytidectomy, 600, 602, 608
Swinging door technique, in deviated nose, 314–318
Sympathomimetics, in turbinate disorders, 89

T incision, of neck, 698
Talwin, preoperative, 41
Tape, waterproof, in chemabrasion, 756, 762
Tattooing, 1, 5
Teeth, filing of, 7
    fixation of, 785–794
        intra- and intermaxillary, 785
Telfa packing, in rhinoplasty, 325, 327
Temple, incision across, 706
Temporal area, dissection of SMAS in, 639, 641
Temporal lift, 620–621, 622
Tension nose, 77
Tethered lip, 247, 252–255
Thigh(s)
    heavy fat, obesity and, 1057
    lateral depressions of, postoperative, 1066
        correction of, 1048, 1049–1053
    medial, ptosis and redundancy of, 1056, 1058
        technique for correction of, 1057, 1058–1064
    plastic surgery of, 1039–1072
        complications of, 1065
        indications for, 1039–1041
        informed consent for, 1040
        postoperative care of, 1065–1066
        preoperative preparation for, 1040
Thiopental sodium, 43
Thrombophlebitis, abdominoplasty and, 1038
Tip of nose, 243–269
    amorphous, rhinoplasty and, correction of, 384, 384
    asymmetric, 373

Tip of nose (Continued)
    augmentation of, 255, 256, 257
    bifid, modification of, 222, 232, 235
    box (square), 222, 231, 392–393
        modification of, 222, 226, 234
        rhinoplasty and, 371, 373
            correction of, 371, 374–376
        surgical plan for, 394–395
    crucified, repair of, 367, 368, 369
    deformities of, implant in, 371, 372
    knuckling of, 222, 223
        rhinoplasty and, 377, 380
            correction of, 378, 379, 380
    plunging, 244, 245, 268, 268, 270–274, 432–433
        rhinoplasty and, 380
        surgical plan for, 434–435
    polly, rhinoplasty and, 361, 363, 364
    preoperative physical evaluation of, 104
    projection of, in non-Caucasian nose, 450
    protruding, resection of, 207, 208–213
        bipedicle alar flap technique in, 199, 205
    ram's, rhinoplasty and, 361, 363, 364
    rhinoplasty and, 371
    rounded, 428–429
        surgical plan for, 430–431
    strong and projecting, 420–421
        surgical plan for, 422–423
    surgery of, 180–181
        alar flap technique of. See Alar flap technique.
        anesthesia for, 181, 182
        approaches to, 177–242
        eversion technique of, 222–243, 224–229
        intercartilaginous technique of, 181–187, 183–184
            dangers of, 181, 185
            results of, 187, 188, 189
        Pitanguy technique of, 239, 242
        Safian technique of, 199, 200–202
        submucous resection in, 240, 241, 242
    thick (beefy), reduction of, 222, 227, 229, 236, 237,
        242
Tip plasty, Joseph, 187, 194–198
    with alar base resection, 278, 283
Tranquilizers, preoperative, 40
Trauma, and alopecia, 866
Triamcinolone acetonide, in augmentation
        mammaplasty, 977
Trichotillomania, 867
Trilafon, preoperative, 41
Trochanteric lipodystrophy, 1041–1065
    evaluation and treatment of, 1041, 1041–1048,
        1063–1064
Tube, endotracheal, 44
Turbinates
    and airflow, 78, 79
    and nasal obstruction, 84(t), 85
    disorders of, 87–98
        medical treatment of, 89
    enlarged, surgical treatment of, 90
    outfracture of, 95
    surgical excision of, 95, 96, 97
Turbinectomy, 95, 96, 97
    for enlarged turbinates, 90
Turbulent airflow, in nasal cavity, 68
Turkey gobbler neck, 664–665, 668–669, 674–675
    in male, 682
Turkey neck, 702

Umbilicus
    excision of, 1015, 1017
    malposition of, abdominoplasty and, 1038
    necrosis of, abdominoplasty and, 1037
    new site for, 1028–1030, 1029
    reconstruction of, 1030, 1031

Umbilicus (*Continued*)
  scars of, abdominoplasty and, 1037
  stalk of, shortening of, 1018, *1023*

Valium, preoperative, 41
  prior to rhinoplasty, 108
Valve
  internal nasal, and airflow, 71, 73(t), *74–76*
    and nasal obstruction, 84(t), *86*
    reconstruction of, 370, *370*
  liminal. See *Valve, internal nasal.*
Vasoconstrictor agents, 42
Vault, osteocartilaginous, 114–176
  reduction of, 128–137, *132*
Vein, jugular, external, *646*
Vestibule of nose
  anatomy of, 60
  and airflow, 70, *71*
  and nasal obstruction, 84(t)
  scarring of, rhinoplasty and, 361, *367*
Vidian neurectomy, 95
Vision, loss of, blepharoplasty and, 534
  intranasal steroid injection and, 93
Vomer, removal of, in nasal obstruction, 292, *294, 295*

Warming, of air, nose and, 67

Wedge removal. See also *Osteotomy, horizontal, of chin.*
  in bimaxillary protrusion, 782
  in micrognathia, *812, 813,* 816
  in retrognathia, *810, 811,* 816
Wound
  dehiscence of
    abdominoplasty and, 1037
    augmentation mammaplasty and, 977
    blepharoplasty and, 564
    plastic surgery of buttocks and thighs and, 1066
  infection of, plastic surgery of buttocks and thighs and, 1066
Wrinkle(s)
  blepharoplasty and, 543, *545*
  facial, chemabrasion in, 509, *750–752*
  lateral orbital (crow's feet), 518, *518*
  of eyelids, chemabrasion in, *509*
  of nose root, *688*
    forehead lift and, 747
  rhytidectomy in. See *Rhytidectomy.*

Xeromammography, and mammaplasty, 989
X-ray, 771
  cephalometric. See *Cephalograms.*

Z-plasty, Lewis technique of, in upper lid blepharoplasty, *483, 484, 484*
Zygomatic area, dissection of SMAS in, *637*